GW00597206

Doctors in Science and Society

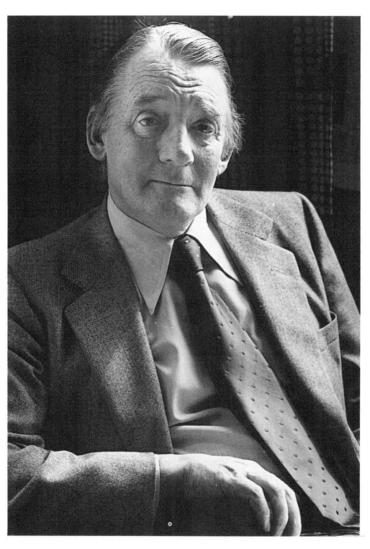

Christopher Booth

CHRISTOPHER C BOOTH

Doctors in Science and Society

Essays of a Clinical Scientist

The
MEMOIR
Club

ISBN 0 7279 0189 3

Made and printed in Great Britain by
Cambridge University Press

For my children

Contents

Illustrations

Introduction

An interest in history is often considered to be the last of the seven ages of a medical scientist. I have never shared that view, nor have I subscribed to the notion, current amongst many social historians, that the biographical approach to history belongs to a bygone age. I have always believed, furthermore, that one need not restrict one's medical friendship to those who live in one's own era.

This collection of essays represents the fruits of historical studies undertaken at weekends, during holidays in the north of England or during those rare idle moments enjoyed by a physician who has been engaged in both clinical practice and research. Many of the essays in this book are derived from formal addresses given to medical and scientific societies. Some were submitted as articles to medical or general journals.

The collection begins with an appraisal of the contributions of the Age of Reason to medical discovery. The century of the Enlightenment was a remarkable era of British history. The inventions of the Industrial Revolution transformed society, Britain established its imperial role, the first of our great modern republics was founded, the remaining unknown areas of the habitable world were explored, and the first settlements in Australia established. The achievements of medicine, in an era generally considered to have been dominated by a lamentable urge to bleed and to purge, were no less significant. By the end of the century scurvy had been conquered amongst seamen, digitalis had been discovered, vaccination introduced and both the nature of oxygen and the anaesthetic properties of nitrous oxide had been described. With such achievements to its credit it is all the more surprising that the medicine of that era has been so universally derided. In the 1930s, a president of the Royal Society expressed the view that there had been no outstanding advance in the theory and practice of medicine during the entire eighteenth century and he quoted Osler, who had written with an equal degree of historical inaccuracy, "What a vast literature exists between Sydenham and Broussais. What a desolate sea of theory and speculation."[1] The first chapter in this book seeks to redress these erroneous perceptions.

The essay on Sir Samuel Garth, the "*Dispensary* Poet," was first stimulated by reading Harvey Cushing's paper, "The Kit Cat Poet," published in the early years of the current century. Garth was an important figure during the reign of Queen Anne, physician to the Duke and Duchess of Marlborough and a member of the famous Kit Cat Club. He was also a poet whose work was an important link between the era of Dryden and that of Alexander Pope. My own interest in Garth was further encouraged when I discovered that he had lived at Harrow-on-the-Hill and that he was buried there in a tomb beside the altar in St Mary's Church. Northwick Park Hospital, where I have worked for the past eight years, commands an admirable view of the spire of that lovely church upon the hill.

Several of these essays were the result of my association with the Yorkshire dales, where I was brought up and where I have lived during summer holidays and any other brief visits that a busy medical life has allowed. My interest in William Hillary was first stimulated by Dr W N Pickles of Aysgarth, within the confines of whose practice in Wensleydale my family lived.[2] Pickles had referred to Hillary's epidemiological studies of infectious disease in his classic book *Epidemiology in Country Practice*,[3] but neither of us knew that Hillary was himself a Wensleydale man until some recently discovered correspondence of his eighteenth century fellow dalesman, Dr John Fothergill, revealed that his family had been an important Quaker family in Upper Wensleydale. Hillary made important medical observations during the course of his work as a physician in the island of Barbados during the 1750s, where he attended George Washington and his brother in 1751. He also witnessed a few years later the extraordinary tidal surges in Barbados that were caused by the Lisbon earthquake.

Dr John Fothergill, a committed Quaker, was born in a seventeenth century Yorkshire farmhouse on whose land I helped with haymaking as a boy. He was a close personal friend of Benjamin Franklin, to whom he had been physician. He was also an ardent supporter of the American cause during the years that led to the War of Independence. It was my collaboration with Betsy C Corner in the editing of Dr Fothergill's letters, a venture initially supported by a grant from the American Philosophical Society, that led to studies of Dr Fothergill's work on coronary artery disease and his involvement in the affairs of the American colonies. It was also Dr Fothergill who introduced me to Benjamin Rush, Robert Willan, John Haygarth, and many others who appear in these pages.

Betsy Corner, editor of William Shippen's London diary,[4] was the wife of the distinguished American reproductive physiologist and medical historian George W Corner. Dr Corner believed that the study of medical history enhanced the career of a medical scientist rather than otherwise.[5] For many years, until his death in 1981 at the age of 90, he gave generous encouragement to my own historical studies, which he was kind enough to introduce to meetings of the American Philosophical Society, the oldest learned society in the United States. My much valued friendship with the Corners was remarkable in spanning both an ocean and a generation.

The place of women in history is becoming an increasingly important feature of modern historical study. The essay on Dr Fothergill's sister, the "Mistress of Harpur Street," owes everything to the preservation for more than two centuries of a collection of her correspondence, as well as her recipe book, which has long been treasured by a later generation of her family. Her letters give a rare insight into the mind and actions of a remarkable Quaker lady of the eighteenth century, as well as describing the domestic life of a London physician of that era.

The study of the Willan family, another story from the

xiii

Yorkshire dales, gives detailed information on the social and economic background of Robert Willan, the founder of modern dermatology in Britain. Willan was an important figure of the late eighteenth century and the early years of the nineteenth, a period when medical men formed a significant element of the emergent middle class. The Willans, like the Hillary and Fothergill families, were Quakers, although later generations were to lapse as members of the Society of Friends.

John Dawson was another son of the Yorkshire dales. A self taught mathematical genius, he was an unlettered surgeon who served his fellow dalesmen as a general practitioner. His prowess as a mathematician, however, was remarkable and during the summer months of the later years of the eighteenth century it was his custom to tutor at his home a succession of distinguished Cambridge undergraduates, many of whom later became wranglers of the university.

It was the discovery of vaccination by Edward Jenner at the end of the eighteenth century that led, during my life time, to the total eradication of smallpox. This achievement must rank as one of the greatest of all time, surely as deserving of a Nobel prize as any series of laboratory experiments. The essay on the conquest of smallpox traces the disease from its earliest appearance as an affliction of mankind to its successful eradication by the united efforts of the World Health Organisation a decade ago.

The development of medical journals in Britain had its origins in the eighteenth century. The story includes the fascinating events that later led to the foundation by Thomas Wakley of the *Lancet*. It illustrates, furthermore, the importance of the radical in the history of both medicine and medical journalism.

The later chapters are concerned with the modern era. Technology has come to play a dominant role in the practice of medicine in recent decades. The piece on technology and medicine was originally given as an evening technology lecture at the Royal Society. It seeks to outline some of the problems currently facing doctors and society.

The history of clinical research under the auspices of the

Medical Research Council and the story of the first 50 years
of the Royal Postgraduate Medical School are complementary
to each other, setting out the way in which two different
organisations, the Medical Research Council on the one hand
and the University of London on the other, have sought to
encourage clinical research in this country during the current
century.

The final chapter on "Clinical Science Today" brings together ideas that were formulated in a series of addresses
which include "Klinische Forschung in einer Zeit vermin-
derter finanzieller Mittel und schwindender Motivation" at
the Ludwig Heilmeyer Symposium of the Gesellschaft für
Fortschritte auf dem Gebiet der Inneren Medizin in Düssel-
dorf in December 1982, "Clinical Research Today" at the
Medical Society of London in January 1986, and the presidential address to the British Medical Association, "Better a
Commitment to Health and Research than to Missiles," at
Scarborough on 25 June 1986. It also draws on an essay
review of the book by R A Hall and B A Bembridge, *Physic
and Philanthropy*, which marks the fiftieth anniversary of the
Wellcome Trust.[6]

I am grateful to Mrs Maureen Moriarty of the word processing group at
the Clinical Research Centre for preparing the manuscript. I am also
particularly indebted to Ms Ruth Holland for her skilful editing of the
text.

NOTES

1 Hopkins FG. Anniversary address. *Proc R Soc B* 1934; **114**: 181–
205.
2 Booth CC, Pickles W N. William Hillary MD (1697–1763). *Br Med J*
1957; i: 102–4.
3 Pickles WN. *Epidemiology in country practice*. Bristol: John Wright
and Sons, 1939: 27.
4 Corner BC. *William Shippen, Jr*. Philadelphia: American Philosophical
Society, 1951.
5 Corner GW. *The seven ages of a medical scientist: an autobiography*.
Philadelphia: University of Pennsylvania Press, 1981: 211.
6 Booth CC. Essay review of *Physic and Philanthrophy*. *Medical History*
1986; **30**: 473–5.

1 Clinical science in the Age of Reason

Eighteenth century medicine is traditionally associated with the lancet and the purge. There was no greater enthusiast for these hallowed methods of treatment than Dr Benjamin Rush of Philadelphia. He thought that there was only one disease process and that was "irregular convulsive or wrong action of the system affected." Treatment was therefore to reduce convulsive and wrong action by depletion and this entailed a murderous regime of bleeding and purgation.[1] Joseph Priestley, visiting Philadelphia at the end of 1800, had the misfortune to encounter Benjamin Rush who diagnosed his malady as a "bilious fever" with pleurisy; seven profuse bleedings did much to prolong his recovery.[2] The influence of Rush probably hastened Washington's end the year before, though it had been the President himself who had insisted, against his wife's better judgment, that he be bled.[3] Since Rush had learnt much of his medicine in Europe it is not surprising that patients fared little better on the other side of the Atlantic, where the old mad King suffered countless indignities at the hands of his physicians.

England in the eighteenth century, as portrayed by Hogarth, Fielding, and Smollett, was unwashed and unsavoury and much of its medicine was little better. It was the England of *Tom Jones*, the *Rake's Progress* or *Marriage à la Mode*. The upper classes – powdered, rouged, and bewigged – flirted at masked balls, played cards until daylight, recited

Fitzpatrick lecture delivered at the Royal College of Physicians of London, 5 December 1979. *Perspectives in Biology and Medicine* 1981–2; 25: 93–114.

scandal to each other, and then retired to take the waters of the spa where Beau Nash presided over the gaming table, and the doctors – obsequious and guinea collecting – hovered discreetly. Old theories, derived from the humoral concepts of ancient times, permeated clinical practice. Evil humours had to be removed from both blood and bowel. The inadequacies of medicine provided endless opportunities for the quack whose patent remedies were officially encouraged by the new patent laws and widely advertised in the newly developing newspaper trade.

It is perhaps for these reasons that many medical historians have dimissed the eighteenth century as a fallow period "sandwiched between two centuries of intellectual excitement" or as the darkness before the dawn.[4] Others have followed Richard Shryock in concluding that modern medicine had its origins in the medical renaissance that followed the revolutionary reforms in France in the 1790s. D'Arcy Power was one of the few who saw things differently, believing that Samuel Johnson had witnessed the replacement of the old medical order by the new. It is doubtful whether in his final illness Johnson himself, reaching surreptitiously beneath the blankets with a scalpel in a vain attempt to relieve his swollen and dropsical legs, could have thought that medicine in 1784 had much more to offer than when he was born in the early years of the century.[5] Lewis Thomas has written perhaps the most severe indictment of the era preceding the nineteenth century. "The history of medicine," he wrote, "has never been a particularly attractive subject in medical education and one reason for this is that it is so unrelievably deplorable...bleeding, purging, cupping and the administration of infusions of every known plant, solutions of every known metal, every conceivable diet including total fasting, most of them based on the weirdest imaginings about the cause of disease, concocted out of nothing but thin air – this was the heritage of medicine until a little over a century ago."[6]

The teachings of the great theorists of the eighteenth century were certainly replete with weird imaginings. Stahl and Hoffman remain obscure to the contemporary reader and much of Boerhaave's teaching is difficult now to understand. Later in the century Cullen was the most influential of the Edinburgh school and the contrast between his system and the theories of Brown provided students with a bewildering choice. It was out of this conflict that Rush distilled his unitary hypothesis. Yet if the eighteenth century was bedevilled by superstition and mystery and with "whymsical hypothesis and conceited imagination,"[7] it was also the century of the Enlightenment. It would be a severe indictment of medicine indeed if during such a century there had been no significant developments in clinical science. In fact, the eighteenth century was not the only era in human history when to be sick at all could mean disaster, and there were during that period many who sought to create order out of the chaos which surrounded them. As this account will show, they have many achievements to their credit.

The Age of Reason is traditionally associated with the eighteenth century but in reality it was the publication in 1687 of Newton's *Principia* and of Locke's *Essay Concerning Human Understanding* in 1690 that heralded the new era. Newton, described by Voltaire as "ce destructeur du système Cartesien," established an experimental philosophy that had major significance for all science but particularly for medicine, for Newtonian experimentalism gradually came to replace the empty theorising that derived from the philosophy of Descartes. John Locke's importance was to define in philosophical terms the scientific outlook of Newton. Locke, himself a physician, regarded Boyle, Newton, and his close friend Thomas Sydenham as the master builders of knowledge, and saw himself as an underlabourer who cleared the ground a little and removed the rubbish that lay in the way of knowledge.[8] His emphasis on the accurate use and significance of language found practical expression in that most famous of all dictionaries, in the preface to whose first edition Johnson wrote, echoing Locke, that he too was "the slave of science...doomed only to remove rubbish and clear obstructions from the path of learning and genius..." Under his entry on "Physick," he cited Locke who had written, "Was it my business to understand Physick, would not the safe way

3

be to consult nature herself in the history of diseases and their cures rather than espouse the principles of the dogmatists..." Perhaps reflecting contemporary thought, Johnson also pointed out that "the people use physick to purge themselves of humours," but his own definition of the word "Physick" is significant. "Physick," he wrote, "is the science of healing."[9]

The concept that the art of healing might be a science received considerable impetus from the changes that took place in medical education in Europe in the early years of the eighteenth century. For European medicine, the appointment of Hermann Boerhaave as lector in medicine at the University of Leyden in 1701 was an event of great significance. Leyden University, founded in 1575 by William the Silent, enjoyed the same religious and intellectual freedom as had Padua in the previous century. There was no religious bar to entry, in striking contrast to the situation in England where the universities of Oxford and Cambridge accepted only members of the Established Church, a limitation to their intellectual development that persisted until well into the nineteenth century. Boerhaave, despite the theoretical nature of much of his teaching, was the first of the great university teachers of practical clinical medicine. An avowed Newtonian, who, in the words of a French admirer, "ne pouvais jamais s'empêcher de rire au nez de Descartes," he sought to inculcate a spirit of scientific inquiry in the training of a physician. He both carried out experiments himself and taught at the bedside. He derived inspiration from the English clinician Thomas Sydenham, whose empiricism he much admired. His students remembered him throughout their lives. The great physiologist of later years, Albrecht von Haller, recalled being "filled with unbelievable delight when I heard him explain for the first time the true medicine."[10] Boerhaave's students came from far and wide. When he died, in 1738, the loss that the city of Leyden sustained from the reduction of his pupils was considerable. A Yorkshire Quaker was a pupil of Boerhaave in the 1720s, and as long as 40 years later he wrote of his mentor that he was "an able philosopher, and the greatest anatomist,

4

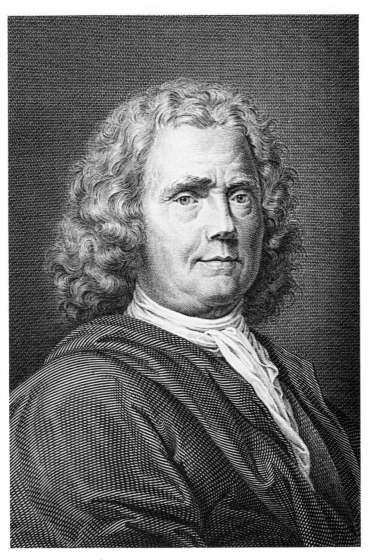

1 Hermann Boerhaave
 (Royal College of Physicians of London)

chemist, botanist, and the most eminent physician of this or any other age."[11]

Yet if Boerhaave was a teacher of the scientific method he was not so much its practitioner, and he made few important discoveries himself. It was through his pupils and the institutions they created that he exercised his influence, and it was these institutions that diffused the new experimental philosophy throughout Europe. Haller, after first returning to his native Switzerland, created the medical school of Göttingen, a university founded in 1734 by an Elector of Hanover who was also George II of England, and a major influence on the development of academic medicine in the eighteenth century in Germany. Another of Boerhaave's pupils was Gerhard van Swieten, physician to Maria Theresa and highly influential in the development of medical teaching in Vienna. His major importance to clinical science in Britain, however, was his influence on Scotland, for he taught the first professors at the medical school founded in Edinburgh in 1726.

It is well known that Edinburgh inherited Leyden's position as the centre of medical teaching in Europe after Boerhaave's death. A succession of brilliant teachers ensured that graduates of this university played a major role in both Britain and the United States throughout the eighteenth century. Edinburgh University enjoyed the same religious freedoms as Leyden and Padua. It was therefore an academic haven for the nonconformist, a situation that encouraged an atmosphere of free thinking ferment in the Scottish capital.

Edinburgh's graduates brought the traditions of their school to many parts of the world but particularly to London. Here, in the capital, there were other developments which helped to establish England as a centre of scientific medicine in Europe in the middle of the eighteenth century, even though at that time the country was unable to boast a single university school of medicine. Oxford and Cambridge had, unlike Leyden, Padua, Paris, or Edinburgh, never interested themselves in clinical studies – a situation that was to persist until well into the twentieth century. In London there was no university and the hospitals provided little opportunity for investigation and research, contenting themselves with clinical activity and an apprenticeship type of training for their students. It was for these reasons that a number of private schools of medicine emerged during the early years of the eighteenth century. William Cheselden, the famous surgeon, was perhaps the earliest to found a school for dissection.[12] In later years it was the school that the Hunters founded that eclipsed all others. William Hunter, friend and collaborator of William Cullen, had arrived in London in 1740 after studies in Glasgow and Edinburgh and in 1746 began a course of anatomical lectures with instruction in the operations of surgery, the application of bandages, and the art of dissecting. His first resident pupil was an American, John Jones of Philadelphia, one of those who was later to become a founder of the New York Hospital in 1771. In 1748 William Hunter was joined by his brother John and they set up their anatomy school in a large house in the northwest corner of the Great Piazza in Covent Garden. Here among the anatomical specimens John Morgan and William Shippen from Philadelphia, future founders of the first medical school in the United States, learnt the Hunters' methods of vascular injection. Here too William Hunter carried out his studies on the gravid uterus. In 1766 the Hunters moved to Great Windmill Street and it was at this famous school in 1770 that the young Edward Jenner, pupil of John Hunter, undertook his first anatomical dissections.[13]

Scientific societies have always played a major role in encouraging research and stimulating interest in new ideas. It was during the seventeenth and particularly the eighteenth centuries that societies with an interest in medicine emerged. The Royal Society, founded in 1660 by Charles II, had been the first in Britain to provide a forum for scientific discussion and debate. During the early years membership was not restricted to scientists – John Dryden was an early member of the society, to which the physician-poet Samuel Garth also later belonged. The Royal Society began the publication of the *Philosophical Transactions* in 1665 and it published Newton's *Principia* as well as the works of that gifted group of early Oxford physiologists who extended the horizon of Harvey's discoveries at the end of the seventeenth century. During the first half of the eighteenth century it was therefore to the Royal Society that any medical man would communicate his work.

The earliest medical society in Britain was founded in Edinburgh in 1731 by the founders of the new medical school, and they published yearly volumes of *Medical Essays and Observations*, dedicated to the Royal Society. It was the Edinburgh graduates in London, debarred from the fellowship of the Royal College of Physicians because they were not graduates of Oxford or Cambridge, who in 1752 emulated their Edinburgh teachers by forming the first society of physicians in England. They met at the Crown and Anchor tavern in the Strand.[14] John Fothergill, a Yorkshire Quaker who graduated in Edinburgh in 1736, was the moving spirit, together with William Hunter, Sir William Watson, Daniel Solander, and others. At Fothergill's expense the society began to publish a selection of the papers read before it and six volumes, entitled the *Medical Observations and Inquiries* were issued between 1757 and 1784.[15] In 1767, however, stimulated by the activities of its licentiates, the Royal College of Physicians began to publish its own *Medical Transactions* at the instigation of William Heberden and his friend Sir George Baker. The early volumes contain both Heberden's description of angina pectoris and Baker's famous work on lead poisoning, the inquiry concerning the cause of "the endemical colic of Devonshire."[16] Baker was a Devonian and his demonstration of the dangerous levels of lead in the cider of the west country led to him being denounced as a faithless son of Devonshire.

The *Medical Transactions* provided a useful forum for the publication of medical papers. It was unfortunate that the Scottish licentiates, led by William Hunter and John Fothergill, refused to submit papers to the college in protest against their continued exclusion from the fellowship. In 1767 a number of disgruntled licentiates, William Hunter among them, employed a blacksmith to break open the lock of the college and stormed into Comitia, causing scenes of unparalled violence.[17] The episode was brilliantly satirised by Samuel Foote in his play *The Devil on Two Sticks*, in which

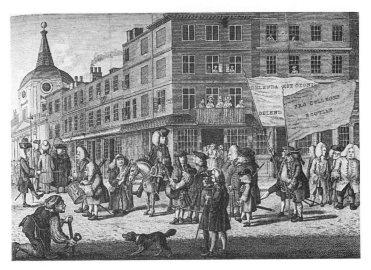

2   The march of the medical militants
(Royal College of Physicians of London)

Dr Fothergill was mercilessly portrayed as the sanctimonious
Dr Melchisedech Broadbrim.[18] This reference to the formidable Quaker's headgear recalls Fanny Burney's remark,
after he had attended her for a putrid sore throat in 1777.
"The hat that he wore," she wrote to Mr Crisp, "was of the
most enormous size you ever beheld."[19]

The Medical Society of London, founded in 1773 by
another Quaker physician and graduate of the University of
Edinburgh, John Coakley Lettsom, provided both a forum
for scientific discussion and, more significantly, a meeting
place for physicians, surgeons, and apothecaries. It was also
the first medical organisation, apart from the Royal Society,
to encourage research by awarding medals for outstanding
contributions. Lettsom founded the Fothergillian medal in
1784 in honour of John Fothergill, to whose patronage he
owed the success of his own medical career. It is to the credit
of the Medical Society of London that in 1793 the medal was
awarded to Robert Willan, another Yorkshire Quaker and
friend of the Fothergills, who had followed the taxonomical

approach of Linnaeus in bringing order to the classification of dermatological disease. The society brought even greater distinction to itself when in 1803 Lettsom ensured that Edward Jenner received the Fothergillian medal.[20]

The university schools of medicine in Leyden and Edinburgh, the anatomical school of the Hunters in London, and the emergence of the new medical societies, all played their role in encouraging a scientific approach to the problems of clinical medicine in the second half of the eighteenth century. There was another important influence: the increase of publishing, and the use of English in medical writing, brought medicine to a far wider readership than ever before. Harvey in 1628 had written in Latin, and published his work in Leyden and Frankfurt. By the middle of the eighteenth century virtually all medical writing was in English and there was a large number of publishers to choose from.

It was perhaps in the military and naval fields that the practical results of improvements in health brought about by scientific endeavour were first discerned. Sir John Pringle's work *Observations on the Diseases of the Army*, published in 1752, was the result of his studies on the use of sanitary measures during the War of the Austrian Succession.[21] As a young man Pringle had been sent to Amsterdam to study business, but he heard a single lecture by Hermann Boerhaave during a visit to Leyden which so impressed him that he determined to study medicine. He graduated at Leyden in 1730, practising first as a physician in Edinburgh and later becoming professor. Although a Scot, he was on the Hanoverian side with Cumberland at Culloden in 1745 and then continued to serve on the Continent until his return in the autumn of 1748 when peace was finally concluded by the treaty of Aix-la-Chapelle. Pringle, an ardent supporter of bleeding and purging in treatment, set out measures dictated by common sense and personal observation that were intended to prevent disease on active service. It is difficult now to determine how effective he was in reducing the numbers of soldiers dying or hospitalised, but there is little doubt that his work was influential not only in bringing him to the attention of medical and scientific colleagues but also to the royal family whom he served as physician. His distinction, and perhaps also his connections, were recognised by the Royal College of Physicians who elected him to the fellowship despite the fact that he had no degree from Oxford or Cambridge, a unique honour which the college did not award to that country practitioner, Edward Jenner. A fellow of the Royal Society, Pringle was awarded the society's highest honour, the Copley medal, for his researches on antiseptics. He was elected president in 1772, serving for six years, and in 1776 he therefore had the opportunity of personally presenting the Copley medal to Captain James Cook in recognition of his success in preventing disease during his remarkable second voyage on the *Resolution*.

It was in fact extraordinary that the Royal Navy had been so slow to recognise how to prevent scurvy. In the early years of the seventeenth century Captain James Lancaster of the East India Company had successfully prevented scurvy in his own ship by feeding bottled lemon juice to the crew, whereas two accompanying ships suffered severely. Woodall had recommended the use of lemon juice in 1617, yet when Anson circumnavigated the globe between 1740 and 1744 he lost more than 600 of his crews which totalled 961 men. This deplorable experience had stimulated contemporary physicians and surgeons to inquire into the causes of scurvy.

James Lind was born in Edinburgh and was a student there before entering the navy in 1739 at the age of 23. Serving at sea in the 50 gun ship HMS *Salisbury* in 1747, Lind studied 12 seamen who had severe scurvy.[23] It would be heartening to relate that Lind's clinical trial, which showed the success of treatment with oranges and lemons, but in a trial group of only two seamen, had the immediate effect of eradicating scurvy from the Royal Navy; but the evidence did not convince, and conservative attitudes died hard both in the Admiralty and in the forecastle. It was not until Cook made his voyages that authority was persuaded that the health of seamen could be preserved by appropriate measures. Cook had been asked by the Royal Society to test out a variety of antiscorbutics. On his second voyage on the *Resolution*, he found that sweet wort was the best, and sauerkraut, vegetable soup, lemons, and oranges were also very useful. The results, by comparison with earlier voyages, were spectacular. His voyage lasted three years and 11 days and took him as far north as 52° and south to 70° in the icy wastes of the Antarctic. He lost only one man during the entire expedition and there was no case of scurvy.

In 1795 Sir Gilbert Blane introduced lime juice for all seamen on naval ships. The effect on the health of crews was impressive. In a two year period from 1781 in the Caribbean, the death rate had been 1 in 7; during the two years before Trafalgar, Nelson found that it was only 1 in 127, an improvement which had an important effect on the health of seamen at his famous victory.[23]

Military surgeons were in general not known for their scientific abilities. John Hunter, however, was one who used his military experience to advantage. He received his commission in October 1760 at the height of the Seven Years' War and left his work at the anatomy school for the next three years. His treatise on gunshot wounds, published posthumously in 1794, was based on his work during the Bellisle expedition and in Portugal.[24] Throughout this period, however, his horizons were far wider than those of a military surgeon, and his interests, which included the organ of hearing in fish and the geology of the Alentejo plateau, were as broad as they were to be for the remainder of his life.

Hunter lived in London after the Treaty of Paris brought an end to the Seven Years' War in 1763, devoting himself to the practice of surgery, teaching and dissecting at the anatomy school, and amassing and developing the extraordinarily rich collections that are preserved at the Royal College of Surgeons in London. He interested himself in an immense variety of activities in biological science, ranging from the transplantation of teeth to the Gillaroo trout and "Observations on the Fossil Bones presented to the Royal Society by the Margrave of Anspach." No man of his time did so much in so wide an area of biology. Committed to earning his "damned guinea," as he put it, as a surgeon, he brought science to an essentially pragmatic area of medical treatment. The experiments that led him to ligate the popliteal artery for aneurysm, together with his constantly thoughtful approach to surgical problems, earned him the largest surgical practice in London and the posthumous reputation of being the founder of scientific surgery.[25]

Yet his contributions to the practice of surgery formed a relatively minor part of his scientific achievements. He is one of the very select band of surgeons who have been awarded the Copley medal of the Royal Society. That body, ever aware of the significance of scientific contribution, made their award not for his surgical work but for his three papers – "On the Ovaria," "On the Identity of the Dog, Wolf and Jackal," and "On the Anatomy of Whales" – which were published in the *Philosophical Transactions* in 1787.[26] It can perhaps be argued that John Hunter's major contribution to those who practise surgery was the demonstration that a surgeon, unversed in the ancients, could be one of the foremost biological scientists of his age. As one of his contemporaries put it, "he alone made us gentlemen."[27]

John Hunter's most famous pupil at the antomy school, Edward Jenner, came to London in 1770 at the age of 21. He impressed his teacher from the start but he was unhappy in London and in 1773 returned to the hills and valleys of his native Gloucestershire, where he worked as a country surgeon.[28] He continued to correspond with John Hunter who was his sponsor for the fellowship of the Royal Society, which he duly obtained in 1788.

Jenner, as a country practitioner, was accustomed to performing the operation of inoculation for his patients. The practice of inoculating material from a case of smallpox into the skin and producing a mild and attenuated attack of the disease had been introduced from Constantinople. Several communications on the operation were made to the Royal Society during the first two decades of the eighteenth century but it was Lady Mary Wortley Montagu, friend of Alexander Pope, who popularised the practice in England after having her son inoculated and persuading the Princess of Wales to have her own children inoculated in 1722.[29] Although the operation had the disadvantage that there was a definite mortality, by the middle of the eighteenth century inoculation was established as a standard procedure for the prevention of smallpox. In the later years of the century John Haygarth of Chester proposed exterminating the "casual smallpox," using inoculation on a wide scale.[30] Although he had considerable success in his own city,[31] it was not until vaccination was introduced that so ambitious a plan could be undertaken.

It was an epidemic of smallpox in his native Gloucestershire in 1778 that encouraged Jenner's further interest, for he found that there were individuals in whom it was not possible to achieve a successful inoculation. He then observed that these were patients who had been previously infected with cowpox. Many years of patient investigation followed. In 1796 Jenner first successfully demonstrated that a boy inoculated in the arm with cowpox could not then receive smallpox by inoculation. At this stage he tried to get his observations published by the Royal Society. Sir Joseph Banks, however, returned his original paper on the grounds that he had not then proved his case. For this reason, Jenner did not give his findings to the public until two years later when, after further experiments, he published the *Inquiry into the Causes and Effects of the Variolae Vaccinae* as a book dedicated to his friend and collaborator, Dr Caleb Hillier Parry of Bath.[32] In Bath the first vaccine institution in England was opened; and it was with vaccine from Bath that the first vaccinations in America were carried out two years later, by Dr Benjamin Waterhouse, first professor of medicine at Harvard.

The discovery that smallpox could be safely prevented by vaccination must rank as one of the greatest in human history. Yet it is interesting that it had its roots in folk medicine and in the beliefs of country people. Throughout the eighteenth century the medicines and practices of contemporary herbalists and quacks interested those of the conventional profession who carried out clinical research. John Fothergill in his early years in London described, in a letter to his old teacher in Edinburgh, Professor Charles Alston, his attempt to extract a powerful purgative from the juice of the squirting cucumber.[35] The crucial step, however, he could not obtain from the woman who prepared it. She told him that "she had been instructed by an old herb woman...and nothing should prevail upon her to divulge so beneficial a secret except to her children, who were to expect this as their only provision." Fothergill, a distinguished botanist in his own right, honoured by Linnaeus in having an American plant named after him, was interested in herbal remedies throughout his life. Writing in 1771 to the American botanist, Humphrey Marshall, he asked whether he knew of any medicines which could operate freely and certainly by producing urine. "We can vomit, purge, sweat to what degree we choose," he wrote, "but we have no certain diuretic. This is much needed in the cure of dropsies..."

William Withering, another Edinburgh graduate, working in Birmingham, was to discover the much sought after diuretic. It was his custom to drive each week to Stafford to see patients referred to him. The journey was about 30 miles so the horses had to be changed at least once. One day in 1775 during the change he was asked to see an elderly lady with severe dropsy whose prospects he pronounced as very poor. When he inquired after her three weeks later he was astonished to find that she had made a good recovery. The lady had been treated with a family recipe for the cure of dropsy kept by an old woman in Shropshire. This herb woman was less fortunate in preserving her secret than Fothergill's friend, for Withering, member of the Lunar Society, one of the leading botanists in England at that time, found it "not very difficult for one conversant in these subjects to perceive that the active herb could be no other than the foxglove." Withering spent the next 10 years carefully recording the effects of the foxglove in cases of dropsy, noting particularly its value when the pulse was irregular, and did not publish his work until 1785, too late to help the aged Samuel Johnson who had died the year before.[34]

The discovery of new remedies is an integral part of medical investigation yet it is almost as important to reject old methods of treatment which have little to commend them other than prolonged usage. A start was made during the eighteenth century at ridding the pharmacopoeia of ancient preparations. Heberden's famous *Antitheriaca*, published in 1745, was a caustic attack on the use of Venice treacle or

Mithradatium, a remedy which at that time contained more than 65 ingredients, including the dried flesh of vipers. In Paris it was publicly prepared during elaborate ceremonies lasting 15–17 days.[35] It is to the ultimate credit of both Heberden and Sir George Baker, then president of the Royal College of Physicians, that in 1786 the question whether the Theriaca should be retained in the pharmacopoeia was put and as the *Annals* of the college record, "determined in the negative".[36] Other practices took longer to change but during the eighteenth century even bleeding and purging came under attack. Fothergill in London and Wall – of porcelain fame – in Worcester both advocated supportive rather than depletive regimens for the treatment of what was then called the "malignant sore throat," the condition which probably killed George Washington. "How many lives were lost," wrote Withering in 1793, "until Dr Fothergill and Dr Wall taught us to withhold the lancet and the purge."[37]

The investigation of popular remedies was also indirectly the stimulus to the development of research in chemistry. The story began with Sir Robert Walpole's bladder stone. In the belief that Walpole had benefited from a medicine invented by a Mrs Joanna Stephens, an Act of Parliament was proposed to reward her with £5000 for her discovery. To meet criticism Parliament appointed a body of trustees to investigate Mrs Stephens's claim. It was a roll call of the most influential in the land, but a group scarcely qualified to adjudicate on a medicine which, when revealed by Mrs Stephens in 1739, was found to consist of "eggshells and snail shells, both calcined, wild carrot seeds, burdock seeds, ashen keys, hips and haws, all burnt to blackness and mixed with Alicant soap and honey."[38] Though eagerly sought by a public plagued by bladder stones, the medicine was mistrusted by many physicians. The Reverend Stephen Hales suggested, however, that lime was the important ingredient.

At the instigation of William Cullen, then working in Glasgow, his assistant Joseph Black began experiments with the object of discovering a milder alkali than lime which might serve the same purpose. In 1751, at the age of 23, Black went to complete his medical education at Edinburgh, where he found Professor Charles Alston experimenting with lime water. Alston, however, as Black told Cullen in 1752, "has neither had practice enough nor is a good enough chemist to be perfect in his profession."[39] Black unquestionably had both attributes. It was as a medical student that he carried out the experiments on magnesia which resulted in his discovery of the gas which Lavoisier later termed carbonic acid. He postponed submitting his work until 1754, when he graduated MD with his thesis written in Latin. During the whole of the eighteenth century there was no other thesis submitted to the University of Edinburgh of such momentous significance. Black's observations were of fundamental importance for the birth of chemistry. By the careful use of the balance he laid the foundations of quantitative analysis and his distinction of carbon dioxide, or "fixed air," from common air founded the science of pneumatic chemistry. Black's work was a stimulus to Priestley's investigation of the nature of air which led to his discovery of oxygen, as well as to the work of Henry Cavendish. Lavoisier acknowledged himself his disciple. Black, however, perhaps influenced by his mistrust of systems such as Cullen's or Brown's, thought Lavoisier's generalisations premature, commenting cautiously in his lectures, "Chemistry is not yet a science. We are very far from the knowledge of first principles. We should avoid everything that has the pretensions of a full system"

Black became professor of medicine in Glasgow in 1756 at the age of 28 but moved back to Edinburgh 10 years later. He was a teacher who had a lasting influence on those he taught. Lord Brougham, subsequently influential in the age of reform, was one of his students. He wrote in later years that although he had heard the "commanding periods of Pitt's majestic oratory" and "the vehemence of Fox's burning declamation," he would without hesitation prefer to have the chance of seeing Joseph Black again performing, with his own hands, the experiments by which he made his discoveries.

It was another pupil of Joseph Black who had the idea of setting up a clinic to investigate the curative powers of the newly discovered gases. Thomas Beddoes had studied under

Black in Edinburgh and had extended his medical education at London and Oxford. He lectured at Oxford from 1789 to 1792 but was then forced to resign because of his radical opinions and in particular his enthusiastic support for the French Revolution. In 1793 he had the idea of using hydrogen as a cure for tuberculosis, a concept that brought him into contact with James Watt, who was then in partnership with Matthew Boulton in Birmingham and whose son Gregory suffered from consumption. Beddoes moved to Bristol in 1794 and soon afterwards married Anne, younger sister of the famous Maria Edgeworth, and daughter of the much married Richard Lowell Edgeworth, another member of the Lunar Society in Birmingham. The marriage produced the poet Thomas Lovell Beddoes, author of that mystical poem *Dream Pedlary* – "If there were dreams to sell, / What would you buy?" Beddoes's Pneumatic Institute, however, did not materialise until 1797 when he received enough money to make a start, some from a grateful patient and the remainder from other members of the Lunar Society, who would have included his father in law.

Meantime, Humphrey Davy was apprenticed to an apothecary in Penzance.[40] He was 19 years old and intending to go to Edinburgh to study medicine. He had no experience of chemistry other than reading Lavoisier's *Traité Elementaire* in the French, but he was already undertaking significant experiments on the nature of light and heat. It was at this time that Davy met Gregory Watt, then seeking the milder climate of the south coast for his convalescence. Gregory Watt wrote enthusiastically to Beddoes about the young Davy but his introduction came through Davies Giddy, a Cornishman who was a mathematician and fellow of the Royal Society, later to be president (he helped Telford with his calculations for the construction of the Menai Bridge), and it was therefore through the influence of these two that Humphrey Davy went to Bristol to become Beddoes's assistant in 1799. The work of the next 18 months was the most concentrated of his career. His attention had been drawn to the dephlogisticated nitrous gas of Dr Priestley by reading a pamphlet published several years earlier by a New

York physician, Dr Samuel Mitchill, who had suggested that the gas, nitrous oxide, was the agent of contagion. It did not take Davy long to show that Mitchill was indulging in fanciful theory, for he simply showed by experiments that both animals and he himself could breathe the gas without ill effect. His subsequent experiments on the effects of nitrous oxide were carried out not only on himself but on a remarkable group of volunteer human subjects who included his close friends and fellow poets, Southey and Coleridge. Southey was wild about the new gas. "Davy has invented a new pleasure for which language has no name," he wrote; "I am going for more this evening..." Perhaps Coleridge's vision of his Abyssinian maid, the damsel with a dulcimer, was induced by Davy's gas rather than by opium, as is often supposed. More significantly, Davy found that the gas would relieve dental pain and it was this observation that led him to the suggestion, published in his book on nitrous oxide in 1800, that "it may probably be used with advantage during surgical operations..." He was 21 years old.

Pneumatics, the study of gases, was essentially a basic scientific activity during the eighteenth century and it was not for another 46 years that nitrous oxide was to be used as an anaesthetic. Clinical medicine in the meantime was making its own contributions. The first description of angina pectoris, by William Heberden, was a classic example of careful clinical observation in practice. Later work led during the eighteenth century to the first recognition of its association with coronary artery disease, now the scourge of Western society (see Chapter 4).

Caleb Hillier Parry of Bath, to whom Jenner dedicated his famous work, typifies the physician of the late eighteenth century. It was an age when medicine often formed only part of the scientific activity of clinicians who were scientists, as is so clearly shown by the careers of both Hunter and Jenner. Parry, an outstanding clinical observer, was sufficiently wealthy through his medical activities to indulge his manifold interests and it was as a farmer that he played a major role in developing the Merino sheep, the breed that was to be so important to the Australian wool trade.

There were also throughout the century non-medical men who had no hesitation in interesting themselves in medical matters in the normal course of developing their concern for what was new or beneficial. That remarkable vicar of Teddington, the Reverend Stephen Hales, apart from his many other activities had an intense interest in the health of his fellow men, and the American philosopher and sage, Dr Benjamin Franklin, attempted to use electricity for the treatment of nervous disorders, notably cases of palsy. He showed a healthy scepticism for the results but one of his apparently successful cases, a young lady with convulsive fits, was reported in the first volume of the *Medical Observations and Inquiries* in 1757.[41]

This account of clinical science in the eighteenth century has included selected histories of individual discoveries. I have not mentioned the work of Dr Haygarth of Chester and Dr Percival, of Manchester, on the prevention of fevers,[42] nor Haygarth's merciless exposure, after he moved to Bath at the turn of the century, of the ludicrous claims made for Perkin's metallic tractors.[43] It was this that led to his recognition of the power of the imagination as a cause of and cure for bodily disorders. Many other topics deserve the attention of modern historians – William Cadogan and the infant welfare movement, the improvement in maternal mortality and its association with better obstetrics, and the activities of the Royal Humane Society, founded in the 1770s, which sought the "recovery of those supposedly drowned."

There is also the work of those who followed trade and empire to far flung corners of the globe – James Kerr in India, Cleghorn in Minorca, Alexander Russell in Turkey. Perhaps the most significant of this group was William Hillary, Boerhaave's pupil who worked in Barbados, where he was consulted by George and Lawrence Washington in 1751. Hillary published his *Diseases of the West India Islands* in London in 1759, the year of the capture of Quebec. His book was considered sufficiently authoritative to be republished by Benjamin Rush in Philadelphia as late as 1811, another year of conflict in North America.

What of the men to whom we owe the achievements of

eighteenth century clinical science? They came predominantly from minor gentry or from the emerging middle class. None was from the aristocracy. Jenner was a son of the church. Joseph Black's father was a Belfast born merchant who worked in Bordeaux, where he enjoyed the friendship of Montesquieu. Long Calderwood, home of the Hunters, is a country property very similar to that of the Fothergills or the Hillarys in Wensleydale. These Yorkshire dalesmen had more in common with Scottish lowland freeholders like the Hunters than with the aristocracy and squirarchy of the shires of southern England.

The characters of some of these men have been described by those who knew them. Joseph Black was said, like Marcus Aurelius, to have had a smooth and inoffensive temper. Of John Hunter, Everard Home wrote that "he hated deceit and was above every kind of artifice." He sometimes spoke harshly of his contemporaries and was disputatious on the question of priority, as the sad difference between himself and his brother William indicates. But his assistant, William Clift, considered that "nobody about Mr Hunter seemed capable of appreciating him," and he thought that he had lived before his time. There was no lack of the normal attributes of human frailty and ambition about the men of the eighteenth century. Writing at the age of 25 to his brother Joseph, John Fothergill had told him: "I could not look upon an overgrown doctor, wealthy at the expense of his fellow citizens' lives, lolling in his chariot, without some envious emotion, and tacitly asking myself if such a state would not mightily become me." Forty years later, when he had achieved his ambitions, the charming Fanny Burney, accustomed to the brilliant circle of Dr Johnson and Mrs Thrale, had at first found the aging Fothergill's manners uncongenial, though after he had cared for her in an illness she admitted his virtues.

There was a strong element of nonconformity and dissent among the clinical scientists of the eighteenth century, and they were not afraid to speak their minds. Fothergill, Hillary, Lettsom, and Willan were Quakers. Fothergill, physician to Franklin and his close friend, was an ardent supporter of the

American cause. Robert Willan the elder, MD of Edinburgh in 1745, a kinsman but not, as popularly supposed, the father of the famous dermatologist, wrote a letter to the Earl of Chatham in 1768 pointing out that the "True cause of the suffering of the people is the immoderate aggrandisement of the Noblesse and the Principal Gentry," a courageous view to put before a nobleman who was the greatest Englishman of his time.[44] Edinburgh, alma mater to both Fothergill and Willan and to so many others, made its own contribution to free thinking. Withering was an Anglican but this did not prevent the mob from threatening to burn his house to the ground during the Birmingham riots of 1791. The house was saved only by judicious bribery. Nothing could have helped his neighbour, Dr Priestley, fellow member of the Lunar Society, whose house and entire laboratory were totally destroyed. It was this episode that led Priestley, an outspoken Unitarian and free thinker, to take refuge in self imposed exile in Pennsylvania for the closing years of his life, where he had the unhappy experience of meeting Rush. Sir John Pringle was also a Unitarian, a form of belief most distasteful to Dr Johnson, who refused to meet him for this reason. Perhaps Johnson would have had less admiration for Heberden, the classical scholar, his *Ultimus Romanorum*, had he known that his physician attended Dr Priestley's Unitarian services at Essex Street during the period that Priestley lived in London. The wayward Dr Beddoes's support for the French Revolution has already been referred to.

Contemporary opinion may still recoil in revulsion from the therapeutic horrors perpetrated, no doubt with the best of intentions, during the eighteenth century. Yet there was also a remarkable thread of scientific activity and achievement. It was early days for clinical science, but as in everything else beginnings were made. Perhaps there was something similar in the state of clinical science in Britain and the development in France of the air balloons of Messieurs Montgolfier, Robert and Charles, an adventure which, like clinical science, owed much to the discovery of the new gases. Benjamin Franklin, then representative of the newly independent United States at the court of Louis XVI, was observing the remarkable sight of a balloon, heavier than air, drifting through the sky when someone asked, "Of what use is that?" To which Franklin gave the immortal reply, "A quoi bon l'enfant qui vient de naître?"[45]

A century which, as its most distinguished achievement, gave vaccination to the world has surely now been vindicated by the total eradication of smallpox within the past decade. This has been achieved not by accident nor by random social change, but because there were men in the eighteenth century who believed that it was the science of medicine that could best contribute to the welfare of mankind.

NOTES

1 Shryock RH. *The development of modern medicine.* London: Gollancz, 1948.

2 Gibbs FW. *Joseph Priestley.* London: Nelson, 1965.

3 Ketchum RM. *The world of George Washington.* New York: American Heritage, 1974.

4 Bynum WF. Enlightenment, medicine and physiology. In: Rousseau GS, Porter RS, eds. *The ferment of knowledge.* New York: Cambridge University Press, 1980.

5 Hibbert C. *The personal history of Samuel Johnson.* London: Longman, 1971.

6 Thomas L. Biomedical science and human health—the long range prospects. Paper presented at Festschrift in honour of Professor Dr Otto Westphal, Freiburg, 1 February 1978.

7 Hillary W. *A rational and mechanical essay on the small pox.* London: G Strachan, 1735.

8 Locke J. *An essay concerning human understanding.* London: Basset, 1690.

9 Johnson S. *A dictionary of the English language.* London: Knapton, Longman, Hitch and Hawes, Millar and Didsley, 1755.

10 Lindeboom GA. *Herman Boerhaave. The man and his work.* London: Methuen, 1968.

11 Hillary W. *An inquiry into the means of improving medical knowledge by examining all those methods which have hindered or increased its improvement in all past ages.* London: Hitch and Hawes, 1761.

12 Cope Z. *William Cheselden, 1688–1752.* Edinburgh: Livingstone, 1954.

13 Peachey G. *A memoir of William and John Hunter.* Plymouth: Brendon, 1924.

14 Fox RH. *Dr John Fothergill and his friends.* London: Macmillan, 1919.

15 *Medical Observations and Inquiries by a Society of Physicians in London.* 6 vols. London: Johnson and Cadell, 1752–1784.

16 Baker G. An inquiry concerning the cause of the endemical colic of Devonshire. *Med Trans Coll Phys Lond* 1768; 1: 175–256.

17 Stevenson LG. The siege of Warwick Lane. *J Hist Med Allied Sci* 1952; 8: 105–22.

18 Corner BC. Dr Melchisedech Broadbrim and the playwright. *J Hist Med Allied Sci* 1952; 8: 122–35.

19 Ellis AR. *The early diaries of Frances Burney.* London: Bell, 1913.

20 Abraham JJ. *Lettsom, his life, times, friends and descendants.* London: Heinemann, 1933.

21 Pringle J. *Observations on the diseases of the army in camp and garrison.* London: Millar, Wilson and Durham, and Payne, 1752.

22 Lind J. *A treatise on the scurvy.* London: Millar, 1754.

23 Ellis FP. Victuals and ventilation and the health and efficiency of seamen. *Br J Ind Med* 1948; 9: 185–97.

24 Hunter J. *Treatise on the blood, inflammation and gunshot wounds.* London: Nicol, 1794.

25 Dobson J. *John Hunter.* Edinburgh and London: Livingstone, 1969.

26 Records of Medallists of the Royal Society. Library of the Royal Society, London.

27 Shryock RH. *The development of modern medicine.* London: Gollancz, 1948: 60.

28 Fisk D. *Doctor Jenner of Berkeley.* London: Heinemann, 1959.

29 Halsband R. *Lady Mary Wortley Montagu.* Oxford: Clarendon, 1958.

30 Haygarth J. *An inquiry how to prevent the small pox.* Chester: Monk, 1784.

31 Haygarth J. *A sketch of a plan to exterminate the small pox from Great Britain and to introduce general inoculation.* London: Johnson, 1793.

32 Jenner E. *An inquiry into the cause and effects of the variolae vaccinae.* London, 1755.

33 Autograph letter, John Fothergill to Professor Charles Alston, London, 22 July 1739. Alston MSS, Library of the University of Edinburgh.

34 Peck TW, Wilkinson K D. *William Withering.* Bristol: Wright, 1950.

35 Corner GW. Mithridatium and theriac. *Bull Johns Hopkins Hosp* 1915; 26: 222–6.

36 *Annals of the Royal College of Physicians of London* 1781–1789; 15: 132–3.

37 Withering W. *Account of the scarlet fever and sore throat.* London: Cadell, 1793.

38 Ramsay W. *The life and letters of Joseph Black.* London: Constable, 1918.

39 MS by J M Alston, "Charles Alston MD, 1685–1776." In the possession of the author.

40 Hartley H. *Humphrey Davy.* London: Nelson, 1966.

41 Anonymous. A relation of a cure performed by electricity from Mr Cadwalader Evans, student in physick at Philadelphia. *Medical Observations and Inquiries* 1757; 1: 83.

42 Haygarth J. *A letter to Dr Percival on the prevention of infectious fevers and an address to the College of Physicians at Philadelphia on the prevention of the American pestilence.* Bath: Crutwell, 1801.

43 Haygarth J. *On the imagination as a cause and a cure of disorders of the body exemplified by fictitious traitors and epidemical convulsions.* Bath: Crutwell, 1800.

44 Autograph letter, R Willan to the Earl of Chatham, 12 August 1768. Chatham Papers. Public Record Office, London.

45 Taurneux M. *Corréspondence littéraire, philosophique et critique, par Grimm, Diderot, Meister, etc.* Paris: Garnier Frères, 1877–1882.

2 The author of *The Dispensary*: a literary fellow of the Royal Society

In the spring of the first year of the eighteenth century fellows of the Royal College of Physicians of London may have been surprised to receive a card desiring them "to accompany the corpse of Mr John Dryden from the College of Physicians in Warwick Lane to Westminster Abbey on Monday the 13th of the Instant May in 1700."[1] Dryden had died in somewhat straitened circumstances in Soho on 1 May and his family had arranged for a simple burial the next day at St Anne's Church. Several persons of quality, hearing of this, decided that Dryden, the great poet and dramatist of the Restoration era and forerunner of the Augustan age, deserved a more imposing funeral, and a subscription was raised for a more appropriate public ceremony with subsequent interment at Westminster Abbey. The body was disinterred, embalmed at Russell's, and then removed on 6 May to the hall of the College of Physicians in Warwick Lane where it lay in state for a week. On 9 May the *London Post Boy* reported that the Latin eulogy was to be assigned to "that learned physician and famous orator" Dr Samuel Garth. After the event, which duly took place on 13 May, there were mixed reactions to Garth's performance. The *Post Boy* wrote of his "eloquent oration in Latin," and another report described how Garth had ascended the pulpit where the physicians make their lectures and had "most rhetorically set forth those eulogies and encomiums which no poet hitherto but the great Dryden

Gideon de Laune lecture of the faculty of the history of medicine of the Worshipful Society of Apothecaries, delivered on 3 April 1985. *Notes and Records of the Royal Society* 1986; **40**: 125–45.

could ever truly deserve." Others, however, commented that Dr Garth had thrown away a great deal of false Latin in praising the poet and they criticised the whole event, deploring the singing of the *Ode to Melpomene* of Horace in place of a Psalm of David as unchristian and describing the subsequent procession to the abbey as unseemly and "mostly burlesque." George Farquhar wrote of Dryden: "He was an extraordinary man and buried after an extraordinary fashion." Whatever the circumstances of the cavalcade, Dryden's body was taken to Westminster Abbey and buried between the graves of Chaucer and Cowley in the Poet's Corner, where he lies to this day.[2]

Dr Samuel Garth, the leading figure in these events, made no scientific contribution to the Royal Society, to which he was later to be elected, since he was essentially a literary man. He came from an ancient Durham family. He was born in 1660, thus being an exact contemporary of Hans Sloane who was born the same year.[3] He was the eldest son of William Garth of Bolam, a small village that lies in lower Teesdale between Darlington and Barnard Castle. He was brought up in this relatively isolated area of England and went to school at Ingleton, County Durham, a small town in the parish of Staindrop which is close to Bolam. Here he seems to have received his preliminary education. In 1676, at the age of 16, he went to Cambridge, where he was admitted to Peterhouse on 27 May of that year.[4] His father must have been a man of some substance, since in his will he described how he had been "at great charges in the education of his eldest son, Samuel Garth, at the University of Cambridge and in his taking his degree there as Doctor of Physick."[5]

Samuel Garth's medical education lasted a long time. He took his BA degree in Cambridge in 1679 and his MA in 1684, but he did not receive his medical doctorate until 1691, 15 years after his enrolment at Peterhouse. By then it is evident that he had spent some time on the Continent, enrolling as a medical student in Leyden in 1687. Other evidence suggests that he may have been on military service, for when he applied to the Royal College of Physicians for admission in 1692, the college annals record that he had spent some years in foreign campaigns and hospitals.[6] He may, therefore, have been abroad at the time of the Glorious Revolution of 1688, when the Catholic James II was obliged to flee to France after the landing of William of Orange, the husband of Queen Mary II, in Torbay on Guy Fawkes day.

By 7 July 1691 Garth, then 31 years old, was back in England for he received his MD at Cambridge on that day. One year later he was admitted as a licentiate of the Royal College of Physicians and after only a further year he was elected as a fellow.[7] He was also nominated as Goulstonian lecturer of the college, an honour given to the most distinguished of the youngest newly elected fellows. He gave his lecture in Latin on 8 March 1694, the subject being "De Respiratione," and despite a promise to the president and censors of the college to publish his lecture in Latin he seems never to have done so. It was the year of the death of Mary II of smallpox, an event which caused widespread national grief. A year later Garth became a member of the college's five man committee on medicines – an important body whose chairman was Garth's close friend, Dr Hans Sloane, who by now had been secretary of the Royal Society for two years – and it was at about this time that he married Martha, the daughter of Sir Henry Beaufoy.

Garth must have made a highly favourable impression on his fellow physicians and on such distinguished colleagues as Sloane, for in 1697 at the age of 37 he was appointed as Harveian orator, the greatest distinction that the college can bestow on one of its fellows, other than to elect him president. Harvey's endowment of a public lecture in Latin had emphasised that the orator should commemorate the benefactors of the college, exhort the fellows and members to search and study out the secrets of nature by way of experiment and encourage the profession to continue in mutual love and affection among themselves. In Garth's oration, delivered on 16 September 1697, he made no reference to the secrets of nature, or the desirability of seeking them out. Instead he launched into a commemoration of all the college benefactors by name, starting with Henry VIII and concluding with Lady Grace Pierrepoint, the daughter of the Marquis of Dorchester whose books she had presented to the college library in 1688.

More than half the oration is taken up with extravagant praise of the King, William III. Garth, in the English version of the oration preserved in the Yale historical library, wrote, "You are not only the guardian of this College, but the deliverer of the Christian world and the restorer of public Peace. From you it is that Europe expects better times: from you it is that the Husbandman hopes for joyful seasons: from you it is that matrons are in a capacity to defend their chastity and maids to maintain their modesty. The English reverence you; the Spaniards respect you; the Germans admire you; the Dutch love you; but the French fear you."[8]

It may seem extraordinary today that a Harveian oration should have been devoted to such an enthusiastic eulogy of a ruling monarch. Yet one must remember the importance of William III in the bolstering of the Protestant succession in England in 1688, as well as the general sympathy felt for him throughout the country because of his bereavement in the loss of his queen. Furthermore, September 1697 was a particularly important month in English history. Only six days before Samuel Garth's Harveian oration, William III's negotiators at his palace near Delft in Holland had reached the agreement with Louis XIV's emissaries that ended the long and costly Nine Years' War with France. The news of the peace of Ryswick had been greeted in London during that same week with the firing of guns from the tower and with wild celebrations all over the capital.[9] Under the agreements made at Ryswick, Louis XIV for the first time recognised William III as the lawful king of England and promised not to give or afford any assistance directly, or indirectly, to any enemy of William III, a veiled direct reference to the exiled James II and his son the Old Pretender. Garth's expression of the nation's gratitude in his Harveian oration was therefore appropriate to the occasion and the college recorded that it had been delivered "to the great satisfaction of the audience and his own reputation."[10]

The oration concluded with a paragraph on a question that was causing considerable discord in the college at that time, the profession's "mutual love and affection" being severely disrupted, and he earnestly entreated fellows to return again to "unitie and concord." He referred to the repository, well furnished with drugs for the help of the poor which the college had decided to establish in 1696, following the advice of its committee of medicines. This repository, or free dispensary, had not only caused friction among fellows, but it also brought the college into direct conflict with the Society of Apothecaries, whose opposition to the whole idea of a dispensary was vociferous and unyielding.

An uneasy relationship existed between physician and apothecary throughout the entire seventeenth century and this occasionally flared into open hostility. The apothecaries had originally belonged to the Grocers' Company, but in 1617, under a royal charter granted by James I, they had established the Society of the Art and Mystery of Apothecaries of London. Under this charter the apothecaries were to restrict their activities to the preparation and sale of drugs, but at the same time they were to be subservient to the physicians, who treated patients, since the new society had to consult with the College of Physicians before it adopted any new drug regulations or admitted new members.[11] There were, however, far too few physicians to deal with the increasing population of London and, as the century went on, growing numbers of apothecaries began to prescribe medicines as well as preparing them. Two other issues were influential in changing the role of the apothecary: politics and plague. During the Civil War, many of the physicians were Royalists, like William Harvey, and during the Commonwealth the Royal College of Physicians fell on hard times. The London apothecaries, therefore, increasingly undertook treatment and there was little that the college could do about what it described as "the daring practices of the apothecaries."[12]

After the Restoration of Charles II in 1660, the college felt better able to assert its authority and in 1663 a new charter enhanced its powers of regulation of the apothecaries' affairs. Two years later, however, the city was struck by the great plague. The few physicians then living in the city, who appeared to believe that they could treat the condition,[13] were woefully inadequate to deal with the disaster which killed a third of the city's inhabitants, and this led to a great increase in the number of apothecaries treating patients, however inadequately, as well as preparing drugs. In later years the apothecaries were able with justification to attack the physicians for leaving the stricken capital since many of them fled, including Thomas Sydenham, along with the court and their wealthy patients. The physicians countered by charging the apothecaries with enriching themselves during the plague at the expense of the sick and suffering.

The battle between physician and apothecary was conducted by tract and countertract for the remainder of the seventeenth century. At the same time there emerged among the physicians the idea, possibly induced in part by a sense of guilt at their behaviour during the plague year, that there should be a public charity clinic supported by the Royal College. This was first suggested in 1670, but it was not until 1687 that the college formally announced that its members would give free treatment to any certified pauper and this was followed by the proposal that there should be a public dispensary at the college, where medicines would be provided free for the sick poor. This was thought by the apothecaries to be a direct threat to their livelihood as well as an intrusion into their work as established by their charter. Some physicians sympathised with the apothecaries and there emerged a group of so called apothecaries-physicians who opposed the college plans. By 1696, however, the college committee on medicines proposed that a dispensary should be established by the college with free medicines for the poor and by the end of the year 52 college members, including Sloane, Garth, and the president of the college, Sir Thomas Millington, had subscribed £10 apiece to the venture. It was the discord in the college between those who supported or opposed the dispensary that prompted Garth's exhortation in his Harveian oration that fellows of the college should seek "unitie and concord." In the spring of 1698, the year after Garth's Harveian oration, the dispensary was opened at the college in Warwick Lane and it was so successful that two more dispensaries were opened, one in St Martin's Lane, and the other in Gracechurch Street. These were the first public dispensaries for the poor to be established in this country.[14]

Opposition by the antidispensarians, however, continued unabated and it was not until a year later that Garth, with the publication of his famous poem *The Dispensary* in 1699, virtually ended all dispute. *The Dispensary* had an importance which went far beyond its virtue as a work of art. It was an immediate and resounding success. Three editions were called for in that first year of its appearance; eight editions were published during Garth's lifetime, and it was reprinted intermittently throughout the eighteenth century.[15] Although two historians of the Society of Apothecaries give Garth the credit for having "chased the opposition from the field",[16] disputes between the physicians and the apothecaries grumbled on until the famous case of William Rose, an apothecary charged before the courts with the illegal practice of medicine in 1703, whose conviction was reversed on appeal to the House of Lords.

The importance of Garth's *Dispensary*, however, lies not only in its undoubted effect on a prolonged and undignified professional quarrel, but also in its unique contribution to English literature. It formed an indispensable link between the poetry of Dryden and the grandeur of the Augustan age and it was the first English poem to be written in the "mock heroic" mode, in which a comic, trivial, or even sordid topic is dealt with in a lofty and classical poetic style. It was later to be immeasurably refined and developed by Alexander Pope. Garth points out in the introduction to the first edition of the *Dispensary* that the idea for the poem was sparked off by a trivial event at the College of Physicians. There had apparently been a scuffle in the dispensary between a member of the college with his retinue – presumably an anti-dispensarian physician – and some of the servants who attended there to dispense the medicines.

The poem begins with a description of the College of Physicians, which was then in Warwick Lane, near the Old Bailey:

> Not far from that most celebrated Place,
> Where angry Justice shows her awful Face,
> Where little Villains must submit to Fate
> That great Ones may enjoy the world in State
> There stands a Dome majestic to the Sight
> And sumptuous Arches bear its oval Height
> A golden globe placed high with artful Skill
> Seems to the distant Sight a gilded Pill.

The poem goes on to describe how the high moral purpose of the college had been disturbed by discord among the physicians and the god Sloth has taken up residence. His slumbers are rudely interrupted by the sounds of the construction of the new dispensary and, complaining bitterly, he sends off his servant Phantom to summon help from the goddess Envy. Phantom finds Envy, who assumes the shape of Colon (an apothecary called Lee). Colon then goes to see a fellow apothecary, Horoscope (Dr Barnard), in his shop. It is full of the nauseous tools of his trade; mummies lie "most reverently stale," and there is a crowd of gullible people promised "future health for present fees" by Horoscope. Envy's news of the building of the dispensary causes Horoscope to faint at the prospect of his loss of income and he revives only when his assistant Squirt gives him vapours from a urinal. Colon breathes a storm of envy against the dispensary movement into Horoscope's breast and leaves it there "like a brood of maggots" to develop. Horoscope spends a restless and sleepless night pondering what response to make. He sends off Squirt to summon the apothecaries to a meeting and in the meantime unsuccessfully solicits the help of the goddess Disease in the struggle he anticipates. The scene changes to Apothecaries' Hall, described by Garth in the following derogatory lines:

> Here where Fleet Ditch descends in sable Streams
> To wash the sooty Naiads in the Thames,
> There stands a structure on a rising Hill,
> Where Students take their licence out to Kill.

The assembly is addressed by Diasenna, a conciliator, Colo-

33

cynthis, who wants a fight to the death, and Ascarides who suggests that they ally themselves with the disaffected physicians in attempting to subvert the dispensary. The meeting is shattered by an explosion, which occurs in the basement laboratory of Apothecaries' Hall.

The action now moves to Covent Garden where Mirmillo has brought together a group of antidispensarian physicians to decide on future action. Mirmillo, who appears to have been the antidispensarian physician Dr William Gibbons,[17] proclaims

> Long have I reigned unrivalled in the Town,
> Glutted with Fees and mighty in Renown.
> There's none can die with due Solemnity,
> Unless his Pass-port first be signed by Me.
> My arbitrary Bounties undenied,
> I give Reversions and for Heirs provide,
> Nor cou'd the tedious Nuptial State support
> But I to make it easy, make it short.

Horoscope, having failed to elicit the help of the goddess Disease, urges caution but the Bard (a figure based on Sir Richard Blackmore, physician and fellow poet of Garth) recites some of his own pedestrian verses and this succeeds in bringing forth Disease, who is now only too willing to help in the fight. It is Mirmillo's turn for a sleepless night worrying about the future confrontation. The goddess Discord, however, assumes the form of Querpo, another antidispensarian physician, and he restores Mirmillo's flagging spirits with an eloquent call to arms. Dawn finds the apothecaries and their sympathisers among the physicians gathering for an attack upon Warwick Lane. Querpo (Dr How)

> A Pestle for his Truncheon led the Van
> And his high Helmet was a close stool Pan.

Happily the goddess Fame has warned the physicians and they are ready to meet the foe. A furious battle ensues, during which syringes, gallipots, and a whole range of medical paraphernalia are used. "Pestles," wrote Garth, "peel a martial Symphony." The apothecaries begin to gain the day and

Querpo is on the point of slaying Stentor – who is thought to be Dr Charles Goodall, the leader of the physicians – when Apollo assumes the form of Fee, at which Querpo instinctively snatches instead of striking the fatal blow. An engraved illustration of the battle was included in the seventh edition of *The Dispensary*, published by Jacob Tonson in 1714. In the final stanzas the fighting ceases when Hygeia, the goddess of health, appears and bids Machaon (Sir Thomas Millington) to send Carus (who is Dr Tyson) to accompany her to the Elysian fields to consult with William Harvey. They meet with the horrifying inhabitants of the underworld: Old Chaos, an awkward Lump of shapeless Anarchy, with dull Night, his melancholy Consort; pale Fear and dark Distress, parched Ey'd Febris,

> Then Hydrops next appears amongst the Throng,
> Bloated and big, she slowly sails along,
> But like a Miser in Excess she's poor
> And pines for Thirst amidst her watery Store.

They meet meagre Phthisis, Lepra the loathsome, as well as other sights that go to make up the frightful horror of the place, but at last they are ferried across the Styx and find the shade of William Harvey. He first addresses himself to Hygeia, referring to the dissent within the faculty:

> Where Sickening art now hangs her Head
> And once a Science, is become a Trade;

then to Carus to whom he turns with the admonition that by attending to science more and to lucre less and by letting Nassau's – that is, King William's or England's – health be their chief aim, the college could once again become restored to the position that it held under Willis and Wharton, Bates and Glisson. The poem ends with Carus and Hygeia returning to the college with this message.

Poetry, like science, is often derivative. In the case of *The Dispensary*, it was indubitably the French poet and literary critic Nicholas Boileau who had the greatest influence on Garth. In 1674 Boileau had anticipated Garth in his poem *Le Lutrin (The Lectern)* and this formed an invaluable model of the mock heroic which had been closely followed by Garth.[18] Like *The Dispensary*, Boileau's *Le Lutrin* had been stimulated by an actual event, a ludicrous argument between clerics on the placing of a lectern in St Chapelle. Garth's Sloth was an exact replica of Boileau's Mollesse and the poem culminated in a battle between two conflicting groups of prelates. It was not surprising, therefore, that some of Garth's contemporaries accused him of plagiarism, Blackmore in particular referring to "felonious Garth who smuggles French wit as others silks or wines."[19] Others disagreed, particularly Voltaire, who wrote in his *Dictionnaire Philosophique* in 1761 that he greatly preferred Garth's *Dispensary* to Boileau's *Lutrin*, Garth's poem having "beaucoup plus d'imagination" as well as "une profonde érudition embelli par la finesse et par la grace."[20]

The success of *The Dispensary*, described by Sir Richard Steele as Garth's nine days' wonder, was due in no small part to the contemporary interest in the thinly disguised identities of the protagonists in the drama. Samuel Johnson, however, attributed a greater measure of its success to its laudable moral stance, and he wrote in his life of Garth that it was on the side of charity against the intrigues of interest, and of regular learning against licentious usurpation of medical authority and was, therefore, naturally favoured by those who read and can judge poetry.[21] There were, of course, others who disparaged Garth's achievement. It was not surprising that Sir Richard Blackmore, who had been caricatured in *The Dispensary* as the Bard, should have rapidly produced his *Satyr against Wit* where "Garth and all the little loit'ring fry that follow Garth" are held up to ridicule. Blackmore, however, attacked not only Garth, but also the whole company of poets and wits associated with John Dryden and who were thought in their satires to mock both religion and virtue.[22] He was naturally countered by his victims and particularly by Garth who replied with his crushing verses *To the Merry Poetaster of Sadler's Hall in Cheapside*:[23]

> Unwieldy pedant let thy awkward Muse,
> With Censure praise, with flatteries abuse,

To lash and not be felt by thee's an art;
Thou ne'er mad'st any but thy schoolboys smart.
Then be advised and scribble not again
Tho'rt fashioned for a Flail and not a Pen.

This was an unkind reference to Sir Richard Blackmore's early career as a schoolmaster. These exchanges took place in the months preceding Dryden's death and although Dryden himself did not take part in the controversy he was no doubt shown the response before publication.

Garth's debt to Dryden went beyond the mere friendship encouraged by belonging to the group of wits who surrounded the legendary poet at Will's Coffee House near Covent Garden. Garth had subscribed to Dryden's translation of Virgil published in 1697 and in the preface to his version of Ovid's *Metamorphoses*, published 20 years later, Garth made clear his indebtedness to the poet.[24][25] It is certain that Dryden himself read *The Dispensary* for in one of the last poems that he wrote in 1699, *To my Honoured Kinsman John Dryden*, he referred to Garth "generous as his muse" and recorded his admiration for the dispensary movement.[26]

Garth's poetic style and the later poetry of the Augustan age owed much to Dryden's introduction of the new satirical method of writing, in which the heroic mode was used to characterise and attack individuals or to describe events. Dryden's highly successful poem *Absalom and Achitophel*, published in 1681, had been a satirical account of the encouragement by Lord Shaftesbury of the illegitimate Duke of Monmouth in his intrigues against the King, his father. *MacFlecknoe*, published the following year, was an attack on Thomas Shadwell who was later to succeed Dryden as Poet Laureate. Both these poems had an important influence on Garth and his followers as did, in terms of verse technique, Dryden's recommendation of "the verse of ten syllables which we call the English heroic" as the most suitable mode for what he termed manly satire. Dryden had further urged the satirist to write with grace, elegance, and wit. "How easy it is to call rogue and villain," he had written, "and that wittily, but how hard to make a man appear a fool, a blockhead or a knave without using any of those opprobrious terms. There is still a vast difference betwixt the slovenly butchering of a man and the fineness of a stroke that separates the head from the body and leaves it standing in its place".[27] It was a technique to reach perfection in the age of Alexander Pope.

When Dryden died in 1700, however, Pope was scarcely 12 years old. With no immediate competitors apparent it was, therefore, not surprising that there were many who saw Garth as the natural successor to Dryden. An anonymous epistle to Sir Richard Blackmore, occasioned by the death of John Dryden, awards his mantle to Garth "by destiny" and as late as 1709 Ned Ward wrote "that all rivals resign the crown when Garth appears." The remarkable Catherine Trotter equated Garth's genius with that of Dryden.[28] In 1704 another author describes how Apollo and the Muses meet to determine which living poet best qualifies to occupy "Witt's throne." Twenty three candidates are considered, including Steele, Rowe, Defoe, and Congreve. All the other candidates are considered and rejected

> Till Clio call'd out for her Garth to appear,
> Rising up with his Works in her Hand,
> And said to the God sh' had a Candidate there,
> Would their Votes and their Wishes command.
> A Bard, that for Judgement, Expression and Thought,
> For sweetness of Style and Address
> Had never yet known such a thing as a Fault
> And that only was fit for the Place.
> *Parnassus* confess'd his approach and each Muse
> At his Entrance transported arose
> Nor was it in *Phoebus* to put by or refuse
> What the General Suffrage had chose.[29]

After such remarkable eulogies as these, Garth's reputation suffered an extraordinary eclipse in subsequent years. This was not only due to the emergence of Pope as the master of wit and epigram, but also because of the fickleness of poetic taste, the acclamation of one generation being quite likely, in Edmund Gosse's words, "to be hooted out of Court by the next."[28] It was also, presumably, because Garth's poetic output remained relatively modest, probably owing to his increasing professional commitments after the year 1700.

At the time that Queen Anne came to the throne, however, Garth's reputation as wit, poet, and physician was unrivalled. He had continued to publish poetic work, his translation of Plutarch's *Life of Otho*[30] having come out in 1700, and in 1702 – the year of Queen Anne's accession – he had translated Demosthenes's *Second Philippick*.[31] In that same year he was elected a censor of the Royal College of Physicians. His friendship with Sloane lasted throughout his life. On many occasions they attended patients together and among the letters written by Garth to Sloane are several requesting medical help.[17] Garth's manner could be brusque. He once wrote to Sloane: "If you can recommend this miserable slut to be fluxed you will do an action of charity." On another occasion he wrote more politely: "Be so good as to call at my house, Mrs Garth is ill." In 1705 he moved from his home near St Martin-in-the-Fields to the highly fashionable area of St James's, near to St James's Palace and around the corner from Marlborough House where the Duke and Duchess of Marlborough lived. In the following year Sloane proposed Garth as a member of the Royal Society, presumably on grounds of friendship rather than scientific prowess, and his election is recorded immediately before the reading of a letter from Mr Leeuwenhoek from Holland concerning the appearance in the microscope of the gut of a woman executed.[32]

England under Queen Anne enjoyed a growing sense of wealth and power, accompanied by a flowering of literary and artistic activity. The lapsing of the Licensing Act in 1695 had brought a remarkable freedom to the press of which full advantage was to be taken by writers such as Defoe, Pope, Addison, Steele, and Dean Swift. In the arts there were distinctive contributions by Wren, Gibbons, Vanbrugh, and Kneller, and Handel's arrival in London preceded that of Queen Anne's Hanoverian successor. A whole style of decorative art and architecture was associated with Queen Anne. The increasing importance of science was recognised by the knighthood conferred on Isaac Newton. Politically the

Act of Union brought together the thrones of England and Scotland. It was also an era of unparalleled military success, the Duke of Marlborough's campaigns during the War of the Spanish Succession successfully challenging Louis XIV and French supremacy in Europe.

Garth, whose amiability and good nature seem never to have lost him a friend or made him an enemy, was on the side of the Whigs throughout his life and it was his admission to the club of honest Whigs, the Kit Cat Club, that brought him into contact with some of the most powerful and influential literary and political men of his time. The club was named after Christoper Catling, a pastrycook in whose shop the first meetings were held. The club subsequently met at the Fountain Tavern in the Strand, later at the Crown and Achor and sometimes in the Upper Flask Tavern in Hampstead. Garth was the only physician in the club and it seems likely that it was Jacob Tonson, Dryden's publisher, who introduced him, for Tonson, a founder member, had published Garth's translations of Plutarch and Demosthenes. The club numbered among its early members the Lords Dorset, Essex, Somerset, Sunderland, Somers, and Clare, the future Duke of Newcastle. More to Garth's literary taste there were Joseph Addison, Richard Steele – who had praised *The Dispensary* – and William Congreve. Sir John Vanbrugh and Sir Godfrey Kneller were also members. Undoubtedly, however, the most valued friendship that he made through his membership of the Kit Cat Club was with the Duke and Duchess of Marlborough who became his patients and were to remain his friends throughout his life.[33]

It was Marlborough's decade. Captain General of the British forces throughout the War of the Spanish Succession, he had marched his polyglot army to the banks of the Danube in 1704 to win his most famous victory at Blenheim. A grateful Queen rewarded him with the gift of the manor at Woodstock, where his palace was to be built by Sir John Vanbrugh. Ramillies followed in 1706 and Oudenarde in 1708. At home he had the support of the Queen's chief minister, his fellow Kit Cat, Lord Godolphin. His wife Sarah was one of the Queen's oldest friends and became her closest adviser,

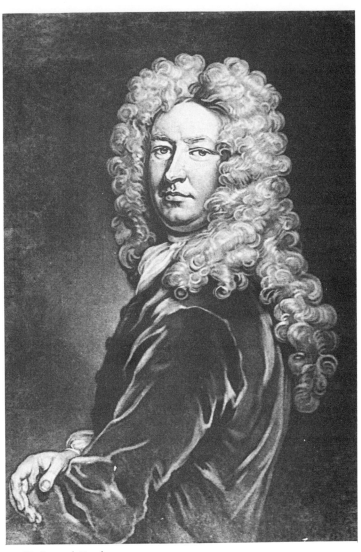

3   Sir Samuel Garth
    (Royal College of Physicians of London)

Groom of the Stole, Mistress of the Robes and Keeper of the Privy Purse. Garth seems to have been smitten by the beauty of the duchess, whom he described as "the best woman in the world, the most generous and compassionate and ready to do good when any cause was rightly represented to her," and he pondered how one of so much merit ever came to be a favourite.[34]

It is a tribute to Garth's literary reputation at the time that Alexander Pope showed him his *Pastorals*[35] before their publication in 1709 and he dedicated "Summer" to Garth with the lines

> Accept O Garth the Muse's early Lays
> That adds this Wreath of Ivy to thy Bays.
> Hear what from Love unpracticed Hearts endure
> From Love, the sole Disease thou can'st not cure.

Pope regarded Dr Samuel Garth as one of his first friends.

To the uninformed observer the Marlboroughs in 1709 must have seemed wealthy, charming, powerful, and unchallengeable. After the carnage of Malplaquet in August of that year, however, the storm clouds began to gather. The losses in that battle were so appalling that Malplaquet has since come to be regarded as an eighteenth century Passchendaele. The Queen herself on hearing the news exclaimed "When will this bloodshed ever cease?" Sarah, the duchess, who had perhaps allowed the famous Mrs Morley/Mrs Freeman correspondence with Queen Anne to delude her into thinking herself the social equal of her monarch, lost her position at court to her cousin Abigail Hill, later Lady Masham. The political manoeuvrings of Robert Harley, later Lord Oxford, and Henry St John, Lord Bolingbroke, led to the Queen's dismissal of Marlborough's political ally Lord Godolphin in 1710. Garth had been one of the medical men consulted during the final illness of Anne's husband Prince George of Denmark in 1708, but he had remained a staunch supporter of the duke, Godolphin, and their Whig political friends. He wrote in 1710 his consolatory 32 line poem to the Earl of Godolphin on his dismissal, praising his conduct in office:

> Whilst weeping Europe bends beneath her ills,
> And where the sword destroys not, famine kills;
> Our Isle enjoys by your successful Care,
> The Pomp of Peace among the Woes of War

But, he went on, "now some star, sinister to our pray'rs, Contrives new schemes and calls you from affairs."[36] Sadly he noted that "Ingratitude's a weed of every clime,/It thrives too fast at first, but fades in time." Some months later Godolphin responded with his own poetic tribute to Dr Samuel Garth upon the loss of Miss Dingle, which apparently referred to the elopement of Garth's only daughter Martha to marry Colonel William Boyle.[37]

In 1711 Garth was again in print with a volume in Latin *Epitaphium Lucretii Editionis*.[38] The same year, in July, he visited Marlborough's Continental headquarters in Holland bringing letters from Whig supporters at home. A dinner guest at Marlborough's table described how the duke "told us very merrily of the letters the doctor brought from Lady Duchess, Lord Godolphin and Mr Craggs. He said that by the colour and smell of them it would seem as if the doctor had made use of no other paper of any occasion during the whole voyage."[39] Garth returned by Ostend to London, where the Tory campaign against Marlborough and the continuation of the war was reaching its climax. Marlborough arrived in London on 17 November and on 27 November Swift, at the instigation of Lord Oxford and his cronies, published his highly partisan and misleading account of the war, *The Conduct of the Allies*, which brought a protest from the Elector of Hanover, the future King of England. By the end of December, however, the invalid Queen had been persuaded to dismiss the Duke of Marlborough from all his offices. He was soon to be accused, together with his secretary, of peculation during the war at the nation's expense.

The government's plans for peace were to be the major contentious issue that divided Whigs and Tories during 1712. It was also to be the year of the first publication of Pope's best known poem in the mock heroic style that Garth had pioneered in England. *The Rape of the Lock* was prompted by the cutting off of a lock of Arabella Fermor's hair by the young Lord Petre. Pope recorded how the addition of the sylphs to later editions was on the advice of Dr Garth "who, as he was one of the best natured men in the world, was very fond of it."[35]

By November of that year the Duke of Marlborough's position had become so insecure that he left England for a period of self imposed exile on the Continent. In February 1713 he was joined by his duchess who, according to Lord Berkley "hath given great presents at her taking leave of her friends, several fine diamond rings and other jewels of great value, to Dr. Garth for one."[40] Later that spring Addison's highly successful play, *Cato*, was presented in London. Pope wrote the prologue and there was an epilogue by Garth on the odd fantastic things that women do in matters of love, written in the light hearted vein characteristic of that period. The piece, a political tract, was remarkable in appealing to Whig and Tory alike.

The Tory party of Oxford and Lord Bolingbroke, with the support of the Queen, achieved the peace they had hoped for with the Treaty of Utrecht, which was finally signed in April 1713. Pope, friend of Oxford and with him a member of the Scriblerus Club, wrote an approving heroic couplet in his poem *Windsor Forest*:

> At length great Anna said, Let Discord Cease!
> She said, the world obeyed and all was Peace.[35]

The treaty was celebrated with a Te Deum and Jubilate at St Paul's, specially composed by the 28 year old George Frederick Handel.

The Treaty of Utrecht was a settlement that was decisively to mark Great Britain's emergence as a world power. The treaty recognised the Hanoverian succession to Queen Anne. Britain became the dominant world power in the Mediterranean and there was expansion of her empire in Canada and the Caribbean. Furthermore, both France and Spain gave the English exclusive rights to the lucrative slave trade within Spanish America for a 30 year period. Nevertheless, the Whigs, and Garth, saw the treaty as being unduly favourable to the French, as well as a gross betrayal of the Continental allies of Great Britain. It was this treaty that gave rise to the term "perfidious Albion." Garth, unhappy with the Peace of Utrecht, contemplated the statue of Queen Anne which had been newly erected outside St Paul's Cathedral[41] and expressed his dissent in verse. The statue has symbolic representations of Britannia, France, Ireland, and the American colonies at her feet.

> Beneath her feet four mighty realms appear,
> And with due reverence pay their homage there.

Each nation looks up in homage to the Queen with the exception of France "who alone with downcast eyes is seen." Garth's poem continues with the following reproof to France, the old enemy:

> Ungrateful coutnry to forget so soon,
> All that great Anna for thy sake has done;
> When sworn the kind defender of thy cause,
> Spite of her dear religion, spite of laws;
> For thee she sheathed the terrors of her sword
> For thee she broke her general and her word:
> For thee, for thee alone what could she more?
> She lost the honour she had gain'd before.[42]

Not surprisingly, this poem was not published until after Queen Anne's death, which took place the following year on 1 August 1714.

The accession of George I marked the triumphant return of the Whigs to power. The Queen's ministers were dismissed and Bolingbroke, fearful for his head, fled to the Continent. Marlborough was restored to all his offices, but was to suffer a series of strokes in 1716 which effectively removed him from public life. For Garth, distinction was to be heaped upon distinction. He was the first knight of the new reign, being at his own request dubbed by the King with the sword of the victor of Blenheim. He was also made Physician in Ordinary to the King and Physician General to the army.[43]

Sir Samuel, however, as we now must call him, continued in active practice as a physician. In 1715 he attended, with his old colleague Hans Sloane, the daughter of one of his Kit Cat friends, Lord Kingston. Lady Mary Pierrepoint had married Edward Wortley Montagu in 1712, after a stormy courtship. She was a friend and admirer of Alexander Pope and herself wrote satirical verses. Sadly they later turned against each other. Lady Mary's attack of smallpox was to have a major influence on preventive medicine during the eighteenth century, since it was she, her beauty ravaged by the illness, who played an important role in introducing the practice of inoculation into this country.

Two years later, in 1717, Caroline of Anspach, the Princess of Wales, was ill with "long swoons and frequent faintings." Earl Grantham sent for Dr Mead, who had treated Queen Anne; the Duchess of St Albans sent for Sir Samuel Garth; some others for Dr Sloane; and the King's German physician and Sir David Hamilton were also in attendance. The star of Dr Mead, however, was now in the ascendant and Garth and Sloane were dismissed and out of favour. The Duchess of Marlborough, however, had no opinion of Mead, whom she described as "the most obstinate and ignorant doctor that we have had in a great while."[44] Despite the attentions of her physicians Caroline of Anspach survived, later to become Queen to George II.

Sir Samuel Garth appears to have played an increasing role in political affairs during his last years. In 1715, during the abortive Jacobite revolt of the Old Pretender, he was sent north to Durham, his birthplace, to assist in preserving the loyalty of the people to the King. It was a long way north of Watford. In a letter to his friend and patient the Duke of Newcastle, then Lord Chamberlain, he wrote, "I am so far northward that there is nothing worth looking on, but the star that bears that name. I have not had any company since I left York till this day, but at present I am with a woman that is deaf and dumb and by consequence is almost the only person that has not heard of your Grace or does not speak well of you. I think I have seen but one tree since I left York and that is one that bears no leafs, and it is of ye same nature with that at Hyde Park Corner so often mentioned in ye monthly martyrology of Newgate, and I hope ere long will

46

beare ye same fruit."[17] He went on to reassure the duke that "the ordinary people are pretty well inclined in ye Bishoprick of Durham and that ye thoughts of ye invasion has brought them to reason."

In that same year Garth was on the Continent, travelling first to Italy and returning through Paris the following spring, where he had meetings with the exiled Tory minister, his one time friend Henry St John, Lord Bolingbroke. Garth, together with Addison and Craggs, was trying to win Bolingbroke over to the Whig cause. Bolingbroke did not succumb to their blandishments, even though he remained on friendly terms with Garth, whom he described as "the best natured ingenious wild man I ever knew."[45]

At the same time Garth did not neglect his writing, and in 1715 Jacob Tonson published his poem *Claremont*.[46] The poem immortalised the country estate near Esher which Lord Clare, his friend the newly created Duke of Newcastle, had purchased in 1714. Sir John Vanbrugh designed the palatial home which he named Claremont. The poem opens with

> What frenzy has of late possess'd the brain?
> Tho' few can write, yet fewer can refrain.

Garth continues with a castigation of adulatory poets, but carefully admits that men of real merit deserve celebration:

> The man who is honest, open and a friend,
> Glad to oblige, uneasy to offend;
> Forgiving others, to himself severe;
> Though earnest, easy; civil, yet sincere;
> Who seldom, but through great good nature errs;
> Detesting fraud as much as flatterers;
> T'is he my Muse's homage should receive;
> If I could write or Holles could forgive.

The reader is then taken back to the Druids, their noble savagery being contrasted with modern decadence. The story of Montano and Echo is told and the poem concludes with a prophesy of the Druid priests on the forthcoming reign of George I.

The idea for a new edition of Ovid's *Metamorphoses*

47

seems to have come from Jacob Tonson, who through the years had been collecting a number of translations of parts of the work from writers such as Dryden, Addison, and a number of other poets. It appears that in 1714 Garth had agreed to become general editor of a comprehensive translation and undertake with others the remainder of the work. The *Metamorphoses* finally appeared in the summer of 1717 with a dedication to the Princess Caroline and a preface by Garth, who criticised Ovid for prolixity and felt his work could have been improved. His own translations bear signs that he consistently abridged the original.[25]

Exactly when Sir Samuel Garth decided on a country retreat at Harrow-on-the-Hill is uncertain. Pope's memoirs contain references to visits to Harrow from Twickenham and presumably Garth's extensive circle of friends came to see him there. Lady Garth died in May 1717 and was buried at St Mary's Church in Harrow-on-the-Hill, so he must have had a home there by then. Garth himself travelled to the Continent a year later in the spring of 1718. He was intending to go on to Italy, but illness prevented him. He wrote again to the Duke of Newcastle: "I have been very much indisposed since I came hither, but I shall have this advantage from it. I shall have ye pleasure of seeing Your Grace soon. If I should go to Rome it would be a real pilgrimage for I can neither eat nor sleep and therefore think of being in England in less than a month."[17] Soon he was back in England and his illness was sufficiently severe to elicit a poem from George Granville (Lord Landsdowne) *To my Friend Dr Garth in his Sickness*.[47] Granville urged Apollo

> Sire of all arts, defend thy darling son;
> Oh save the man whose life's so much our own.

Garth spent his last months at Harrow-on-the-Hill. He knew that he was dying and shortly before his death sent a message to Congreve, who was himself seriously ill, to let him know he was going on his journey and desired to know how soon he would follow him. Congreve sent back word that "he wished him a good journey but did not intend to take the same road."[48]

It seems that Garth derived little solace from religion in his final hours. Thomas Hearne wrote that "when he was on his deathbed and the subject of another life was mentioned to him he said he had done what good he could and he did not trouble himself with what was to come." Pope, however, later defended his old friend from charges of impiety, writing to Charles Jervas: "If ever there was a good Christian, without knowing himself to be one, it was Garth." By the middle of January 1719 the London newspapers were carrying the news of Garth's serious illness and on 14 January he was "given over by his physicians."[49] He died on 18 January, and on 22 January his body was lowered into the tomb beside the altar at St Mary's Church, where his wife had been buried less than two years before.[50] Who attended him to his grave is not known, nor whether any of his literary friends spoke a eulogy at his funeral, as he had done for John Dryden. He had, however, expressed his views on death 20 years earlier in the poem for which posterity remembers him. These lines, written nearly 300 years ago and much admired in their day, may serve as his own epitaph:

> To Die is Landing on some silent Shoar,
> Where Billows never break, nor Tempests roar;
> Ere well we feel the friendly Stroke, 'tis o'er.
> The Wise thro' Thought th' Insults of Death defy;
> The Fools thro' bless'd insensibility.
> 'Tis what the Guilty fear, the Pious crave;
> Sought by the Wretch, and vanquished by the Brave.
> It eases Lovers, sets the Captives free;
> And, tho' a Tyrant, offers Liberty.

That same liberty gives to all the opportunity of judging whether that is great poetry or a descent into mere sentimentality.

NOTES

1 An illustration of the original card was published by Harvey Cushing in his paper, Dr Garth: the Kit Kat poet. *Bull Johns Hopkins Hosp* 1906; **17**: 14–56.

2 Cook, RI *Sir Samuel Garth*. Boston: Twayne, 1980: 16–20. Hereafter referred to as Cook.

3 There is no trace of Samuel Garth's birth in the local parish records, where his young brother's baptism is recorded, nor has the family home at Bolam been identified. Cornog WH. Sir Samuel Garth: a court physician of the eighteenth century. *Isis* 1938; **29**: 30–42.

4 The Peterhouse admission book under the date Maii 27 1676 contains the following entry: "Samuel Garth, Dunelmiensis, in Schola publica Ingeltoniensis (sita in Dunelmensi agro) institutus, currente jam 17 aetatis suae anno, per Praefectum, Decanoret Praelecti deput, examinatur, aprobatur, admittiturque Pensionarius sub Tutore et fidejussore M^{ro} Pern."

5 Cook, p 11.

6 Ellis FH. *Poems on affairs of state*. Vol 6. New Haven and London: Yale University Press, 1970: 60.

7 The college *Annals* record that on 25 June 1692 "Dr. Samuel Garth being proposed to being elected Candidate was chosen Nomine Contradicente, gave his ffaith the Statutes of the College and was admitted."

8 An original version of the oration in English is preserved in the Yale University Medical School Library. Ellis FH. Garth's Harveian oration. *J Hist Med* 1963; **18**: 8–19.

9 Gregg E. *Queen Anne*. London, Routledge and Kegan Paul, 1984: 108–9.

10 *Annals of the Royal College of Physicians of London* 1697; **7**: 121.

11 Wall C, Cameron CH, Underwood EA. *A history of the Worshipful Society of Apothecaries of London*. Vol 1. London: Oxford University Press, 1963: 41–59.

12 *Annals of the Royal College of Physicians of London* 1655; **4**: 55a.

13 In the plague year the Royal College of Physicians published *Certain necessary directions as well for the cure of the plague as for preventing the infection with many easie medicines of small charge very profitable to his Majesties Subjects*. London: John Bill and Christopher Barker, 1665.

14 Clark G. *A history of the Royal College of Physicians of London*. Vol 2. Oxford: Clarendon Press, 1966: 427–47.

15 Garth S. *The Dispensary: a poem*. London: John Nutt, 1699. After the seventh edition of 1714 Jacob Tonson was the publisher.

16 Cook, p 58.

17 Sena JF. The letters of Samuel Garth. *Bull NY Public Library* 1974; **78**: 81–94. The identities of the prominent characters in *The Dispensary*

are given by Garth in an undated letter to Arthur Charlett, Master of University College, Oxford. The same identities are given in a contemporary hand in a copy of the second edition of *The Dispensary* in the Library of the Royal College of Physicians of London.

18 Boileau-Déspreaux N. *The Lutrin*. Translation by N Rowe, 4th edn. Dubin: G Risk, 1730. The copy in the library of the Royal College of Physicians is appropriately bound with an edition of *The Dispensary* of 1730.

19 Cook, p 64.

20 Voltaire. *Oeuvres complètes*. Vol 37. Paris, 1821: 407–8.

21 Johnson S. Cited by Cook, p 75.

22 Blackmore R. *A satyr against wit*. London: S Crouch, 1700.

23 Garth S. To the merry poetaster at Sadler's Hall in Cheapside. In: *Commendatory verses on the author of the two Arthurs and the satyr against wit*. London, 1700.

24 *The works of Virgil...translated into English verse by Mr Dryden*. London: J Tonson, 1697.

25 *Ovid's Metamorphoses in fifteen books: translated by Dr Garth and others*. 5th edn. London: J and R Tonson and S Draper, 1751.

26 Dryden J. To my honoured kinsman John Dryden. In: *Dryden's Poetical Works*. London: Frederick Warne, 1912: 215.

27 Cook, p 73.

28 Gosse E. *Some diversions of a man of letters*. London: William Heinemann, 1920: 50; 10.

29 Cook, p 125.

30 Garth S. *Life of Otho*. Cited by Cook, p 162.

31 The second Philippick. In: *Several orations of Demosthenes...English'd from the Greek by several hands*. London: Jacob Tonson, 1702.

32 *Journal Book of the Royal Society*. Vol 10. London: Royal Society, 1706.

33 Cushing H. Dr Garth: the Kit Cat poet. *Bull Johns Hopkins Hosp* 1906; 17: 14–56.

34 Cook, p 22.

35 Pope A. *The poetical works of Alexander Pope*. Ward AW, ed. London: Macmillan, 1908: 17; 69; 38.

36 Garth S. To the Earl of Godolphin. In: *The works of Sir Samuel Garth*. Dublin: T Ewing, 1769: 104–5.

37 Godolphin. *The Earl of Goldolphin to Dr Samuel Garth, upon the loss of Miss Dingle*. Cited by Cook, p 26.

38 Garth S. *The dedication for the Latin edition of Lucretius*. London: J Roberts, 1714.

39 Cook, p 29.

40 Cook, p 23.

41 The original statue, by Francis Bird, was erected in the forecourt of St Paul's Cathedral in 1712. It was restored in 1825 but removed in 1886

in a state of dilapidation and replaced with a copy by the Victorian sculptor, Richard Best. The original statue is preserved in the grounds of Holmhurst near Hastings. Hayward CM. Story of a statue. *Dome* 1983–84; **21**: 10.

42 Garth S. On her Majesty's Statue in St Paul's Churchyard. In *The Works of Sir Samuel Garth*. Dublin: T Ewing, 1769: 105–6.

43 Churchill WS. *Marlborough: his life and times*. Vols 1–4. London: Harrap. 1983: 1020.

44 Brook, E St J. *Sir Hans Sloane*. London: Batchworth, 1954: 82.

45 Cook, pp 35–6.

46 Garth S. *Claremont: address'd to the Right Honourable the Earl of Clare*. London: Jacob Tonson, 1715. The original house by Vanbrugh was demolished in 1768 by Lord Clive, who erected the building now to be seen at Claremont.

47 Granville G. *The genuine works in verse and prose of the right honourable George Granville, Lord Lansdowne*. London: J Tonson and L Gilliver, 1732.

48 Cook, p 39.

49 Cook, p 38.

50 The tombstone, which is on the floor to the right of the altar in St Mary's Church, carries the following inscription, somewhat defaced: "In this Vault lies ye body of ye Lady Garth late Wife of —muel Garth who dy'd ye 10th of May in ye year 1717. Dr. Samuel Garth obijt jan^e the 18th 1718." The date of Garth's death is given in the old style so that in modern terms it was 1719.

3 A pupil of Boerhaave

When Boerhaave died at Leyden in 1738, the *Gentleman's Magazine* in London wrote, "The University has lost its chief glory, and the City of Leyden, at a moderate Computation, twenty thousand pounds sterling a year, which she gained by his pupils from Great Britain, without reckoning those from most other Nations in Europe."[1] This estimate, as is usual with the popular press, was something of an exaggeration but it serves to illustrate the extraordinary reputation of the greatest clinical teacher of the eighteenth century, Hermann Boerhaave, professor of medicine at Leyden University from 1714 to 1738. It has been demonstrated that during his years at Leyden he taught nearly 2000 medical students, of whom as many as a third were English speaking.[2]

Not all his pupils achieved the immortality of Haller, van Swieten, or his Scottish pupils who founded the Edinburgh medical school. Many became competent physicians, too busy perhaps for literary endeavour, too obscure to influence the history of their time. There were others, however, whose works reveal to this day, as do those of Haller, the influence and encouragement they derived from their teacher at Leyden. Among these was an Englishman, Dr William Hillary, a physician who enjoyed no outstanding reputation in his lifetime, but who is remembered today for the book that he wrote on the *Diseases of Barbados*. This book is one of the first treatises written by an English physician which deals specifically with tropical diseases. Of greater significance, it contains what appears to be the earliest account of tropical sprue.[3]

From *Medical History* 1963; 7: 297–316.

William Hillary was a Yorkshireman. He was born in Wensleydale, the loveliest and broadest of the Yorkshire dales, on 17 March 1697.[4] He came from a Quaker family. His father, John Hillary, born in 1666, appears to have become a Quaker as a young man and his position among the Friends must have been much strengthened in 1692 when he married Mary Robinson, daughter of Richard Robinson of Countersett, head of the leading Quaker family in Wensleydale.[5] George Fox had stayed in his house at Countersett on the second of his visits to those parts.[6]

John Hillary and his bride lived for the early years of their married life at the farmhouse called Birkrigg, an isolated and lonely spot at the head of Wensleydale. In summer it is a lovely place. The grey stone farm buildings stand in a group of trees on a high bank above the river Ure. The river here is a rushing stream passing from its wild moorland beginning to the wide green valley of Wensleydale beyond. The green meadows and dry stone walls around the farmhouse stretch upwards to the moors of Widdale Fell above. Eastwards there is the long view down Wensleydale, Wether Fell and Addleburgh outlined against the sky on the south, and northwards the ridge of Stags Fell, Abbotside, and Ellerkin separating the valley from Swaledale. In winter it is bleak and cold, the fields empty, cattle kept close and warm in the barns. During the long winter evenings, when snow had drifted round the lonely farm buildings and blocked the road from Hawes, the isolation of Birkrigg must have been complete.

The Hillarys had several children during those early years at Birkrigg, Ann born in 1693, Isaac, the eldest son, born the following year, two other girls who did not survive, and then in 1697, William, the future physician, named after his grandfather. Within two years of William's birth, however, the Hillarys had moved from Birkrigg. Probably they needed a larger house for the growing family. It is also likely that they wanted to be in a less isolated place, nearer to Mary Hillary's relations at Countersett. This may have been the reason for their choice of Burtersett, a small village on the south side of Wensleydale, four or five miles down the valley from Birkrigg and only two miles from Countersett.

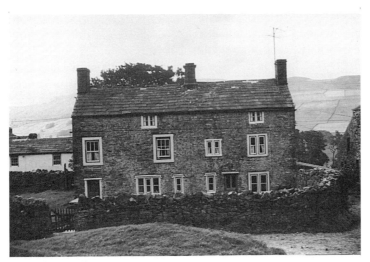

4   Hillary Hall

Four more children were born to the Hillarys in Burtersett:
Margaret in 1699, Mary in 1702, and another son, Richard,
in 1703. Rachel, the youngest, was born in 1705.[7] William
Hillary's early years were therefore spent as a member of a
large family, in this small Yorkshire village where the family
home is known as Hillary Hall to this day.[8] Nothing is
known of his schooling. He must have learnt the Latin then
essential for a physician, yet his name does not appear in the
register of Sedbergh School, the best school in the north
country and only 20 miles away.

By 1715 he had decided on the customary first step towards
a medical career. On 29 December he was apprenticed to an
apothecary, Benjamin Bartlett, for a period of seven years.[9]
Benjamin Barlett was a Quaker who was a leading citizen of
the growing town of Bradford in Yorkshire.[10] He was an
excellent master. His house, wrote Gilbert Thompson later,
might be called "The Seminary of Ingenious Physicians."[11]
John Fothergill of Carr End, the famous London physician,
was among those who were later to serve their apprenticeship
with Benjamin Bartlett at Bradford.[12] Here Hillary would
learn about the actions of drugs and how to prepare them; he

would visit patients in their homes, bringing medicines from his master, getting experience of sickness, suffering, and death. How long he stayed in Bradford is uncertain, but it is likely that he was released before the end of his seven years. Some time between 1720 and 1722 he went on to Leyden University to take his medical degree, an essential step if he was to become a physician.

Leyden was a long way from the Hillary home in Wensleydale. Yet it was a natural choice for a Quaker who wanted to study medicine. The universities of Oxford and Cambridge were closed to him as a dissenter but there was no religious bar to entry at Leyden. The story of its foundation in 1575 is well known. William the Silent offered the citizens of Leyden either a university or relief from taxes for 10 years as a reward for their courageous stand against the Spaniards in a desperate siege the year before. The far seeing citizens had chosen the university and it is to their credit that it came to enjoy a degree of academic and religious freedom similar to that of Padua.

In 1720 the Leyden medical school was at the height of its fame, its reputation world wide. This was predominantly due to the influence of Hermann Boerhaave. A graduate of the University of Harderwyck in 1693, Boerhaave had been appointed lector of theoretical medicine in 1701 and became professor of medicine in 1714. But he was a great deal more than that. A master of mathematics, chemistry, botany, and physics, as well as the leading physician of his age, Boerhaave was a clinical teacher who sought to inculcate a scientific spirit of inquiry into the practice of medicine. He emphasised the importance of the primary sciences in the training of a physician and encouraged the practice of correlating pathological changes found by dissection with clinical observations. As a clinical teacher he derived great inspiration from physicians such as Sydenham, whose careful descriptions of disease at the bedside recall the observations of the Hippocratic school.[13][14]

It was in the environment of such ideas that William Hillary studied at Leyden. No record of his life there has survived; but he no doubt found the flat country of Holland very different from the hills and valleys of his native dales. He probably took advantage of the students' privilege to obtain his wine and beer tax free. He would certainly have visited the famous public anatomy hall, full of extraordinary objects collected from various parts of the globe. At the entrance he would have seen, among other oddities, two elephants' heads, a pair of Laplander's breeches, two East Indian tigers, a parturition chair, and a "great Knife taken from a Rioting fellow." Within, he would find things more gruesome. There were "some monstrous bones." He had a large variety of skeletons to choose from – among them "an Asse upon which sits a Woman that killed her daughter's child," or "a French Nobleman who ravished his sister and afterwards murthered her, and was beheaded at Paris, and given to the Anatomie." He could also see a "Mumie of an Egyptian Prince about 1800 years old," a "Japan letter of a Whore," the "skin of a man dried like parchment," "some mens gutts," and a wide variety of pathological specimens such as "Preserved Fingers with Nails on 'em." These items are chosen at random from the English edition of the catalogue.[15]

On 24 July 1722 he had to defend his thesis in public and afterwards entertain the professors and students. It was written in Latin and entitled *Dissertatio Medica Inauguralis Practica de Febribus Intermittentibus*. His thesis, as was then customary, was published and copies are preserved in both the University of Leyden and the British Museum. The dating of his thesis provides a clue to some of his medical friends at Leyden. He must have known Andrew Plummer, a Scotsman who graduated on the day before he did with a thesis entitled *De Phthisi Pulmonali*.[16] Andrew Plummer was to become first professor of chemistry and materia medica in the new medical school at Edinburgh in 1726.

Hillary's father had not lived to see his son graduate. He died in 1721. For a yeoman farmer he was relatively wealthy, well able to afford the expense of educating his second son at a foreign university. He left the bulk of his estate to his eldest son Isaac.[17] William's share was £300, "*including* the moneys he has had." As this probably refers to the expense of his education at Leyden, it is clear that William did not start life with much capital. He had then to put his education to good account.

About 1723 or the year following, William Hillary settled as a physician in the small cathedral town of Ripon in Yorkshire, only 30 miles from the family home at Burtersett. The town was a market centre for the surrounding countryside – rich, rolling farmland which was very different from the wildness of the upper part of Wensleydale. Ripon then, as now, was renowned for its proximity to Fountains Abbey. It is also famous for the horn which is sounded at night in the Market Square, a custom dating from the time of Alfred the Great. When Hillary lived in Ripon he would have heard the horn blown at 9 o'clock each evening, as it still is today.

In this pleasant country town he started practice. By 1726 he had begun to record the changes in the weather and the epidemics he encountered in an attempt to correlate weather and disease. He was one of the first physicians in England to attempt to do this. A year later, in 1727, Dr Wintringham of York published his *Commentarium Nosologicum*, a similar study in which he gave a careful record of the relationship of weather to disease in the nearby city of York where he practised.[18] Hillary was much discouraged when this work came out, as he felt himself forestalled. But in the interest of comparing results, he decided to carry on his researches and he continued them until the end of 1734, when he left Ripon. His account was published some years later. This work makes it possible to study the pattern of disease as Hillary saw it in a country physician's practice more than 200 years ago. In 1726, for instance, he saw more than 60 patients with smallpox, nearly as many as he had seen in an epidemic two years earlier. In 1731 he encountered a curious epidemic disease which he had not seen previously. Children or young people under 20 would develop a fit of shivering followed by swelling of the face and neck. The swelling was occasionally unilateral but usually it affected both sides and sometimes it was remarkably severe. All his patients recovered completely in two or three weeks. This is a clear description of mumps and it seems curious that Dr Hillary, with several years' practice behind him, should never have seen it before. In 1734 he described his experience of a world pandemic of influenza. According to the papers, it had occurred in Europe, Asia, Africa, and America. Few escaped it in Yorkshire, writes Hillary, and in the city of Leeds at least one third of the population were affected. He made no important discoveries and no clear relationship between weather and disease emerged, but his observations represent a worthwhile attempt to study this problem in a scientific manner, and they illustrate the energy and enthusiasm that he brought to his work in a small country town.

The disease which interested him most during this period was smallpox, one of the scourges of eighteenth century life. It was a disease that attracted a great deal of attention. The practice of inoculation had recently been introduced into England and its value was hotly debated during the first half of the century. Hillary had made notes of the epidemics that he had seen in his practice and in 1732, at the instigation of his friends, he was encouraged to prepare his notes for publication. The result was his first book, *A Rational and Mechanical Essay on the Small Pox*, which was first published in 1735.[19] This book is not remarkable for its description of the disease, nor for its treatment. Hillary adopts the current methods of his time, duly acknowledging his debt "to the sagacious and learned Boerhaave." He enthusiastically recommends the customary regimen of bleeding and purging, thought from time immemorial to remove evil humours from the body. It is alarming to read the amount of bleeding that his patients might have to endure. Several were ordered to lose as much as 120 or 140 ounces of blood, an amount likely to be fatal to all but the fittest and most phlegmatic. But there are two noteworthy statements in the preface. The first deals with the recently introduced practice of inoculation. Hillary states, with an unusual clarity and simplicity, the nature of the problem. Its success, he wrote,

in this...Climate, remains somewhat doubtful, and must be so, 'till the following Propositions are clearly proved, and confirmed by just Observations or their Contraries: viz. 1. That having the Smallpox by inoculation, is less hazardous than having them in the natural Way is. And 2. That the having them that way is as sufficient a Security against the having them a second time as the other is.

These propositions are put forward so clearly that they warrant the practical trial which he should himself have carried out. Hillary's style is characteristically forthright and to the point. The reason why it is so difficult to come to clear conclusions is, he tells us, "that in most cases (even in the greatest concerns of Life) Men first form to themselves Opinions, and then think and argue with too strong Prejudices for those Opinions..."

The second and more striking extract from his preface is as clear a plea for the importance of a scientific approach to medicine as has ever been written.

It appears how necessary it is for a Physician who would be Successful in his Practice, or make any tolerable Figure in his Profession, to be well acquainted with the structure of the Human Body, the use of all its Parts, the Principles of Mechanical Powers, the Laws of Motion and Hydraulics, with a sufficient skill in geometry and Mathematics, to apply them; as well as a knowledge of Chymistry, Pharmacy, and the Virtues and Doses of Medicines. For it is by a proper Use and Application of these, both in our Practice and Reading, that we can account for the Causes and Effects of Diseases, and the manner of the Remedies acting, so as to produce their saluterious effects. It is by these and accurate observations in Practice, that we must improve our Knowledge in the State of Physic and Disease; it is this Knowledge, and these Abilitys, that must be the distinguishing *Characteristic* of a true *Physician*, from an Empiric; it is by this Method of reasoning from Data, founded upon Observations and real facts, that the *Healing Art* must be improved and brought to a State of Perfection; for if we once quit our Reason for Mystery, and abandon a just Method of Mechanical and Geometrical Reasoning, for the unintelligible terms of Occult Faculties and Qualities, with all such like Metaphysical and Chymical Jargon and Nonsense, heretofore too much used in the Schools; we must wander through endless Mazes, and dark Labyrinths, playing at Hazard with Men's Lives, and suffer ourselves to ramble wherever conceited Imagination, or whymsical Hypothesis will lead us.

These words are written in the forthright language characteristic of a Yorkshire dalesman, but the ideas clearly derive from Boerhaave's teaching at Leyden. They illustrate the philosophy of medicine that was to activate Hillary throughout his life.

The Rational and Mechanical Essay on the Small Pox was published as a second edition in 1740 and it was in this edition that Hillary added the "Principal variations of the Weather and the Concomitant Epidemic diseases as they appeared at Rippon and the circumjacent parts of Yorkshire." In this edition also he described how he was induced to leave Ripon, in August 1734:

> About this time dy'd the eminent Dr Bave of Bath, and being weary of the Fatigue of Country Practice, I was advised by some of my Friends to remove thither, in which Place chronical Distempers are so frequent, and acute Epidemical so seldome appear, that I could not pursue these observations, or carry them on longer.

These comments justly describe the differences in Hillary's work that would result from a move to Bath. Yet there were other differences more important. Bath, the most fashionable watering place in England, frequented by royalty and the nobility, was a whole world away from the peaceful country town of Ripon. It attracted some of the most successful physicians in the country, with whom the young Yorkshireman would have to compete.

There may, however, have been other reasons why he left Ripon. September 1734 found him in Leeds where he applied to the Brigghouse monthly meeting for a certificate. This was duly given on the sixth of the month, by eight weighty Friends who included "Jon Robinson" and "Jo Fothergill," family connections from the Countersett meeting. There is an implication in the certificate, which is preserved among the Fothergill family papers, that Hillary's behaviour in Ripon had not been entirely to the liking of his fellow Quakers. The document recorded that:

> he inclined more to Frds than when he lived at Ripon, where perhaps he met with some Discouragement rather than any advantage upon a Religious Act…Now as he was born of believing Parents and had his education in Truth's way and was never publicly disowned by Frds, nor ever given to vice or Intemperance (that we heard of) save only of his being modish or

fashionable in his Conversation and Conduct (a thing by no Means to be Incouraged)...[20]

However, the certificate continued, "notwithstanding his failure in that respect," the question that required a "serious thoughtfullness on Fr[ds] part" was whether by "taking some notice of him" he would be obliged to be "more Circumspect and Conformable to the purity & plainness both in habit & speech which Truth Leads the obedient unto." Despite his moments of weakness, he was, the certificate concluded, "worthy of regard."

It was with such cautionary encouragement that the young physician set out on the next stage of his career. It would be a major change in his life. Hillary must have been only human to have had qualms as he embarked on his journey southwards.

Dr Hillary arrived in Bath when it was at the height of its fame, in its golden age. The waters of Bath had been known since before the Romans built their baths there and were renowned throughout England in medieval, Tudor, and Stuart times. But until the early eighteenth century it was essentially a resort for the sick, for those genuinely seeking a cure. In 1702 and 1703, however, Queen Anne visited Bath. As the natural leader of English society, she was followed by an immense crowd of people seeking diversion and entertainment. Among these people was a professional gambler, the famous Beau Nash, who obtained the position of Master of Ceremonies. Richard Nash was a magnificent organiser, a social genius. He reorganised the Pump Room, arranged dances at the Assembly Rooms and insisted on rules of conduct, drawn up as a Code of Behaviour, which set standards for "polite society" which have endured to this day. His activities earned him the titles of "Uncrowned King of Bath," the "Arbiter of Elegance," the "Dictator of the Manners of Polite Society."

At this time the leading physician was Dr William Oliver, the inventor of the Bath Oliver biscuit, another Leyden student, who had started practice in Bath in 1725. In 1740 he was to be appointed physician to the Bath General Hospital, in whose foundation he had played a leading part. The architect John Wood the elder, another Yorkshireman, was transforming Bath into the lovely city it remains today. The Royal Cresent and the Circus belong to the second half of the eighteenth century, but when Hillary arrived Queen Square, the "true consummation of English Palladian architecture" was almost completed. Prior Park, the incomparably magnificent home of Ralph Allen, was being built. Here Allen entertained Alexander Pope, Dr Warburton, Gainsborough, and William Pitt. David Garrick and his old rival Quin met at this house. For the first four decades of the eighteenth century, the cream of English society took itself to Bath for the summer, there to divert itself with the waters, conversation, music, dancing, the theatre, and the pleasure of being seen in the company of the most distinguished people in the land.

It was a very different world for the young physician from Yorkshire, to whom as a Quaker the pleasures of society were sinful and therefore to be shunned. But he no doubt started his practice among the numerous members of the Society of Friends, with whom he seems to have been successful. Then, in 1737, he heard of an interesting incident. Charles Melsom, a cooper, had some labourers working near a place called Lincomb, a small village in a valley a little to the south of Bath, and he used some water from a local spring to make a bowl of punch for his workmen. Unfortunately there seemed to be something strange about the water, for the punch turned to a blackish purple colour and some of the workmen refused to drink it. William Hillary heard about this incident from a neighbour and at once concluded that the water must be a chalybeate water, a mineral water which contains iron. "Some time after," he wrote later, "going to see the Spring, I presently found from its smell and taste, and a few slight experiments, that it was so, but that it differed very much in several respects from every other spring of that kind, which I had hitherto seen." In the summer following, in 1738, he began to make experiments on the water, and this "being taken Notice of, led great numbers of People to the Place." He described these experiments together with his views on the uses of the waters, in his book *An Inquiry into the Contents and Medicinal Virtues of Lincomb Spaw water near Bath*, published in 1742.

In this book he dignifies Lincomb with the name of a Spa. He describes it as "a pleasant little valley on the South side of, and about half a mile distant from, the City of Bath. The natural agreeableness of the Place is increased by the conveniences made for the Accommodation of those who resort to the Spaw." There had evidently been some development of the site. Though claiming to be disinterested, he advocated the waters of Lincomb with unabashed enthusiasm. The spring produced 1800 gallons per day, enough for all, although a mere nothing compared with the half million gallons put forth in Bath each day. The smell was variable before the spring was covered in. "It might sometimes have been perceived by a Nice Organ at a distance of 30 or 40 yards," he wrote. The water contained "large quantities of elastic Air," a "subtile chalybeat, principle" and a "Quantity of an alkaline Earth." It contained an "alkaline, Lixivial Salt" and a portion of iron. It differed from other waters, such as those of Harrogate, Croft, and Tunbridge. The Bath waters contained only one tenth of the steel of the Lincomb water. It most clearly resembled the waters of the Continental spa, Geronster. Its uses, were, according to the custom of the time, legion. It could be prescribed for "Disorders of the stomach and Bowels arising from Loss of Appetite and Indigestion, i.e. Heartburn and Belchings. Inert viscid Phlegm, Nausea and Vomiting, flatulent oppression, with pinching colic pains. Obstructions of the Liver, Gravel and Stones of the gallbladder, preventing and curing the Jaundice" and "Gravel and Stones of the Kidneys..." It would clear and heal ulcers, "take off Strangury and Incontinence of Urine" and in "obstructions of the Menses" was "no less effectual." It was also useful in cachexias, in "hard Drinking and high Living, attended with swelled legs, and an icteral Complexion..." and would "restore the Constitution more than the Bath waters do." It could bring "the Anomalous Gout to be regular, when the Bath waters have failed" and externally it was effective in curing scrophulous ulcers among a host of other skin disorders. He concluded his account with seven case histories. Thomas Harley, of Whitstable near Canterbury, for instance, was so crippled with rheumatism between 1736 and 1738 that he lost the power of one side completely. He tried the Bath waters without effect and finally, in the summer of 1739, took the Lincomb water for two months, at the end of which time he was so much relieved that he was able to walk home to Canterbury. A military gentleman, aged 50 or more, provides another example. He had made an extensive trial of the Bath waters in a vain attempt to cure recurrent abdominal pain and vomiting. He took the Lincomb water from March until July and went away from Bath perfectly recovered. "I saw him some months afterwards," wrote Hillary, "when he was grown fat, jolly and hearty as ever, and I hear continues so."

His general conclusions as to the value of the Lincomb water are as follows:

It seems a very natural Method to obtain these effects, to recommend the Use of cold Chalybeat Waters, after the warm ones have been sufficiently used; which method the German physicians judiciously practice in advising the Patients to drink the Geronster water at Spa, after a competent stay at Aix-la-Chapelle. What resemblance there is betwixt the Geronster water and the Lincomb has been importunely inquired into above. We shall therefore submit it to the Judicious, whether after a proper use of the warm Waters at Bath, this cold Chalybeat may not be of like Advantage in chronical Cases.

It is interesting to speculate how much these conclusions had been influenced by the distinguished nobleman to whom Dr Hillary dedicated his book. Philip Dormer Stanhope, fourth Earl of Chesterfield, had been to both Aix-la-Chapelle and Geronster in 1741 and was well aware of the advice given by German physicians, for he had taken it himself.[21] It is also evident that the earl, a frequent visitor at Bath, had tried the Lincomb water, for in his dedication Hillary states that his book "cannot be more properly addressed to anyone, than to a Patron, who has experienced its virtues, and seen its good Effects in some remarkable cases." Such patronage must have enhanced the reputation of Hillary's spa.

He no doubt did well during the next few years. In 1744, John Fothergill, fellow dalesman and Quaker, Hillary's junior by 15 years, then in the early years of his practice in London, visited Bath to see his ailing father, friend and neighbour of the Hillary family in Wensleydale and one of those who had signed Hillary's certificate in Leeds 10 years before. Dr Fothergill advised his aging parent to make a trial of the Lincomb water. "Dr Hillary," he wrote to a colleague in Staffordshire, "was well; he has pretty good business." But Bath was anathema to the Quaker Fothergills. "It's a place," Dr John went on, "that I should choose to reside in the last of all others. The people are accustomed to behave well to everybody when present, but more than that they don't seem to think is expected or necessary."[22] His father, a famous Quaker preacher, thought Bath "a miserable poor place" where "the enemy of Mankind had attempted in various ways to draw attention off from their deepest Interest, by all sorts of temptations, but had lamentably succeeded in that place. Religion of any kind seems to be banished from thence with as much solicitude as Judaism or heresy from Portugal or Spain."[23]

The environment of Bath must have been alien to William Hillary as a member of the Society of Friends. But during the next two years there were developments which made the city even more uncongenial to him and which led to his leaving Bath. There had been a hint of trouble ahead in the dedication of his book on the Lincomb Spa Water. It had been his aim "To rescue this medical water from Neglect and Obscurity and to render it more extensively useful" – a laudable intention. Nevertheless it clearly represented a possible threat to other physicians in the neighbourhood whose livelihood depended, as was inevitable, on the waters of Bath. He had gone on: "If my Endeavours are favoured with the Approbation of his Lordship...the partial Censure of those who are interested in opposing them, will have less weight with the benevolent." This sentence suggests that he had enemies in 1742. And by the summer of 1746, for reasons which remain uncertain, he was making plans to leave Bath. His dilemma is clearly stated by his friend, John Fothergill, writing from

London on 11 September 1746 to his elder brother Alexander Fothergill at Carr End in Wensleydale.[24] The letter was no doubt shown to Isaac Hillary, living with his sisters at nearby Burtersett.

Dear Bro[r]
I met with thy kind letter at my return from Scarbro' relating to Dr. Hillary's intended voyage, and now sit down to acquaint thee what I know of it. As S. Bevan did not write to him I had no occasion to say much, and indeed I could not, till I knew from the Dr. himself his principal reasons. He set out from hence to Bath on 2nd day last. During his stay in town he conferred several times with S. Bevan and several persons of note who mostly discouraged him from going thither, so that all thoughts of that place have been laid aside. Whilst he was here, news arrived of the Death of the only eminent Physician at Barbados: I procured him an interview with a person who gave him an exact account of the affairs of that Island, he likewise spoke with several others who jointly recommended the place as much preferable to Jamaica. His relations I doubt not will be averse to his leaving England at any rate, but as his situation at Bath is not the most agreeable nor the prospect very pleasing and at the same time one half of life may perhaps be over whilst he sees himself unfortunately stript of what might have rendered the remaining part pleasant, can one avoid listening to any proposals that may tend to remove any inconveniencys. I was always averse to Jamaica: At Barbados there are several meetings, the Island pleasant and healthy; the people much more humane and polite than any where else with a prospect of good employ: I have been far from urging him to go to either, yet was I in the like situation, I own I should be strongly drawn to this last place: and if he should apply to his relations for their consent, I think they should not too positively refuse him. The galling situation he is in at present, I see renders life a burthen to him, but this betwixt ourselves.

It is clear from this letter that some remarkable circumstance had radically affected William Hillary's position in Bath. Had jealous colleagues succeeded in ousting him? Or had the spring dried up? Certainly his livelihood was jeopardised and he had to seek alternative employment. He was 49 years old and unmarried, so had no ties to limit his choice. Jamaica was evidently his first thought. It was fortunate that he was dissuaded, for had he gone there he would never have seen a case of tropical sprue, a condition which for mysterious reasons has never been described on that island. For a Friend, Barbados was a better choice. John

Fothergill had good reason to recommend it: his father had made religious visits there in 1723–4 and 1737–8 and had related his experiences in letters to his son.[25] There were many Friends and five different meetings on the island.

By November 1746 Dr Hillary's mind was made up. On the third of that month, he applied to his monthly meeting in Bath for the certificate customarily taken by a Quaker when he moved to a new place. He asked for a "Certificate of his removal to Barbados." On 9 November, at a special meeting called at Bath for the purpose, "John Corbyn and Toby Walker there reported that Dr Wm Hilary appeared clear on ye account of Marriage and of an orderly Conversation in consequence thereof have drawn and brought a Certificate for his removal which was then signed by many Friends."[26]

He must have travelled to Barbados in the spring or early summer of 1747. No doubt he was disappointed that Bath had failed to realise his hopes. In fact, it was the most important step in his life. Had he stayed in Bath, dosing the chronic sick with the waters, he would perhaps have made a fortune but he would have made little contribution to the medicine of his day. In fashionable Bath Hillary had given up his practice, started in Ripon, of observing the changes in the weather and the related epidemic diseases. Working entirely on his own in Barbados, he would take up this practice again and obtain data "founded upon observations and real facts" which would be of lasting value.

The West Indian island of Barbados lies farther out into the Atlantic than any of the islands of the Leeward group, directly in the path of the prevailing northwest trade winds. Barbados was entirely uninhabited at the beginning of the seventeenth century. In 1624 John Powell, returning home from Brazil, had landed there. He was struck by the beauty and fertility of the place and took possession in the name of King James. Returned to England, he succeeded in persuading Sir William Courteen, a London merchant with Dutch connexions, to back a settlement of the island. By 1631 the population numbered around 4000 persons. At first, attempts were made to grow tobacco and cotton, but the quality of the tobacco was too poor to compete successfully on the London market and there was too little available land to lay out the extensive plantations that cotton would have required. It was the Dutch merchants who encouraged the West Indians to grow sugar, and in 1637 the first canes were brought from Brazil. By 1640 the population of the island had risen to the remarkable figure of more than 30 000, but at that time, before sugar production had seriously got under way, there were only a few hundred negroes. To grow sugar profitably it was necessary to have some form of cheap labour, and this led to the importation of armies of negro slaves, bought on the coast of West Africa in increasing numbers. When Hillary reached Barbados the island was entirely covered with sugar plantations, each with its quota of slaves. The negro population was more than 50 000, the whites between 10 000 and 15 000. The years 1748–56 were the golden age for the sugar plantations. Prices remained steady and fairly high and both production and demand were increasing all the time.[27]

Ann Austin and Mary Fisher, the first Quakers on the island, had landed there in 1655. They were followed soon after by Henry Fell, and in 1671 George Fox himself paid a visit.[28] By 1747, when Hillary presented his certificate in Bridgetown, there were five meetings. His own meeting was in Tudor Street, Bridgetown.[29] Dr Hillary seems to have taken an active part in the affairs of Friends in Barbados. In the summer of 1748 he rode up the coast road, the clear blue sea sparkling in the sunshine beside him, to attend the quarterly meeting near Speightstown. His signature, in a flourishing but easily legible hand, appears on the "Epistle to the Friends and Brethren of the Yearly Meeting in London," sent from there in June 1748. But Friends at that time had slipped from the ways of their forefathers, a fact deplored in a report of the quarterly meeting:

It must be lamented that a remission even in profession is so observable here among many that are joined in Society with us, which the sensible justly consider as a declension in degree from the Evangelical Foundation and Power of Godliness. This hath bound the hearts of the sincere under an humble and fervent concern on their accounts, not without hopes what good thing remains may yet be strengthened, and that a just regard may at

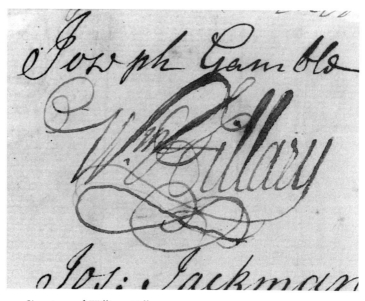

5   Signature of William Hillary
    (Library Committee of the Religious Society of Friends, London)

length prevail with them for the prosperity of truth in themselves and others.[30]

It was in fact a period of decline of the Society of Friends in Barbados. By 1760 the meetings for discipline were no longer being held and succeeding years witnessed a progressive loss of the society's properties.[31]

As a physician in Barbados, Hillary would find himself consulted by planters and their families, by military personnel stationed on the island, and no doubt also by seafaring men whose vessels called at Bridgetown. He would see negro slaves on the plantations and perhaps witness the unloading of this unhappy human cargo from the slave ships newly arrived from West Africa. These ships made a triangular voyage – first to the slave coast with goods, across from there to the West Indies laden with slaves, then the final leg back to England with a cargo of sugar for the London market.

Nothing is known of Hillary's day to day work during his

early years in Bridgetown. But one visitor to Barbados has left an account of a professional visit from Dr Hillary in 1751. The writer was a young Virginian, aged 19, who had brought his elder brother to Barbados for his health. The elder brother had developed ominous signs of consumption and had been ordered to spend the winter in a warmer climate than Virginia. They arrived in Bridgetown on 3 November, where they met Major Gedney Clark who was Collector of His Majesty's Customs and a member of the island's council. The writer recorded in his diary for 5 November 1751:

Early this morning came Dr. Hilary, an eminent physician recommended by Major Clarke, to pass his opinion on my brother's disorder, which he did in a favourable light, giving great assurance, that it was not so fixed but that a cure might be effectually made. In the cool of the evening we rode out accompanied by Mr. Carter to seek lodgings in the country, as the Doctor advised, and were perfectly enraptured with the beautiful prospects, which every side presented to our view – the fields of cane, corn, fruit trees, all in a delightful green.[32]

The patient referred to in this passage was none other than Lawrence Washington, of Mount Vernon in Virginia who had a connection by marriage with Gedney Clarke. The young diarist was his stepbrother, George Washington, inheritor of Mount Vernon, commander of the armies of the American colonies in the War of Independence, first President of the United States of America. Dr Hillary's favourable prognosis is at first difficult to reconcile with his patient's subsequent progress. Lawrence spent three months in Barbados, then went to Bermuda. He arrived home in Virginia in the following June, a shadow of his former self, and died on 24 July 1752. But the modern physician would approve Hillary's cheerful approach. He must have been familiar with pulmonary tuberculosis, must have himself known what the prognosis might be. Yet no physician will readily leave his patient without hope, whose therapeutic effects are mysteriously effective, and there is therefore much to commend in Hillary's encouragement.

The Washington brothers stayed in Barbados in a house on Carlisle Bay belonging to Captain Crofton, commander of

James Fort. Here, George fell ill with smallpox and from 17 November until 12 December was under the care of a Dr Lanahan. He does not record whether Hillary, whose book on the smallpox would make him an expert on this disease, was called in. Fortunately the attack was mild and George Washington came through relatively unscathed, having achieved an immunity to the disease which was no doubt valuable in later years.

William Hillary's next book had the somewhat heavy title *Observations on the Changes of the Air and the Concomitant Epidemical Diseases in the Island of Barbados; to which is added a Treatise on the putrid Bilious Fever, commonly called the Yellow Fever; and such other Diseases as are indigenous or endemical, in the West India Islands or in the Torrid Zone.* This was first published in London, by C Hitch and L Hawes, in 1759, the same year as his return. It is disappointingly lacking in autobiographical detail and tells little of his life in Bridgetown. He records an unfortunate accident to his barometer which prevented him starting his *Observations on the Changes of the Air* until 1752. He used Fahrenheit's mercurial thermometer, a barometer, and a hygrometer, and all his observations were made at Bridgetown. A narrative account follows of the weather and the recurrent epidemics of fever, throat infections, skin diseases, and diarrhoea that he encountered. The preface and introduction contain two other passages which are worth quoting. He cannot resist a few words of advice to some of his professional colleagues:

For those who neither read, nor yet know how to reason on the Causes or their manner of Production of Diseases, and yet will boldly practice by rote, and prescribe by guess at a Venture, though the Life of the Patient depends on the right or wrong method of prescribing; I must seriously advise them at least to peruse the sixth Commandment.

He was equally forthright in condemning local sartorial fashions. "Fashion and Custom," he wrote, "are two prevailing Things, which enslave the greatest Part of Mankind, though often both contrary to Reason and Conveniency, and particularly in our Dress." For the hot climate of the West

Indies he advised a "thin loose gown or Banjan," the dress of the Mandarins, immensely more comfortable than "a thick rich Coat and Waistcoat, daubed and loaded with Gold" under which he had seen men melting, preferring the "Character of a Fop" to that of a "Man of Sense and Honour."

Hillary recorded that November 1755 "was much drier, and some Days were much warmer than any in the last Month." It was on the first day of that month, All Saints' Day, that he described an extraordinary series of events whose cause he was perceptive enough to determine, although he did not receive confirmation of his theory for a further two months. The story of what happened on that fateful day is best told in his own words:

On the 1st of November 1755, which was three Days before the new Moon, a very extraordinary Phaenomenon happened at *Bridge-town* in *Barbados*. At 20 Minutes after 2 o'Clock after Noon, above an Hour after it was High water there, the sea suddenly flowed and rose more than two Feet higher than it does in the highest Spring Tides, and in three Minutes time it ebbed so as to be as much lower than the usual lowest Ebb; and then it flowed again as high as it did before: And thus it continued to ebb and flow to this uncommon Height, and to fall to that unusual Lowness, every five Minutes, so as to leave the Sides of the channel dry to a considerable Distance; but the Times between its Ebbing and Flowing decreased, so as to be a little longer, and the Water to rise a little less each Time, almost in an arithmetical Progression, after the first four or five Times, till near seven o'Clock in the Evening, when I returned out of the Country, and had this Account of it from several Gentlemen who carefully observed it: And it then continued ebbing and flowing, though it did not then rise above one Foot higher, and fall one Foot lower, than its usual Ebbing and Flowing in the common Tides, and it was then about twenty Minutes between each time of Flowing; and so it continued gradually to abate in each oscillation, till after nine o'Clock in the Evening, when the Return of the usual tide put an end to this extraordinary Motion of the Sea. This Day was remarkably serene, warm, and dry; we had little Wind, and that from the East; the Face of the Sea was calm and smooth before it came, and the Ships in the bay were not moved by it; but the small Craft in the Channel over the Bar, were driven too and fro with great Violence, and some of them up against the Bridge: And the Water flowed in and out of the Harbour with such a Force, that it tore up the black Mud in the Bottom of the Channel, so that it sent forth a great Stench; and caused the Fishes to float on its Surface, and drove many of them onto dry Land, at a considerable Distance, where they were taken up by the Negroes. Many People were Witnesses of this uncommon Phaenomenon, which could not be accounted for, from the known Cause of the Tides, nor from any other natural Cause, unless we supposed that an Earthquake was at some Distance in the Sea, as I then said: Though no Motion of the Earth was perceived here by any person on the Land, or in the Ships in the Bay; neither was any Noise heard, either from the earth, or in the Air.

But two Months after this, we received an Account of a most dreadful Earthquake, which happened on the same Day at Lisbon in Portugal, and destroyed the greated Part of the populous rich City.

The first shock of the earthquake had hit Lisbon at about a quarter to ten in the morning and a second more violent earthquake occurred about half an hour later. It was a major catastrophe. The churches, which were crowded with people for All Saints' Day, were totally destroyed, and the mortality was fearful. At least 30 000 lives were lost. From a knowledge of the timing of the initial shock and the time difference between Portugal and Barbados, Hillary was able to calculate that the shock wave had crossed the Atlantic at approximately seven and a half miles a minute, which, as he put it, "is a very swift Motion to be communicated by Percussion, through so soft a Medium as Water is."

In the second half of the book he described "Such Diseases as are most frequent in the...West India Islands." He started with a good though not original account of yellow fever. It was on account of the description of this disease that Dr Hillary's book was republished in Philadelphia in 1811 by Benjamin Rush. Rush followed Hillary's method of treating the disease and agreed with his view that the yellow fever could be taken more than once.[33] He found the "dry gripes," the abdominal colic of lead poisoning, common in the West Indies, and gave a clear description of the neuritis which may complicate this condition. "Dysenteries" were so frequent that he considered diseases of the intestines to be the commonest disorders in Barbados. The "opisthotonus and Tetany" were much commoner than in England. He did not know what caused tetanus but emphasised the difficulty of conceiving "how such a small Puncture or Wound, and such a trifling cause as a small Puncture with a Pin, a small bone of a Fish, or a Nail, or a small slight cut with a Sharp Stone, but little more than Skin deep, in such remote parts of the Body, should produce such violent Symptoms, and so fatal a Disease." Other diseases described were rabies canina, yaws, nyctalopia and leprosy. A hint of homesickness is included in his description of this last: "O the happy Climate of England, which is totally a stranger to this and some other miserable Diseases."

He also made some interesting observations on the pathology of elephantiasis, a common condition in those parts. With Mr Hickes, an "ingenious Surgeon in the Navy," he had the opportunity of dissecting an immensely swollen leg affected by this disease, which had been amputated. They discovered that the muscles and bones of the leg were entirely healthy and that the morbid matter was present only in the subcutaneous fatty tissue. Their conclusion that this matter was produced by a fevered condition involving the glands and tissues of the leg was not far wide of the mark.

It is Hillary's description of tropical sprue, given in this book, that has earned him an assured place in medical history. Tropical sprue is a form of intestinal malabsorption associated with nutritional deficiencies that has a very curious and striking geographical distribution. It occurs all over the Far East. Physicians in the Indian services have repeatedly encountered it. Manson saw it in China,[34] Bahr in Ceylon.[35] But no certain case has hitherto been described in Africa, and although occurring in Barbados and Puerto Rico, it has never been recorded in the neighbouring island of Jamaica.[36] Where it occurs, it is usually endemic and liable to sporadic epidemics. Hillary was not in any position to define its geographical distribution, though this is implied in his statement that he had never seen it in England. But he did note its epidemic nature. "After I came there in 1747," he wrote, "I did but see one Person who had it, in the first four Years of my residing there; and three more in the next three Years: But within the four last Years past, it is become so frequent that I have seen some Scores of Patients labouring under it... " In his description of the disease, which he called the "Aphthoeides chronica," Hillary emphasised the cardinal clinical features of tropical sprue – the chronic nature of the disease, subject to relapse and remissions, the troublesome glossitis, now known to be due to folic acid deficiency, the recurrent diarrhoea, which as he states, gradually wastes the patient, depriving him of his nourishment, leading to anaemia, progressive wasting, and death.

Hillary has not been credited by some writers with the first description of tropical sprue. This is because until recent years the tropical form of sprue has been confused with its non-tropical counterparts, coeliac disease and idiopathic steatorrhoea, which are entirely different disorders. Descriptions which may possibly be of the latter condition were published in Europe in the seventeenth century, but such descriptions are ambiguous and uncertain and bear no relation to the purely tropical condition that Hillary saw in Barbados. Hillary's description is authoritative and complete. He had watched and recorded at the bedside of many of his patients, and he no doubt remained as puzzled about aetiology as the physician of today. The first edition of Hillary's book on the *Diseases of Barbados* is rare today and the second edition, published in 1766, is often quoted as the date of his description, by which time he had been dead for three years.

Hillary returned to England after a stay of 12 years in Barbados, in 1759. It was the most remarkable year of the Seven Years' War. William Pitt's military strategy had gained great victories for England in every corner of the globe. In America there were triumphs at Niagara, Ticerondoga, and Crown Point. Madras was taken, the Battle of Minden won. And war crept close to Barbados too. In the spring of 1759 a British force attacked and took the French island of Guadaloupe. Perhaps Hillary decided that discretion was the better part of valour. He was now over 60 and perhaps the climate taxed his increasing years. He seems also to have been financially successful. A contemporary stated that he had made £6000 during his 12 years on the island. Whatever the cause, by the late autumn of 1759 he was back in London, probably in time to hear the firing of the park and tower guns, to see the flags displayed from steeples everywhere and the greatest illuminations ever known, with which on 12 October the city of London celebrated the fall of Quebec.

Dr Hillary lived for the remaining years of his life in London, apparently at first in East Street, off Red Lion Square in Bloomsbury. Although then in retirement, he was by no means idle. He must at once have been busy preparing his *Diseases of Barbados* for the press. Soon afterwards he was occupied with another literary venture. This was entitled *The Nature, Properties and Laws of Motion of Fire – discovered and demonstrated by Observations and Experiments*.[37] His preface, dated East Street, 14 November 1759, describes how he had first made attempts "to discover the subtile and mysterious nature of fire by Experiments...above twenty years since; but the great difficulty of carefully examining such an intractable being, and sometimes the want of proper instruments for that purpose, and more frequently the avocation of my profession, often put a stop to my proceedings therein, and several times obliged me to lay them aside for several years." It was addressed to the Earl of Macclesfield, president, and to the council and fellows of the Royal Society of London, probably because he wished to bring himself to their notice. The book is interesting in indicating the curiosity, breadth of knowledge, and erudition of an eighteenth century physician. It contains no startling discoveries or observations. Fire is consistently confused with heat; but Hillary emphasises its fundamental importance to living things. If there were no fire, he argues, to "penetrate, pervade, rarify and expand all other bodies," there would be no fluids, hence no vegetable juices, no nutrition, no growth, no life itself. He again gives due credit to the scientific methods of his old teacher, Dr Boerhaave, who "wisely and judiciously pursued that excellent Method of investigating the causes of things by Experiments and Induction, recommended by the great Lord Verulam...and this is the Method by which Newton, Boyle, Locke and Boerhaave, and all other great Philosphers since his Lordship's time, have made discoveries..."

Hillary remained throughout his life an advocate of the

scientific method and his idealism does not seem to have been dulled by increasing years. His last book, published in 1761, was in some ways his most ambitious and idealistic venture. *An Inquiry into the Means of improving Medical Knowledge, by examining all those Methods which have hindered or increased its improvement in all past ages* was no less than an examination of the art and practice of medicine since the earliest times, with a view to determining what had either aided or hampered its progress.[38] It is of particular interest to the medical historian, since it is in fact an eighteenth century history of medicine, an account of medical practice through the ages that illustrates the very extensive knowledge and wide reading of the writer. His introduction again stresses the author's indebtedness to Boerhaave, who, writes Hillary,

was blessed with great Penetration, a sane Judgement, and the strongest Memory; all of which he early applied with indefatigable Industry, to obtain a perfect knowledge of all the learned, and many of the modern Languages, and all the Sciences; an able Philosopher, the greatest Anatomist, Chemist, Botanist and the most eminent Physician of this, or any other Age.

No teacher of medicine could wish for a more handsome tribute.

His book starts at the very beginning of things with the Creation, and first takes the reader up to the time of Hippocrates. He then gives an account of the improvement of medicine after this period, describing the work of Celsus and Galen. He displays an astonishing knowledge of the work of the Arabians, in particular Mohammed ibn Zakariyya al-Razi (Rhazes), emphasising how medicine flourished in Arabia during the dark ages in Europe. These ideas certainly reflect the teaching of Boerhaave. He recognises to the full the importance of the "Restoration of Learning," and again pays his most ardent homage to

Francis Bacon, Lord Verulam, one of the greatest Genius' that any Age ever produced; and although he was not a Physician, but a Lawyer and a Philosopher, yet *he* first discovered and taught Mankind the right way of Thinking, and the true method of discovering Truth, and obtaining true

Knowledge and Certainty, both in Philosophy and in Physick, and all other Sciences...

It was to this method of reasoning, for example, that William Harvey owed the demonstration of the circulation of the blood, and Boerhaave his success. Hillary's "General Remarks on the Improvements and Hindrance of its Improvement" follow. They include an enthusiastic recognition of the significance of the *vis medicatrix Naturae*, of which he would be well aware after a lifetime of practice. He disapproved of Galen and the long period during which acceptance of his ideas had hindered progress, and he was surprisingly critical of Aristotle. He quoted a number of specific errors made by practising physicians, for example the curious story of how the use of blisters on the head in a patient with gout had brought the disease to that site and led to death within 30 hours. It is difficult in some of these instances to follow the line of argument. His approval of the Hippocratic method of careful clinical observation of disease, which Boerhaave had so admired in Sydenham and which Hillary had himself practised in Barbados so successfully, again gave him the opportunity of a word of critical advice.

I am sensible that this Method of observing Disease in Nature, and strictly following and assisting her, may probably be objected to by some of the Faculty, especially by those who think it too tedious and laborious a thing, so strictly to observe Diseases and Nature, and too servile a thing to follow and assist Nature in that Manner; especially if they are used to hurry over their Patients, and are in a haste to grow rich...

On the use of medicines likewise:

It is not our having a great Number of choice Prescriptions, or a great Variety of Formulae, however neat and elegant...that will make either the most able or the most successful Physician; but his truly Knowing the Disease, and what the Cause really is, and when and how he should assist Nature by administrating suitable Medicines, and when not...

His objections to polypharmacy have a remarkably modern ring; and his words on those who haste to grow rich relate to one of the age old problems of medical practice, as true today as when his book was written.

William Hillary died on 25 April 1763.[39] He is described in the records of the Friends as "of St Dunstan in the West" and had been a member of the Peel meeting, which met at St John Street, Clerkenwell. He was buried on 1 May in the Friends' Burying Ground at Bunhill Fields. The cause of his death was stated to be "fever," and it may have come on him suddenly for he left no will. An administration was granted to his younger brother, Richard, "one of the next of kin," but there is no record of what his "goods, chattels and Credits" comprised.[40] Did his old friend John Fothergill, now at the height of his fame as a London physician, attend him during his last illness? History has left no record of those last days, nor was his grave marked by a stone, for this was not the practice of the Quakers at that time. The *Gentleman's Magazine* of April 1763 merely recorded briefly the death of "Dr. Hillary, well known for his many ingenious treatises on physic."[41]

These "ingenious treatises" deserve the attention of all physicians who today seek to improve the practice of medicine by scientific methods. Hillary has a forthright style which is attractive to read. The clarity of his thinking, his careful bedside descriptions of disease, his condemnation of bigotry and preconceived ideas are refreshing reminders of the scientific renaissance that began to influence clinical medicine in Britain during the eighteenth century. The most impressive feature of his work is the wholehearted enthusiasm of his belief in the value of a scientific approach to medicine. In an age when much remained mysterious and unknown, when ignorance was glossed over by "whymsical hypothesis" and "conceited imagination," he believed that rationalism could replace empiricism, that mystery could be dispelled by science. "It is by this Method of reasoning from Data, founded upon observations and real Facts, that the Healing Art must be improved and brought to a state of Perfection," he had written in 1735. Nearly 30 years later, the scientific idealism inculcated at Leyden by Boerhaave was in no way diminished.

NOTES

1 *Gentleman's Magazine* 1738; **8**: 491.

2 Innes-Smith RW. *English-speaking students of medicine at the University of Leyden.* London: Oliver and Boyd, 1932.

3 Major RH. *Classic descriptions of disease.* Springfield, Illinois: CC Thomas, 1939.

4 In the records of the Society of Friends, Willaim Hillary's date of birth is given as the 17th of the first month 1696/7. *Yorkshire Births.* Library of Society of Friends, London. Until the introduction of new style dating in 1752 the first month in the Quaker calendar was March.

5 "John Hillary of Birchrigg, Aigarth, Yorkshire" was married to Mary Robinson at John Robinson's in Countersett on the 22nd of the fourth month, 1692. *Yorkshire Marriages.* Library of Society of Friends, London.

6 Pontefract E. *Wensleydale.* London: JM Dent, 1936: 96–7.

7 The births of the Hillary children are recorded in *Yorkshire Births* at the Library of the Society of Friends, London. The initials RH and the date 1773 can with difficulty be recognised on a gravestone preserved in my garden at Worton. This stone marked the resting place of Rachel Hillary in the Friends' burial ground at Hawes and is one of the only remaining traces of the Hillary family in Wensleydale today.

8 The family home at Burtersett passed out of the hands of the Hillary family in the early nineteenth century when it was sold by Sir William Hillary, second son of Dr William Hillary's younger brother Richard. Sir William Hillary is remembered for the part he played in the foundation of the Royal National Lifeboat Institution.

9 Among a file of notes on the Hillary family in the records of the Society of Genealogists in London, the following has been preserved: "1715 Dec. 29. William son of Jno Hillary yeom appt. to Benj. Bartlett of Bradford apoth. for 7 years." William Hillary's apprenticeship to Benjamin Bartlett is also attested by JC Lettsom in *The Works of John Fothergill MD...with some account of his Life.* London: C Dilly, 1784: iv.

10 Scruton W. *Pen and pencil pictures of old Bradford.* Bradford: Thomas Brear, 1889.

11 Thompson G. *The life and character of Dr Fothergill,* London: Cadell and Phillips, 1782: 6.

12 Tuke JH. *A sketch of the life of Dr Fothergill.* London: Samuel Harris, 1879.

13 Neiret G. *Etude sur Hermann Boerhaave.* Paris: Henri Jouve, 1880.

14 Sigerist H. *Great doctors.* London, Allen and Unwin, 1933: 185.

15 Schuyl F. *Catalogue of all the chiefest rarities in the publick anatomie hall of the university of Leyden.* Leyden: Widow Hubert van de Boxe, 1719.

16 Plummer A. *De phthisi pulmonali.* MD thesis, University of Leyden, 1722.

17 Under John Hillary's will, Isaac received property at Hawes, Gayle, and Appersett, as well as the Birkrigg farm. He also inherited Rigg House and the family home at Burtersett. These properties indicate the extent of the Hillary estates in Wensleydale. The inventory listed "household property, wooll, six horses and two calves, four stirks, thirteen steers, two fat steers, 147 old sheep, fifty four hoggs, Hay and husbandry gear." The total value was £980 0s 6d, of which the major part, £730 0s 0d, was made up of "Money's owing." MS Will of John Hillary. City Library, Leeds.

18 Wintringham C. *Commentarium nosologicum morbus epidemicos et aeris variationes in urbe Eboracenci logisque vicinis, ab anno 1715 ad finem anni 1725 grassantes complectens.* London, 1727.

19 Hillary W. *A rational and mechanical essay on the small pox.* London: G Strachan, 1735.

20 Certificate in the possession of Mrs Winifred Fothergill Quinlan, of Townbank, New Jersey.

21 Mahon, Lord, ed. *The letters of Philip Stanhope, Earl of Chesterfield.* Vol III. London: Richard Bentley, 1845: 139.

22 MS autograph letter, Dr John Fothergill to Dr Robert Key, Leek, Staffordshire, dated 6 August 1744. Toft MSS No 42. Library of the Society of Friends, London.

23 MS autograph letter, Dr John Fothergill to Tabitha Horner, Leeds, Yorkshire, dated 6 August 1744. Portfolio 22/94. Library of the Society of Friends, London.

24 MS autograph letter, Dr John Fothergill to Alexander Fothergill, at Carr End, Wensleydale, Yorkshire, dated 11 July 1746. Library of the Society of Friends, London.

25 Letters written from Barbados by John Fothergill, Snr, to his son are published in *An account of the life and travels in the work of the ministry of John Fothergill.* London: Luke Hinde, 1753: 290.

26 *Records of North Somerset Monthly Meeting, 1741–1772,* pp 105, 106. Library of the Society of Friends, London.

27 Parry JH, Sherlock PM. *A short history of the West Indies,* London and New York: Macmillan, 1956.

28 Anonymous. Friends in Barbadoes. *The Friend* 1887; 60; 178–80.

29 Sturge CD. Friends in Barbadoes. *J Friends Hist Soc* 1908; 5: 43–9.

30 This epistle is preserved in Portfolio 28:135 at the Library of the Society of Friends, London.

31 Anonymous. The decline of Friends in Barbadoes. *The Friend* 1887; 71: 275–80.

32 Toner JM. *The daily journal of Major George Washington in 1751–2, kept while on a tour from Virginia to the island of Barbadoes, with his invalid brother, Major Lawrence Washington, proprietor of Mount Vernon on the Potomac.* Albany, NY: Joel Munsell's Sons, 1892.

33 Butterfield LH, ed. *Letters of Benjamin Rush;* Vol II. Princeton; Princeton University Press, 1960: 698; 1045.

34 Manson, P. Notes on sprue. *China Imperial Maritime Customs Medical Reports* 1880; **19**: 33–44.

35 Bahr [afterwards Manson-Bahr] PH. *A report on researches on sprue in Ceylon.* Cambridge: Cambridge University Press, 1915.

36 Manson-Bahr PH. *Manson's tropical diseases.* London: Cassell, 1954.

37 Hillary W. *The nature, properties and laws of motion of fire – discovered and demonstrated by observations and experiments.* London: L Davis and C Reymers, 1760.

38 Hillary W. *An inquiry into the means of improving medical knowledge, by examining all those methods which have hindered or increased its improvement in the past ages.* London: C Hitch and L Hawes, 1761.

39 *Middlesex Burials.* Library of the Society of Friends, London. The entry reads: "William Hillary, of St Dunstan in the West aged about 63 years, 25/4 1763, of a fever."

40 The administration is preserved at Somerset House and a copy is among the Hillary papers at the Society of Genealogists, London. It records: "on the eleventh day [of May 1763] Admin. of the goods Chattels and Credits of William Hillary, late of the parish of St Dunstan in the West, London, a batchelor decd was granted to Richard Hillary the natural and lawful Brother and one of the next of Kin of the said decd, he having been first sworn duly to administer." No other details are given.

41 *Gentleman's Magazine* 1763; **35**: 202. The date is here given as 22 April, three days earlier than the date recorded by the Society of Friends (see note 39).

4 Angina pectoris and the coronary arteries

Dr John Fothergill was an exceedingly modest man. His biographer and pupil John Coakley Lettsom wrote of him after his death: "Few men of distinguished reputation pass through life with more silent admiration... Dr Fothergill was more desirious of doing good than of having it known."[1] It is perhaps for this reason that relatively little is known of him or his work today. His contributions to the understanding of angina pectoris have, however, received some recognition from historians who have recorded John Hunter's discovery of ossified coronary arteries in a patient of Dr Fothergill's who died with angina pectoris, the first recorded instance of coronary artery disease in this condition.[2] But the extent of Fothergill's observations and their significance in directing attention to the heart in this disorder have not been fully recognised.

Dr Fothergill's self effacing modesty may have been in great part the result of his upbringing as a member of a strict Quaker family. Son of a famous Quaker preacher, he came, like William Hillary, from Wensleydale in Yorkshire where the Hillary and Fothergill families were close friends. He was born at Carr End, the family home, in 1712. Like so many other eighteenth century nonconformists, he received his medical training in Scotland, where he graduated MD at Edinburgh in 1736. He went to London in the same year, and after two years' further study at St Thomas's Hospital set up in practice. His reputation gradually increased, particularly after the publication in 1748 of his treatise on the *Malignant*

From *Medical History* 1957; 1: 115–22.

Sore Throat, which won him international renown and assured his success. He remained one of the leading physicians in London until his death in 1780. He wrote, during an exceptionally busy life in practice, on a wide variety of medical subjects. But his achievements were by no means limited to medicine. A strict Quaker throughout his life, he was an active member of the Society of Friends and in his last years took the leading part in founding the famous Quaker school at Ackworth. He was an ardent botanist, friend of Peter Collinson, correspondent of Linnaeus. He maintained a garden at Upton in Essex which was said to be second only to Kew in the whole of Europe, and collectors from all over the world sent specimens to him. He collected minerals, butterflies, shells and corals, animals, and insects of all kinds. A close friend of Benjamin Franklin, to whom he had been physician, he worked with him and the Quaker merchant David Barclay in a vain attempt to avert the final breach with the American colonies in 1775.[3] He kept up a correspondence with many American friends, and he was associated with the early days of the medical schools in America. He never married, living in Harpur Street, Bloomsbury, with his sister for most of his life.

Fothergill moved little in social circles, but he was a keen member of a small and select medical society, whose members included William Hunter and Daniel Solander, and of which he was himself president at the time of his death. It was to this Medical Society of Physicians, whose meetings were held at the Mitre Tavern in Fleet Street on alternate Monday evenings, that most of Fothergill's original medical observations were communicated. The proceedings, the *Medical Observations and Inquiries*, were published between 1757 and 1784. Fothergill's two papers on angina pectoris were given to the society. These papers were read a few years after Heberden's remarkably accurate description of angina pectoris was first published, at a time when the aetiology of the painful affection of the breast was still unknown. Fothergill's observations on the disease were highly original and of considerable significance, for he was the first physician to suspect on clinical grounds that the heart might be affected in this

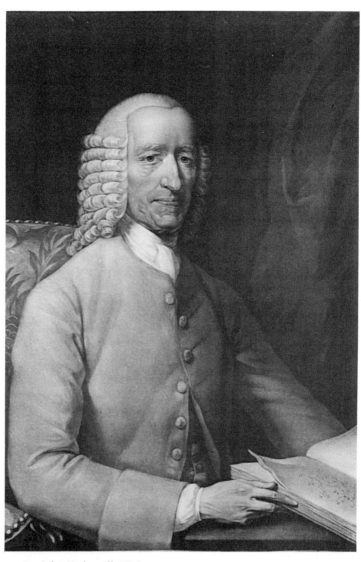

6   Dr John Fothergill, FRS
     (Medical Society of London)

condition, and he was the first to record abnormalities in the myocardium and coronary arteries of patients who died suddenly with this disease. His observations, which were read to the Medical Society in 1774 and 1775, were, however, preceded by the reports of two patients who had died with angina pectoris, in both of whom a postmortem examination had been performed. These case reports were read by Heberden in 1772, the first being the only one he had himself seen at necropsy, and the second being a case of Dr Wall of Worcester. To illustrate the significance of Fothergill's observations it is necessary to describe these cases in some detail, and also to consider at greater length the extent of Heberden's contributions to the understanding of this condition.

On a July day in the year 1768 Dr William Heberden had read to the College of Physicians in London his observations on the new disease to which he had given the name "Angina pectoris."

Those who are afflicted with it are seized while they are walking (more particularly if it be uphill, and soon after eating) with a painful and most disagreeable sensation in the breast, which seems as if it would extinguish life if it were to increase or continue; but the moment they stand still, all this uneasiness vanishes...

The termination of the angina pectoris is remarkable. For if no accident intervene, but the disease go on to its height, the patients all suddenly fall down and perish almost immediately.

Heberden's paper on the "Angina pectoris," published later in the *Medical Transactions* of the Royal College of Physicians, is a classic piece of descriptive medical writing.[4] In it he summarised his experience of a disease whose course he had carefully watched and recorded in more than 20 patients in his practice. His description of the characteristic pain in the chest, the radiation of the pain, the age and sex incidence, has not been bettered by any writer since. Yet it must be admitted that Heberden had little idea of the cause of the pain which he had called angina pectoris. It belonged, he said, "to the class of spasmodic, not of inflammatory complaints;" and he continued, "but though it be most probable that a strong spasm be the true cause of this disorder, yet there is some reason for thinking, that it is sometimes accompanied with an ulcer, and may partly proceed from it; for I have seen two of these patients, who often used to spit up blood and purulent matter, one of whom constantly asserted, that he felt it came from the seat of the disorder." He had no reason to believe that the heart was at fault, because "the pulse is, at least sometimes, not disturbed by this pain, and consequently the heart is not affected by it; which I have had an opportunity of knowing by feeling the pulse during the paroxysm: but," he went on, "I have never had it in my power to see anyone opened who had died of it."

An opportunity for performing a postmortem examination in a case of angina pectoris came to him, however, soon after the publication of these observations in 1772. A worthy and benevolent gentleman "who had been troubled with that disorder," left his body to Dr Heberden to be opened and examined. He died suddenly, and Heberden arranged for the dissection to be carried out by "that experienced and accurate anatomist, Mr J. Hunter." After a careful examination no cause for the sudden death could be discovered. The thoracic contents were examined "with peculiar attention, particularly the heart with its vessels and valves, and were all found to be in a natural condition..."[5] Edward Jenner, however, at that time a surgical student working with John Hunter, seemed to doubt the "peculiar attention" with which the heart was dissected, for in a famous letter written more than 20 years later to Caleb Hillier Parry, he referred to this necropsy and wrote, "There, I can positively say, the coronary arteries of the heart were not examined."[6] At this time, in the year 1772, neither Heberden nor Hunter seems to have seriously considered that there might be any significant lesion in the heart or coronary arteries of patients dying with angina pectoris.

Fothergill's observations were antedated by one other case report. Dr Wall, a physician of Worcester, sent his notes on a patient who had died with angina pectoris to Dr Heberden in a letter written in May 1772. This letter was read to the College of Physicians by Heberden in November of that year, but it did not appear in print until the third volume of the *Medical Transactions* was published in 1785.[7] The case that Dr Wall recorded was that of a man of 66 who for six or seven years had suffered increasing tightness across his breast and arms on walking. He had, "in the former part of his life," had several attacks of rheumatism. At the postmortem examination he was found to have a heart "of uncommon size," but there was no apparent abnormality "till we opened the left ventricle; and there, the semilunar valves, placed at the origin of the aorta, were found to be perfectly ossified." He did not think that the induration of the semilunar valves was necessarily always the cause of the disease, but suggested that "some malformation in the heart and vessels, immediately proceeding from it, may be so." His case appears to have been one of rheumatic aortic stenosis with anginal pain, and is the first recorded instance of a cardiac lesion in a patient dying with angina pectoris.

Within a year or two of Heberden's original paper Fothergill had also reached the conclusion that the heart might be affected in angina pectoris. In 1776 he published, in two papers, detailed case reports of two patients who had died with angina pectoris, together with the postmortem findings. The first of these papers, read in 1774, included his reasons for supposing that the heart might be affected. He makes no reference to Dr Wall's unpublished case, and it is quite likely that he had not heard of it. He had seen one case, he said, with the "constriction which the thorax suffers upon accelerated motion," where a postmortem examination had revealed a "generalized anasarca," though the heart was normal with the exception of a small ossification in one of the mitral valves. Another circumstance inducing him to interest himself in the heart was "that I have very seldom met with this disease, but it was attended with an irregular and intermittent pulse, not only during the exacerbations, but often when the patient was free from pain and at rest."[8] These reasons, though incomplete and not in all respects correct, were sufficiently cogent to stimulate him to make further and more detailed observations in the cases that came under his care.

The first case that he described was that of RM, aged about 58, who consulted him in the autumn of the year 1773. In July of that year he had been attacked "with a spasm in the breast, which at first affected him only when he used exercise, and chiefly when he walked up hill."

Dr Fothergill advised him "to abstain from everything heating, not however to drink less wine than usual, and to observe caution in respect to quantity of proper food." He went to take the waters at Bath, and seemed a little improved by the journey and the waters, but "they did not alleviate the original pain in his breast, which sometimes came so suddenly and violently, towards the morning especially, as to alarm those about him with fears of his immediate death, and which at length happened, very suddenly, in the morning of the 10th of May."

It is a measure of Fothergill's interest, enthusiam, and influence that he was able to arrange for a postmortem examination on a patient dying in Bath while he was himself occupied in London. The dissection was carried out by the Langleys, "judicious surgeons of the neighbourhood," and they approached their task armed with instructions from Fothergill "to attend to the condition of the heart with all possible accuracy."[8] The findings of this necropsy have previously been dismissed by historians as "inconclusive," but there was one observation that Dr Fothergill thought worthy of note, though its significance not unnaturally eluded him. The Langleys found the heart in the following condition: "The auricles and ventricles with all the vessels and valves perfect; not the least ossification or appearance of disease, except on the outward muscular part, near the apex, a small white spot, as big as a sixpence, resembling a cicatrix." Commenting on the case, Fothergill drew attention to this "scar-like appearance of the heart." This seems most likely to have been due to a previous episode of cardiac infarction in the case of the unfortunate RM, and it appears to be the earliest occasion on which a myocardial scar has been described in a case of angina pectoris. As to the causation of the pain in the chest, Fothergill suggested that the immense amount of fat found in the abdomen and chest of his patient could have impeded the flow of blood in the heart and lungs, but this he thought not the only cause of the distemper. "Time and further opportunities must inform us of the rest," he concluded.

The "further opportunities" came in the summer of the same year, 1774, when HR, aged 63, "a gentleman rather inclined to corpulency, but active, and of a very irritable habit..." consulted Dr Fothergill. For three or four years he had been unable to walk up a moderate ascent because of a painful sensation of constriction in the breast. He took the waters at Buxton that summer, "and though it did not appear that much ground was being gained, the same constriction returning if he attempted any exercise beyond a certain point, which his experience had taught him, yet he perceived no increase of the disease." The end, however, was exactly as had been predicted by Dr Heberden, and "on the 13th of March, 1775, he fell down and expired immediately."

It may have been easier for Fothergill to arrange the post-mortem examination on this occasion, for the patient died in London. But in the eighteenth century it must have taken considerable influence to persuade relatives to grant permission for the removal and dissection of a body. In addition, Fothergill was exceptionally busy, quite apart from his medical commitments, in the early spring of 1775. He was engaged on work with the naturalist John Ellis, describing the mangostan and breadfruit.[9] He had been long occupied with Benjamin Franklin and David Barclay in formulating proposals for a conciliation between Britain and her American colonies. In March 1775, when his patient HR died, he was busy with other Quakers subscribing money to help the needy in Philadelphia, and preparing a petition which he later presented to the King on their behalf. In a letter written four days after HR's death, and sent by Benjamin Franklin's hand, Fothergill complained to James Pemberton in Philadelphia that he was "exceedingly straitened for time by almost increasing applications in the duty of my profession."[10] Nevertheless he found time to prevail upon the family of HR to allow the body to be opened by John Hunter, who did the dissection on the following day.

Fothergill's report of this case forms the substance of his second paper, and it contains the first description of calcification of the coronary arteries in a patient suffering from angina pectoris.[11] It might be supposed that the calcification of the coronary arteries was a chance finding in the course of the examination of the heart by the brilliant and skilful John Hunter, and that Fothergill played a relatively minor part in this discovery. A study of the evidence presented in this paper, however, suggests that this was probably not the case. Fothergill had in fact suspected previously that the heart might be affected in angina pectoris. In addition, he found an unexplained abnormality in the previous case whereas John Hunter's examination of Heberden's single case had revealed no abnormality, nor had he examined the coronary arteries, and it seems most likely that it was Fothergill himself who suggested that Hunter take particular note of the condition of the heart in this case.

We can imagine Fothergill's intense interest in what was to be found. We can see the suppressed excitement in his stern old Quaker eyes as he described his previous cases to John Hunter. Perhaps he gave Hunter instructions similar to those he had given the Langleys nearly a year before. History leaves no record of their conversation, but the postmortem findings set out by Hunter fully justified Fothergill's expectations:

The heart to external appearances was also sound; but, upon examination, I found that its substance was paler than common, more of a ligamentous consistence, and in many parts of the left ventricle it was become almost white and hard, having just the appearance of a beginning ossification.

The valvulae mitrales had a vast number of such appearances in them, and were less pliant than in the natural state; but did not appear to be unfit for use.

The semilunar valves of the aorta were thicker than common, but very readily filled the area of the artery.

The aorta had several small ossifications on it, and several white parts, which are generally the beginning of ossifications, and which were similar to those found in the heart and valves.

The two coronary arteries, from their origins to many of their ramifications upon the heart, were become one piece of bone.

The significance of these findings may have escaped John

Hunter. He himself never attempted to explain them. Parry, in his *Syncope Anginosa* published in 1799, wrote: "In a person dying of angina pectoris in the year 1775, Mr Hunter found the coronary arteries ossified; but, as far as I can learn, did not consider this state as having any important influence on the patient's health, and says nothing of it in any of his lectures or publications." In Hunter's later years there was a very good reason why he should have said nothing of it, for he was himself a sufferer from angina pectoris. Jenner avoided discussing the subject with him for this reason, and he postponed publishing his own theories on the subject, "as it must have brought on an unpleasant conference between Mr Hunter and me."

Parry, however, made no reference to Fothergill's conclusions, which were published 23 years before the *Syncope Anginosa* appeared in print, and some years before Jenner accidentally discovered ossification of the coronary arteries in another patient dying with angina pectoris. Fothergill had not missed the significance of Hunter's findings. While he did not fully understand them, he commented: "The state of the parts about the heart fully shows, that under such circumstances, it is impossible to bear with impunity the effects of sudden and violent agitations, whether they arise from gusts of passion, or suddenly accelerated muscular motion."

Fothergill was one of the first physicians to attempt to correlate the clinical features with the pathological findings in cases of angina pectoris, and he was the first to look specifically for cardiac lesions when the bodies of his patients were dissected. Heberden, to whose brilliant clinical description little has since been added, went so far as to say that the heart was not affected, and, perhaps a little unluckily, Hunter found no lesion in the heart of the one patient whose autopsy Heberden was able to arrange. But, as Jenner pointed out, the coronary arteries were not examined in that case. Fothergill was not the first to find a cardiac lesion in angina pectoris, for Dr Wall had correctly surmised that the ossification of the semilunar valves that he found in his case might have been connected with the pain in the chest. But the observations that Fothergill made, and the establishment of the link between angina pectoris and diseased coronary arteries were entirely original and represented a major contribution. For these observations much of the credit belongs to Dr Fothergill. No doubt he would never have claimed it.

NOTES

1 Lettsom JC. *The works of John Fothergill, MD... with some account of his life.* London: C Dilly, 1784: 100.
2 Major RH. *Classic descriptions of disease.* Springfield, Illinois: CC Thomas, 1932: 459.
3 Corner BC, Singer JW. Dr John Fothergill, peacemaker. *Proc Amer Phil Soc* 1954; 98: 11–32.
4 Heberden W. Some account of a disorder of the breast. *Med Trans Coll Phys Lond* 1772; 2: 59–89.
5 Heberden W. A letter to Dr Heberden, concerning the angina pectoris; and Dr Heberden's account of the dissection of one, who had been troubled with that disorder. *Med Trans Coll Phys Lond* 1785; 3: 1–11.
6 Parry CH. *An inquiry into the symptoms and causes of the syncope anginosa, commonly called angina pectoris.* Bath: R Crutwell, 1799.
7 Wall J. A letter from Dr Wall to Dr Heberden on the same subject. *Med Trans Coll Phys Lond* 1785; 3: 12–24. The "same subject" refers to the subject of the previous paper on angina pectoris by Heberden (see note 5).
8 Fothergill J. Case of an angina pectoris, with remarks. *Med Obs and Inq* 1776; 5: 233–50.
9 MS letters, John Fothergill to John Ellis. Ellis MSS, Linnean Society, London.
10 MS autograph letter, John Fothergill to James Pemberton. Etting MSS, Historical Society of Pennsylvania.
11 Fothergill J. Further account of the angina pectoris. *Med Obs and Inq* 1776; 5: 252–8.

5 Three doctors and the American revolution

Practising doctors are today rarely active in politics. Perhaps they feel less driven to political activity than their predecessors, whose consciences must have been constantly pricked by exposure to the social problems which were a major cause of disease 100 or more years ago. In the past, however, doctors were often enthusiastically active in contemporary politics, frequently pioneering unpopular causes. The careers of three such men, all of whom played an important part in the political affairs of their time while also practising the art of their profession are examined in this chapter. In British eyes they were all rebels, for they were concerned in the American revolution. The first was the English doctor John Fothergill, who lived in London and who was physician to Benjamin Franklin. The other two were Americans – Joseph Warren of Boston, who died at the Battle of Bunker Hill, and Benjamin Rush, a Philadelphian who signed the Declaration of Independence.

In the spring of 1775, when the war with America broke out, John Fothergill was 63; he was a distinguished senior member of the medical profession and had a highly successful practice. His patients included Lord Dartmouth, Secretary of State for the American Colonies; the Chancellor, Lord Hyde; and the Speaker of the House of Commons, Sir Fletcher Norton; and he had attended John Wesley and Lord Clive of India. But he was as nonconformist in his attitudes as his background had made him. As a Quaker, he belonged to the most nonconformist sect of the day, and as a dalesman he

From the *Lancet* 1967; ii: 358–64.

came from an area of England where the inhabitants had not been enervated by subservience to a leisured, aristocratic ruling class. They themselves farmed their land; they had themselves reclaimed their fields from rough moorland and drained them from bog. They were freeholders, and they developed a sturdy independence of thought and spirit which persists to this day. They never tip their caps to the gentry, and they have always, like the Celts, had a healthy respect for education. At their local school at Sedbergh, young lads like John Fothergill could learn the Latin and Greek then essential for a university education.

Dr Fothergill's background played a large part in deciding that, successful though his practice was and distinguished scientifically as he became, he never really joined the medical establishment of his day. This was predominantly because of his education. As a Quaker, he could not go to the universities of either Oxford or Cambridge; as a graduate of Edinburgh, where he took his MD in 1736, he could not be elected a fellow of the Royal College of Physicians of London, for this distinction was at that time reserved for graduates of Oxford and Cambridge only. Thus he, along with other Scottish graduates, remained throughout his life an opponent of the distinguished but often dull and unimaginative pillars of his profession who ran the affairs of the royal college. His education at the medical school in Edinburgh was in fact far better than he would have received at either of the English universities. Fothergill knew this and his adverse opinion of one of those universities is clearly stated in a letter to the Bodleian librarian at Oxford in 1769. He wrote: "I do not know of anything that would give me more pain than to reside a few months at Oxford. There I should discover men of the first rate of understanding, partly from want of opportunity, but much more from indolence, absorpt in an insignificant round of doing that which the lowest mankind enjoy as much as themselves: eating, drinking and sleeping."

With this background and these forthright ideas, Fothergill was a natural rebel. Although financially dependent on their goodwill, for many of them were his patients, he was an active opponent of the ruling hierarchy in England at the time of the American revolution and, like Chatham and Burke, he admired, encouraged, and actively supported the rebellious colonists in America until his death. He had a long association with America and in particular with the Quaker colony of Pennsylvania. In 1738, at the age of 26, he had been appointed London correspondent for the members of the Society of Friends in Pennsylvania, a task that brought him into constant contact with colonial affairs. His father and his brother had both travelled widely in America on journeys in the ministry for the Society of Friends. He had American relations in Rhode Island. He was also physician to the American philosopher and scientist, Benjamin Franklin, and his close friend. In 1751, some years before they first met, he had been instrumental in getting Franklin's early experiments on electricity published in London, and in 1757, when Franklin arrived in London to discuss taxation with the Penn family on behalf of the colonists of Pennsylvania, one of his first visits was to Dr John Fothergill. Fothergill was physician to the Penns, the proprietories of the colony of Pennsylvania, and he at once used his influence to arrange meetings with Franklin. The friendship between the two men was warm and personal and it lasted until Fothergill's death in 1780, during the American war, when Franklin had become the distinguished representative of the rebellious American colonists at the court of Louis XVI of France.[1]

The trouble between Britain and America was originally sparked off by the passage of the Stamp Act by the English Parliament in 1765, the notorious Act by which the British government sought to raise taxes from the Americans to pay for the cost of colonial defence, but it was another 10 smouldering years before the real conflagration began. Fothergill's attitude at this time, 10 years before the outbreak of war, shows how consistent were his views. A few days after the Act was passed he wrote to a correspondent in America: "A resolution at the House of Commons has within these last few days given America a dreadful stab and hurt..." and he at once set about lobbying and campaigning for the repeal of the Act. He wrote to the Earl of Dartmouth in July pointing out that "it is too well known that some late acts and regulations have spread universal discontent and produced some very unjustifiable proceedings on the other side" – a reference to the rioting and violence with which the Americans greeted the news of the passage of the Stamp Act. He recommended to the Earl of Dartmouth sending commissioners over to America to investigate and then went on to the heart of the matter: "That the Colony's aspire at Independency has been asserted, but if we treat them with mildness, yet firmly securing the connection by making it their interest cheerfully to obey, this prospect must be at a very great distance."[2]

But he did not only write letters; he also wrote a pamphlet, *Considerations Relative to the American Colonies*, which was published in the summer of 1765. It was sent to the Earl of Dartmouth and to the Prime Minister, the Marquess of Rockingham, also Fothergill's patient. This pamphlet is a remarkable document for an Englishman to have written, for in it Fothergill reveals an extraordinary understanding of the geographical and social distinctions of a society he had never seen. Repeal of the Stamp Act was essential, he wrote. Repeal and only total repeal would "convince the Americans so fully of British equity and moderation that they would no longer suspect designs against their freedom, their privileges and their interests." What could be expected from people "bred up almost in independency, and full of republican principles," when without consultation, or application to the duly elected Houses of Representatives in each colony, taxation reaching down to their everyday expenditure was suddenly imposed by parliamentary Act? Then, at the end of the pamphlet, he suggested: "If we promote scholarships for Americans in our universities, give posts and benefits in America to such Americans who have studied here, preferably to others...the Americans, by mixing with our own youth at the University, will diffuse a spirit of enquiry about America and its affairs; they will cement friendships on both sides, which will be of more lasting benefit than all the armies Britain can send thither."

In response to the clamour on both sides of the Atlantic,

and in large measure as a result of the efforts of the British merchants threatened by the American non-importation agreements, the Act was repealed in 1766. But in Philadelphia a storm broke out and a rumour circulated that Franklin had given his support to the Act. It was to Fothergill he turned for an attestation to clear his name. Franklin had been, wrote the doctor to the Philadelphia colonists, "an able, useful advocate for America in general and the province of Pennsylvania in particular." From first to last he had done all in his power to oppose the Stamp Act. During three hours of grilling by the entire House of Commons (the episode referred to by Burke as "a schoolmaster catechising his pupils"), he had given an extraordinary exhibition, fully exposing the mischievous tendencies of the Stamp Act.[3]

If things had been left there, with the Act safely repealed, all might have been well. But from 1768 onwards Parliament sought to establish its right to tax the colonists by imposing duties on goods brought into America. These Acts, the Townshend Acts, were also repealed in response to objections on both sides of the water, with the regrettable exception of the tax on tea. And when the East India Company in 1773 sought to land its Bohea tea in Boston, the inhabitants of that city reacted by tipping it into the harbour.

Throughout these troublesome years, from 1766 to 1774, Fothergill had steadfastly opposed the measures of the British government. He saw the vital importance of maintaining Britain and America united. In September 1768 we find him writing to a friend: "I speak of Great Britain and America, but write as an Englishman who knows no difference between their mutual interests. What one loses, both lose – and what they lose their enemies gain."

His attitude at the end of this period is best summarised in his own words, written in a letter to a friend in India in the autumn of 1774, six months before the war began:

I must in the first place inform my friend that I have been on the side of America from the time the Stamp Act was first proposed, and have therefore beheld with much anxiety the subsequent measures of administration which have brought us to the brink of a gulph, which without the most consummate prudence and the interposition of Providence, will swallow up the honour, wealth, power and consequence of the British Empire irrevocably...

I do not therefore hesitate to say that these measures have been uniformly oppressive – I do not think they have been so, as the Americans suppose, systematically, but merely from that kind of disposition which leads John Bull always to think of his own importance in the first place, and to hate most heartily any other person who dares think he may be mistaken; the right and wrong of the thing never makes part of his consideration when his supposed consequence is doubted...

And, he went on:

They begin to find the infant grows too much a man to be whipped like a schoolboy, and see with amazement, what they ought long since to have known, that between two and three million of people in a country abounding with all the necessaries of life, cannot easily be kept in subjection by 8 millions of people at a distance of more than 3000 miles...

And then, prophetically:

I should not doubt that a confederacy of the 13 colonies would bring into the field near 100000 men. What force have we to oppose to such an army of Englishmen, rendered desperate by the prospect of oppression?

During the winter of 1774–5 Fothergill took part in one last effort which might possibly have prevented the outbreak of hostilities. It is uncertain how these negotiations began, but they took place in the study of Fothergill's house in Harpur Street, Bloomsbury, just off Red Lion Square. Lord Hyde may have played a part, for he knew of Fothergill's friendship with Franklin. Whatever its origin, the meeting included Fothergill, Franklin as the representative of the American colonists, and another Quaker, David Barclay, representing the commercial interest. On 4 December 1774 Franklin produced 17 propositions which he called *Hints for Conversation*. At a later meeting, in January, the title of his paper was changed to *A Plan which 'tis believed would produce a permanent Union between Great Britain and her Colonies"*. This plan included Franklin's famous gesture, his offer to reimburse the East India Company for the tea out of his own private fortune. The *Hints*, and the later plan, were shown, presumably through Fothergill, to the British government, which found the terms totally unacceptable. As Fothergill put it, the difficulties arose from the American Acts – the Boston Port Bill, which had closed the port of Boston after the Boston Tea Party, and the Government of Massachusetts Act, which had suspended the government and legislation of that colony. A concession by the Americans to pay a tax was demanded by the British, and the Americans would accept nothing less than the repeal of the obnoxious Acts. It was a final impasse, which wrung from Fothergill in the spring of 1775 a last despairing cry. He is writing again to the Earl of Dartmouth:

I scarcely know how to attempt to write, nor yet am wholly at ease to be silent on the present interesting situation of this Kingdom... America is now grown too great to be humbled by this country without such an exertion of force as might, like what happens in the human frame, bring on such a haemoptysis as would end in a fatal consumption. We might harrass, vex, destroy a large country, retard their progress to greatness, but never never subject them to Great Britain... Do, my Noble, much esteemed Friend, forget the trifling quarrels fermented by mischievous people for the men of this great Empire, and give America *all* she asks. Was my life worth the pledging, I think I could do it safely, that she will amply repay the condescension.

This was written at the time Franklin finally left London, the negotiations a failure. News had just arrived that Franklin's wife had died in Philadelphia, and with a heavy heart, full of foreboding, but convinced of the rightness of America's cause, he left for home. He carried with him a letter from Fothergill to a Philadelphian friend, which contained the rebellious and cynical comment that, "whatever specious pretences are offered [by the British government] they are all hollow and that to get a larger field to batten a herd of worthless parasites is all that is regarded."

By the time Franklin reached America with Fothergill's letters in his pocket in May 1775, the first skirmishes of the War of Independence had been fought at Lexington and Concord, and the first major battle, at Bunker Hill, was only a few short weeks ahead. At this early stage of the war few Americans had made their mark. Geoge Washington was not well known; to many people, Hancock and Adams were not even names; the aging Franklin was undoubtedly the most talked of man of this period, but he was no romantic figure. Perhaps subconsciously, the Americans sought a hero in the classic mould; and they found him in the young Boston physician Joseph Warren. Young, gay, debonair, always immaculately dressed, he was a symbol of American liberty to the Bostonians during his short life, and he achieved immortality after he met his death at the Battle of Bunker Hill.

Joseph Warren's background was in many ways more conformist than John Fothergill's.[4] His father was a respected and highly esteemed farmer who married a doctor's daughter, and their son was born in the Boston suburb of Roxbury on 11 June 1741. Warren's father is remembered for having introduced into the Boston area an apple known as the "Warren Russett." They were apparently Congregationalist by religion. Joseph Warren therefore spent his early years in the pleasant surroundings of a New England farm, in confortable circumstances, and as a barefoot boy he delivered apples to the market in Boston. At the age of 14, in 1755, he went to Harvard College. Here he met, during the turbulent period of the Seven Years' War, others who later played their part in the War of Independence. John Hancock was a year ahead of him. In his own year were fellow revolutionaries such as John Adams and Josiah Quincey. But Warren at this time exhibited none of the rebelliousness of his later career. In 1761 he is even said to have won a prize for writing the best poem on the death of George II and the accession of George III.

After leaving Harvard, Warren took a post as a schoolmaster, but he only did this for about a year and in 1762 he became apprenticed to Dr Joseph Lloyd of Boston for his medical training. Unlike Fothergill he took no medical degree, but by 1764 – the year before the passage of the Stamp Act, and when he was only 23 – he had settled in the town of Boston as a practising doctor, and he soon had a flourishing practice. He became a freemason, and remained an active mason throughout his life. That same year he married Miss

Elizabeth Hooton, a merchant's daughter, who was described as "an accomplished young lady with a handsome fortune." And so he might have continued, a pillar of respectable colonial society, if it had not been for the passage of the Stamp Act in 1765. Warren was converted by this Act – and his conversion was maintained by what happened later – from a relatively contented and unthinking royalist to an enthusiastic republican who was prepared to give his life for his principles. Although most members of Warren's profession took no sides when the Stamp Act was passed, or even later, Warren at once began to take an intense interest in political affairs. In the evenings, after a long day with his patients, he sat down to read heavy volumes on constitutional law, trying to discover by what right the English Parliament could directly tax the American colonies. He understood at once the nature of the conflict. He was a loyalist still, but wrote to a friend, "I believe the people of this country may be esteemed as truly loyal in their principles as any in the universe; but the strange project of levying a Stamp Duty and of depriving the people of their privilege of trial by jury, has roused their jealousy and resentment." He went on, "You are sensible that the inhabitants of this country have ever been zealous of their civil and religious liberties," and pointed out, "in all new countries there is a more equal division of property amongst the people; in consequence of which their influence and authority must be nearly equal, and every man will think himself deeply interested in the support of public liberty. Freedom and equality is a state of nature..."

Warren first played an active part in events when he joined in the popular uprising of August 1765, with which the people of Boston demonstrated their opposition to the Stamp Act. During the next two years he became increasingly associated with the popular leaders whose ideas were often expressed at public meetings at Faneuil Hall. They were mostly young men: the two Adamses, Hancock, James Otis, Josiah Quincey, Paul Revere. And for the next 10 years, until his death in 1775, Warren was one of this group of young men whose ideals helped to create the first of our modern republics. His practice suffered as a result, a contemporary once referring to his pecuniary affairs being greatly deranged.

He continued throughout these years to work as a doctor during the day. In the evenings he wrote. In 1767 and 1768 he was correspondent for the *Boston Gazette*, the leading liberal newspaper in Boston in the prerevolutionary era. He was whole hearted in his enthusiasm for the American cause, and its outspoken supporter. "The mistress we court," he wrote in 1768, "is Liberty; and it is better to die than not to obtain her." Between 1767 and 1770 he was a member of the town committees and meetings which were set up to decide how to retaliate to the later Acts of the British Parliament, those which substituted external taxation for the internal duties originally proposed in the Stamp Act, imposing duties on a variety of goods imported into America, including that vital commodity, tea. And Warren was also on the committee which later refused to have tea landed in New England, even though the duties on all other goods had been rescinded.

The response of the British government to these activities of the Boston citizens was to quarter an army on their city. This did not intimidate the Americans, however, who insisted on their rights in law of not quartering the troops, thereby forcing the British authorities to build their own barracks. And the quartering of this army led directly to the affair of 5 March 1770, when a file of redcoats, infuriated one night by the taunts of an unarmed mob, opened fire, killing five Bostonians. Warren was a member of the provincial committee set up to inquire into this affray, and which ultimately engineered the withdrawal of the offending army. It is a measure of the esteem in which he was becoming held by his fellow citizens that two years later, when the Bostonians kept the anniversary of what had come to be known as the Boston Massacre, Warren was chosen as the orator. His ringing phrases are reminiscent of Burke: "This is undeniably true, that the greatest and most important Right of a British subject is, that he shall be governed by no laws but those to which either in person or by his representatives, he has given his consent. This is the grand basis of British freedom."

Between 1771 and 1773 political affairs were quiescent in

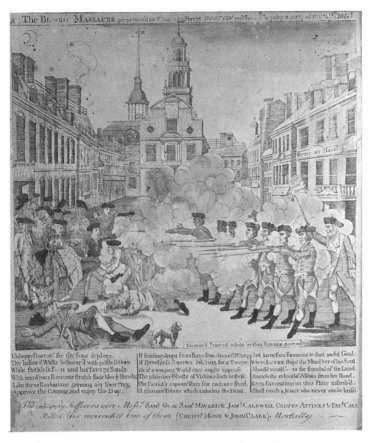

The Bloody Massacre perpetrated in King Street Boston on March 5 1770 by a party of the 29th Regt.

BUTCHER'S HALL

Unhappy Boston! see thy Sons deplore,
Thy hallow'd Walks besmear'd with guiltless Gore.
While faithless P——n and his savage Bands,
With murd'rous Rancour stretch their bloody Hands;
Like fierce Barbarians grinning o'er their Prey,
Approve the Carnage and enjoy the Day.

If scalding drops from Rage from Anguish Wrung
If speechless Sorrows lab'ring for a Tongue
Or if a weeping World can ought appease
The plaintive Ghosts of Victims such as these;
The Patriot's copious Tears for each are shed,
A glorious Tribute which embalms the Dead.

But know Fate summons to that awful Goal,
Where Justice strips the Murd'rer of his Soul:
Should venal C——ts the scandal of the Land,
Snatch the relentless Villain from her Hand.
Keen Execrations on this Plate inscrib'd,
Shall reach a Judge who never can be brib'd.

The unhappy Sufferers were Mess.rs SAM.l GRAY, SAM.l MAVERICK, JAM.s CALDWELL, CRISPUS ATTUCKS & PAT.k CARR
Killed. Six wounded two of them (CHRIST.r MONK & JOHN CLARK) Mortally

7   The Boston Massacre: contemporary print by Paul Revere
(Courtesy of The Bostonian Society/Old State House)

Boston. But in September 1773 news came that the Americans were again to be provoked.[5] The East India Company was to land its tea, duty prepaid in England, in Boston, despite the Boston committee's refusal to have anything to do with it. On 28 November the first ship laden with tea, the *Dartmouth*, arrived, and on 7 December two more came in to lie alongside the *Dartmouth*. The committee of action, Warren a leading member, placed a guard alongside the ships to prevent their being unloaded, and representation was made to the governor by Joseph Warren, John Hancock, and Samuel Adams, not to allow the landing of the tea. The owners were asked to send the tea back to England. This they refused to do, and in any case they had to get the permission of the governor to sail out of harbour with dutiable goods, the permission, of course, not being given. Furthermore, if dutiable goods were not landed within 20 days, they were liable to seizure and forcible landing. So that by the nineteenth day, 16 December 1773, a memorable day in American history, the town committee was faced with the threat that the customs officers with naval help would forcibly land the tea, which would have led to bloodshed with the Americans guarding the ships. In a last effort, the owner was sent back to the governor to see if he could send the ships out of port. The meeting finally convened to hear the reply at the Old South meeting house at 6 pm. Everyone in Boston was aware that something was in the air. The shops were closed. It was a wet winter's night but this did not quench the enthusiasm of the people who crowded out into the streets. The meeting house was dark and there was only a feeble light from the flickering candles as the Bostonians gathered. In later years people remembered the silence of that crowded meeting as Samuel Adams put the fateful question to the owner of the tea ship, "whether he would send his vessel back with the tea in her." He answered that "he could not possibly comply as he apprehended a compliance would prove his financial ruin." Adams then spoke the words that may have been a message to his waiting countrymen: "This meeting can do nothing more to save the country." As these words were spoken, a war whoop was heard in the gallery and at the entrance to the hall. Between 30 and 60 men dressed as Mohawk Indians gathered in the street, went to the wharf and tipped 342 chests of tea into the waters of the harbour. The identity of the Mohawks remains to this day one of history's best kept secrets. This escapade led directly to the British Parliament closing the port of Boston, suspending the Massachusetts provincial government, requesting payment for the tea by the citizens, and quartering an army on the town of Boston. As Dr Fothergill and Benjamin Franklin found, it was these acts which led to the final impasse.

Warren was still busy at his work as a physician when the army came, and he acted as medical adviser to many of the British officers, even attending the wife of the commanding officer, General Gage. On 5 March 1775, however, he was again chosen by the patriots to deliver the oration on the anniversary of the Boston Massacre, and here he spoke his mind. In the meeting house where he spoke, the first four rows were reserved for the officers of the British occupying force. It took courage to deliver what he had to say that night. He started with an inflammatory description of the affair. Then went on, "An independency of Great Britain is not our aim; no, our every wish is that Britain and the colonies may like the oak and the ivy grow and increase in strength together..." and he stressed the need for conciliation. These remarks, from one of America's most ardent revolutionaries, are so much in accord with the sentiments expressed at the same time by John Fothergill in London, that they fully justify the abortive meetings held in Fothergill's study during the previous three months.[6] But then, with a prophetic reference to the battles to come, Warren continued: "But if these pacific measures are ineffectual and it appears that the only way to safety is through fields of blood, I know you will not turn your face from our foes but will press forward until Tyranny is trodden underfoot, and you have placed your adored goddess Liberty...on the American Throne." It was during this purple passage that a British officer increased the tension in the hall by bringing out five bullets from his pocket and holding them out on his open palm. The tension subsided as Warren calmly dropped a lace handkerchief on the outstretched hand.

Things were now moving to a climax. Warren was on the committee of safety, which had the task of watching the movement of the British troops. On the evening of 18 April he was informed of a movement of British troops to capture American stores at Concord, 20 miles from Boston, and also possibly to capture Hancock and Adams, both living near there. Warren at once sent Paul Revere to warn the minutemen of the Massachusetts militia. And so it was that when the British troops reached Lexington Green at 4 30 the next morning, they found the provincial militia drilling. The Americans have always contended that the British fired first. Whoever it was, within minutes there were 10 Americans lying dead upon the green, the first heroes of the revolution. There was now a response of the militia throughout the whole area, and when the British troops reached Concord at 7 am they found the stores gone and large numbers of Americans waiting. There was a further skirmish. Things might have gone well for the British troops if they had returned to Boston at once. But they rested until noon, and by then the American militia was ready to line the whole 20 miles back to Boston. It was a running fight all the way and the weary, demoralised redcoats lost nearly 300 men.

Warren was informed of what was happening just as he was attending a woman in labour.[7] We do not know who she was, nor what became of the child destined to be born on the day of Lexington and Concord. Warren called a student to take care of his patient, mounted his horse and rode away. He was among the most active of the Americans that day. A shot took the pin out of the hair of his earlock. He was described as "perhaps the most active man in the field ... people were delighted with his cool, collected bravery." Four days later, on 23 April, he was elected president of the Massachusetts provincial congress, the illegal body set up by the province to look after its affairs. He did not go back to medicine in the few weeks of life that remained to him.

It is now time to examine the strategic position. At this stage the British troops, joined by those who had struggled back from Concord, were virtually besieged in Boston. They occupied the town – which was almost an island, joined to the mainland only by a narrow neck of land – and the American militia were encamped all around them on the mainland. To the north, Bunker Hill and Breed's Hill overlooked the town across a short stretch of the water of the Charles River, and to the south were Dorchester Heights. It was evident that anyone who could occupy either the Bunker Hill promontory or Dorchester Heights with cannon would make the British position untenable. During May, American hotheads such as Israel Putnam and Colonel Prescott were all for putting a force on Bunker Hill at once, since they argued that this would make the British fight. Others, supported by the provincial president, Dr Warren, favoured less radical measures. Matters came to a head in the middle of June when it was learned, through an agent, that the British troops were to march out to occupy Dorchester Heights, a move that would consolidate their position. The committee of safety, Warren in the chair, decided to act, and on 15 June 1775 resolved to take possession of Bunker Hill. The day before, the provincial congress had appointed Dr Warren the second major general in the Massachusetts army.

At 6 pm the American troops paraded on Cambridge Common, took off their hats in a moment of prayer and then marched out silently to fortify Bunker Hill; the next morning, 17 June, the British awoke to see the Americans entrenching on the top of Breed's Hill, just beside it.[8] General Gage knew at once that he had to act. It took some time to get the British attack ready. But by 2 30 pm 28 barges were landing nearly 2000 seasoned British redcoats on the beach before the American positions. By this time the Americans under Colonel Prescott had completed their redoubt on the top of Breed's Hill, but the men there were thirsty from lack of water and exhausted from a night's digging. To their right and front was the small town of Charlestown, where the flames started by the British in a wanton act of destruction were beginning to rise. To their left there was a breastwork, behind which the Americans waited. Beyond that there was a rail fence stretching down to the beach on the Mystic River, where a hastily erected stone wall protected the defenders. The Americans, watching from their improvised defences, saw the redcoats form up for the attack.

It was at this time that Israel Putnam, behind the breast-work, caught sight of the president of the provincial congress, Dr Joseph Warren. Warren was a striking figure, dressed in his finest clothes. He refused to go back to safety and refused also to take any command, his right as a senior officer. He just asked where he could be of most use and went at once to the redoubt on the top of Breed's Hill, where Prescott's men, tired and thirsty, demoralised by the non-arrival of their promised reinforcements, were at once inspired and encouraged by the presence of their most popular leader. From here Warren must have watched General William Howe's first attack along the beach, his attempt to turn the left flank of the American position. He must have heard the disciplined fire of Colonel Stark's New Hampshire militia, may have witnessed the agony of the British fusiliers as their ranks were mown down by the American volleys, so that the shattered survivors did not just retreat but ran all the way back to their boats. He must then have seen the two successive vain attacks by the lines of Howe's grenadiers against the main American position in the heat of that June afternoon, the British troops overloaded with their heavy packs, struggling through the long New England grass, laboriously climbing the fences that barred their way, finally meeting the murderous volleys of fire from the American positions, and wilting before them. He probably saw Howe, standing alone, his staff all dead around him, his white breeches red with blood – "A moment," as he said, "that I never felt before." So much, then, for General Wolfe's comment during the Seven Years' War that "The Americans are in general the dirtiest, the most contemptible, cowardly dogs you can conceive. There is no depending on 'em in action..." And so much for the Earl of Sandwich. "Suppose the colonies do abound in men," he had said in the House of Lords, "what does that signify? They are raw, undisciplined, cowardly men."

It was after those two fearful repulses by these steadfast cowards that Gage sent General Clinton over from Boston with reinforcements; and as the British again attacked, the watchers on the Boston rooftops heard the last American volley sputter away "like an old candle" as the ammunition ran out. The redcoats broke into the American positions with a great roar, and the rebels had no choice but retreat. It was some time during this last ghastly melee, among the confusion, smoke, and murderous physical conflict, that Warren met his destiny; mercifully shot through the head, he must have died instantaneously.

During the first days after the battle, the Americans had no information about the fate of Dr Warren. Then news came from the British, who had discovered his body on the battlefield and who were delighted to have killed so eminent a rebel. They showed him scant respect. Captain Laurie, in charge of a British burial party, found him and said later that he "stuffed the scoundrel with another rebel into one hole and there he and his seditious principles may remain." So, at the age of 34, died Dr Warren. It was this event, this battle, and, in particular, the burning of Charlestown that stimulated Franklin's famous letter to his erstwhile English friend Mr Strachan, Dr Johnson's publisher:

You are a member of Parliament, and one of that majority which has doomed my country to destruction. You have begun to burn our towns and murder our people. Look upon your hands! They are stained with the blood of your relations! You and I were long friends. You are now my enemy and I am
                    Yours,
                Benjamin Franklin.

To the Americans the death of Warren, their first popular hero, at Bunker Hill was an event of great importance, affecting the minds of many who had until then played little part in events. This is illustrated by the words of a young Philadelphian who in later life recorded how, when he told the famous Virginian Patrick Henry of Joseph Warren's death, Henry replied, "I rejoice to hear it. His death will do a great deal of good. We wanted some breaches to be made on our affections to awaken our patriotism still more, and prepare us for war."

The Philadelphian who recorded this conversation was Dr Benjamin Rush, a physician who is best known today as one of those courageous men who signed the Declaration of Independence.[9] He also achieved fame in another way – by befriending an English writer who had arrived in Philadelphia in 1774 and whose pamphlet *Common Sense* became the literary touchstone of the American revolution.

Benjamin Rush was born in Philadelphia in 1745, and so was an almost exact contemporary of Joseph Warren. He went to school in Philadelphia, and during the same period that Warren was learning his trade in Boston Rush was apprenticed to Dr John Redman for his early medical training. Unlike Warren, however, he did not at once settle to practise, but in 1766 travelled abroad to do a medical degree, and being a dissenter, like Fothergill, he went to Edinburgh. It is interesting that although he had witnessed the riotous reaction in Philadelphia to the Stamp Act the year before, he was not introduced to republican principles there, but in the ultra-conservative city of Edinburgh. He met, soon after he arrived in Scotland, a fellow medical student called Bostock, whose political ideals were coloured by the fact that an ancestor of his had served as a company commander in Cromwell's army. Rush also claimed a paternal ancestor who had served in the same army, so there was a bond between the two men and Bostock appears to have opened his heart to the young American medical student. It was a memorable occasion for Rush who recorded later:

Never before had I heard the authority of kings called in question. I had been taught to consider them as nearly as essential to our political order as the sun is to our solar system. For the first moment in my life I now exercised my reason on the subject of government. I renounced the prejudice of my education upon it; and from that time to the present all my reading, observations and reflexions have tended more and more to show the absurdity of hereditary power, and to prove that no form of government can be rational but that which is derived from the suffrages of the people who are the subject of it. This great and active truth became a ferment in my mind. I now suspected error in everything I had been taught...

The suddenness of Rush's conversion may have been exaggerated, for in 1768, after two years in Edinburgh, he travelled to London and there he lived with Benjamin Franklin, and breakfasted regularly with Dr John Fothergill. It would be surprising if during the discussion of the Townshend duties the ideas of these two arch rebels had not also influenced the young Rush. He tells in his auto-biographical writings how Fothergill, true to his Quaker principles, spoke with horror about war, and how his conversation always dwelt on philanthropic topics. "His manner of discussing them," he wrote, "was animated but methodical. With the strictest conformity to the phraseology and manners of the people called Quakers, he was a perfectly well-bred gentleman."

In 1769 Rush returned to Philadelphia. His friendship with Franklin was no doubt of value to him as a doctor seeking professional advancement, for Franklin had been one of the founders of the Pennsylvania Hospital. Fothergill's friendship had perhaps greater practical significance. When Rush left England he carried with him a testimonial from Fothergill, recommending him as suitable for the chair of chemistry in Philadelphia, which he duly obtained. No doubt in another age he would have settled down quietly to the usual battles of academic life. But during the next few years he was in the thick of some of the most important events of the eighteenth century. By 1773 he, like Warren, was an active revolutionary correspondent writing for the Philadelphia newspapers. In 1774 the first continental congress met in Philadelphia to discuss what measures were to be taken against the British. Rush made it his business to meet all those who attended: he spoke with the Massachusetts delegates, Hancock and Adams, as well as with the eminent delegation from Virginia. The following year, in May 1775, the second continental congress was assembled. Rush, 30 years old now, was again among the revolutionary leaders, and he attended a dinner given for General George Washington at a tavern on the banks of the Schuylkill River by the delegates and by the citizens of Philadelphia. They included Thomas Jefferson and Benjamin Franklin. The first toast after dinner was to the commander in chief of the American armies. Washington, Rush remembered later, stood up in some confusion to thank his hosts; and then, unexpectedly but with great solemnity, the whole company rose and drank the toast standing and in silence.

Rush was a spectator at these events. But during the winter of 1775–6 he was deeply concerned in the publication of Tom Paine's pamphlet, *Common Sense*, and in fact it was Rush who suggested the name for it. Tom Paine was an unusual and unruly fellow. Born at Thetford, Norfolk, in 1739, he was a little older than Rush. After working in his home country as an exciseman and staymaker, he went to Philadelphia in 1774 with a letter of introduction that he had somehow obtained from Franklin in London. He wrote for the newspapers between 1774 and 1776. Sometime in 1775 Rush met Paine at Mr Aitken's bookstore in Philadelphia, where he was at once impressed by Paine's attitude to American independence. Rush tells us that it was he who suggested that Paine should write a pamphlet on the subject. *Common Sense* was published in January 1776.

It was remarkable that Paine, within little more than a year of arriving in Philadelphia, could have written this pamphlet which captured the imagination of a continent. It started from the premise that all government is a necessary evil. Paine went on to attack George III, castigating him as the "Royal Brute of Great Britain", and the "greatest enemy that this continent hath or can have." He attacked the institution of monarchy: "Of more worth is one honest man to society than all the crowned ruffians who ever lived." He pointed out that all Britain's vaunted protection of America, her trading laws, were selfishly designed for her own benefit. America should not have to depend on a small island 3000 miles away. She should forget Britain "and claim brotherhood with every European Christian." He finally stressed the need for a new American government and called for a constitutional conference to discuss how this could be set up.

There were two points of the greatest political importance in *Common Sense*. The first was the plan for calling a constitutional conference, which played its part in stimulating the constitutional ideas that were discussed by the delegates to the vital third continental congress in Philadelphia in 1776. And the second was that it was the first publication, written in the popular style, to call for out and out independence. Both these attitudes led directly to the Declaration of Independence on 4 July 1776. The pamphlet was an immediate success. "It was read," wrote Rush, "by public men, repeated in clubs, spouted in schools, and, in one instance, delivered from the pulpit instead of a sermon by a clergyman in Connecticut." Its effect on the American forces who continued to surround Boston after the Battle of Bunker Hill was heartening to say the least. An officer observed "that a reinforcement of 5000 men could not have inspired the troops with equal confidence than this pamphlet did, in the justice of their cause, and the probability of their ultimate success..."

The other great episode in Rush's life was the signing of the Declaration of Independence, a matter of far greater importance to him. In May 1776 Rush had been elected a member of the delegation to the third continental congress by the Pennsylvanians, and in July he took his seat. It was to this crucial congress that Thomas Jefferson presented the declaration. "We hold these truths to be self evident," it ran, "that all men are created equal, that they are endowed by their creator with certain inalienable Rights, and among these are Life, Liberty and the pursuit of Happiness." It was the first time in human history that anyone had pointed out in a political statement that happiness is a purpose of life. It remains a revolutionary document. It stimulated the activities of the French revolutionaries nearly 20 years later and the principles inscribed in it have served as a justification for the rebellious behaviour of all colonial territories ever since. Rush signed this document along with 40 others on 2 August 1776. His signature, written in a clear, firm hand, is beside that of his London landlord, Benjamin Franklin. And that signature has secured him an honoured niche in the annals of American history.

These three men, Fothergill, Warren, and Rush, were all idealists; and their views on the subject of American independence form only part of the spectrum of motives, ranging from the meanest to the highest, that inspired the American patriots. Fothergill, it might be said, achieved very little. Yet he did what he could and the mutual regard built up between him and Franklin was something that probably encouraged that wily philosopher to trust similar minded Englishmen when in Paris in 1783, after Fothergill's death, the time came to make peace. Franklin held Fothergill in the highest regard. His glowing tribute to his old friend and physician after he died in 1780 is included in a letter to Fothergill's cousin, Dr Benjamin Waterhouse, who became the first professor of medicine at Harvard. "I think that a worthier man never lived," wrote Franklin; "for besides his constant readiness to serve his friends, he was always projecting something for the Good of his Country and of Mankind...and his incredible Industry and unwearied Activity enabled him to do much more than can now ever be known, his Modesty being equal to his other virtues."

Warren undoubtedly stands out not only as the most vivid personality of these three doctors; he was also one of the best loved of the American revolutionary leaders. He was attractive, honest, and sincere, sought no personal glory, and was able to give leadership and guidance to the men of Massachusetts at a crucial period of their history. His death was truly heroic.

Rush was the only one to live on into the nineteenth century. He died in 1813, having seen again, in the war of 1812, British troops burning and pillaging in his native land. Rush was an acid, rather vinegary character, with a great propensity for getting himself embroiled in controversy. But he had great courage, as is shown by his signature on the Declaration, and subsequently in the great yellow fever epidemic in Philadelphia in 1793, when he did not leave the city but worked day and night with his patients, to the detriment of his own health. Perhaps his best epitaph is his own. At his death he left among his papers a series of character sketches of the men who signed the Declaration of Independence. There he wrote on Jefferson, Franklin, and the rest. Of himself he merely wrote these words: "He aimed well." So did they all.

NOTES

1 Fox RH. *Dr John Fothergill and his friends*. London: Longmans, Green, 1919.
2 Corner BC, Booth CC. *Chain of friendship. Letters of Dr John Fothergill 1735–1780*. Cambridge, Massachusetts: Harvard University Press: 191. The letters of Dr Fothergill quoted in this chapter are from this source.
3 Corner BC. Dr Fothergill's friendship with Benjamin Franklin. *Proc Am Phil Soc* 1958; 102: 413–9.

4 Carey J. *Joseph Warren, physician, politician and patriot*. Urbana: University of Illinois, 1961.
5 Labaree BW. *The Boston tea party*. New York: Oxford University Press, 1964.
6 Corner BC, Singer DW. Dr John Fothergill, peacemaker. *Proc Am Phil Soc* 1954; **98**: 11–30.
7 Frothingham R. *The life and times of Joseph Warren*. Boston: Little, Brown, 1865.
8 Ketchum RM. *The battle for Bunker Hill*. London: Cresset Press, 1962.
9 Corner GW. *The autobiography of Benjamin Rush*. Princeton: Princeton University Press, 1948.

6 The mistress of Harpur Street

In the autumn of 1768 a young American physician arrived in London bearing letters of introduction from Philadelphia to Dr John Fothergill. The young man, as was customary, was invited to breakfast at the doctor's house in Harpur Street whenever it suited him. It was through this invitation that Benjamin Rush met Fothergill's lifelong companion, his sister Ann, a lady whose Quaker simplicity and integrity impressed all whom she encountered. Rush described her as a "woman of good sense and great worth who added to the pleasure and instruction of her brother's table."[1] Other contemporaries remembered Dr Fothergill's sister. Franklin, in letters to the doctor, sent his "best Respects to your good Sister" and Quakers on both sides of the Atlantic held her in esteem and affection.[2] On one young English Friend she made a lasting impression. "When I attended Gracechurch Meeting," wrote Sarah Shewell to Ann, "I sat a small distance from thee. Thy sollid countenance and aweful sitting much affected my mind."[3] To her family she appeared less formidable. Her brother Samuel, travelling in the American colonies in 1755, told her how much he rejoiced that he had so affectionate a sister.[4]

Like her doctor brother, Ann came from the small valley of Raydale in north Yorkshire. She was born at the family home in 1718 and it was here that she was brought up. It was a close knit Quaker community in that isolated area of the north of England. Ann's friends included the Robinsons who lived at

From the *Proceedings of the American Philosophical Society* 1978; **122**: 340–54.

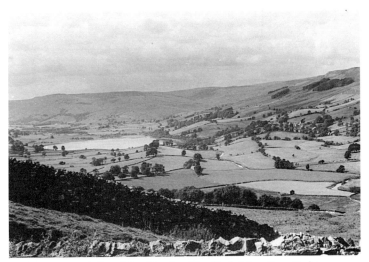

8   Semerwater in Raydale, Wensleydale, Yorkshire. Carr End is
beyond the trees to the right of the lake

nearby Countersett Hall and the Hillarys at Burtersett, home
of her great friend Rachel Hillary. These families met
regularly at the meeting house at Countersett, newly built in
1710. Ann hardly knew her mother, who died in childbirth
when she was a year old, and she was brought up first by a
family friend, Ruth Gorton, then by her stepmother whom
her father married in 1729 when Ann was 11. She was the
only girl in the family, her four surviving brothers being
Alexander, who farmed the family property at Carr End;
John, the doctor to whom she was to devote her life; Joseph,
in business in Warrington; and Samuel, one of the most
famous preachers of his age.

Dr Fothergill had settled in London as a physician in 1736
at the age of 24. By 1749, when he was 37, he had made, as
he put it to his brother Samuel, no progress towards matri-
mony but advancing years.[5] An oblique approach had been
made to an unknown lady, but her behaviour at a meeting
had determined his resolution "not to think about her any
more in that light." A lady denoted in his correspondence by
the letter "P" had come to nothing and some distant over-

tures to the family of a "JD" had not even received the courtesy of a reply. So although Dr Fothergill had not, as he put it to his friend Betty Bartlett, "willfully chosen to be called an old bachelor," that is how it had turned out. In later years he was to tell his patient, Fanny Burney, "My dear, never marry a physician. If he has but little to do, he is very unhappy. If much, it is a difficult life for his companion."

Meantime Ann, too, had remained single. She had looked after her father before his death in 1744 and had then cared for her stepmother until her death two years later, after which she joined her brother Joseph and his family in Warrington. There was apparently some divergence of opinion on her mother's side of the family over the disposal of her stepmother's effects. Ann, in the generous way that was to be one of her life's characteristics, told her brother Alexander at Carr End that she had written to her uncle's family, saying that "it wo'd be more satisfaction to me to return whatever it was than to detain anything t'was my mothers mind they should have." To Alexander she reported that she expected to have a reply "dipt in as much oyl as ink" in return.[6] There was very little for Ann from her father in his will, but her brother John in London now settled £100 on her since "dear father had not in his power to provide so well for her as I could wish." It was in no sense enough to keep her and so she settled into the Warrington household. There was a faint chance of a change in her circumstances in 1746, when she had an unidentified suitor. In 1748 she seems to have been in Leeds. Her brother Joseph wrote to Alexander at Carr End in January:

I am very desirous of getting over to see you butt cannot affix a time. I have some very large concerns on stand in the manufacturing of Hinges that of late has took much of my time having abt 140 Family to find work & wages for in that branch – I should be very glad thou could gett over to see us I hear thou has been at Leeds to see Sister who I hope is fixt there for the Present to her Satisfaction.[7]

By the end of the 1740s, however, she was still single. She had turned 30 and there was no prospect of marriage ahead. At the same time, her doctor brother urgently needed a housekeeper. He was established as a leading medical figure in the metropolis, his classic work on sore throat having been published the year before.[8] He had just taken over the house in Gracechurch Street where previously he had been a tenant. As he told his brother Samuel, however, he was "determined to know as little of housekeeping as possible." He had servants, was "lavish in coach," but he lamented that he had no mistress for the house, his faint hearted approaches having not surprisingly won him no fair lady.

What precipitated his invitation to Ann to come to Gracechurch Street is uncertain, but it may well have been an illness. A letter written by the doctor in November 1749 to his old friend, the botanist Peter Collinson, describes what was evidently a serious indisposition, although he reported that it became daily better "by dint of bleeding, blisters, and a long use of bolus draughts and other pharmaceutical artillery." Whatever it was, by 1750 Ann was established in the doctor's household where she was to stay for the rest of her life.

It was a dramatic change from the simplicity of life in the rural north of England. Ann looked upon herself at first as "wholly unequal to the situation in which I am placed." She wrote to Alexander in Wensleydale in early 1750, soon after her arrival, describing her apprehensions:

I have my health at present full as well before I came here; Being under the care of a kind affectionate Brother and Physician; who often orders some little thing or other to recruite my constitution; and endeavouers to inspire with Cheerfullness and ease as he apprehends, and not without grounds; my spirits has longe been borne downe by various causes to my he thinks great disadvantage; as it has made me quite Cowardly and fearfull; the latter I would not quite loose as fear is said to preserve us, and here as well as other places their is need of Care and Watchfullness; a new scene of life it is to me whear a multitude of ocorances atend to ingage divert or amuse... Singulear I am and so I hope to continue in my dress; the antice folly I observe does not excite me to imetate; Brother's extensive acquaintance and esteem exposes me at present to a pretty deal of company.

At the same time the world around her seemed threatening. The city was twice alarmed by an earthquake which "shouck the house and waked all of us with the trembling motion of our beds, 2 houses were thrown down and severall chimneys."

Some even left the city for fear of worse to come. But soon she was settling in, attending to her brother's comforts in the way she had learnt in Yorkshire, and using the age old culinary approach to the heart of man. She sent to brother Alexander for oatmeal and then borrowed a bakestone "scarce expecting to see such a thing in town." Then, in the manner that derives from the Norsemen who settled those northern dales, she made oatbread, still called haverbread, the Old Norse word.[9] "Several thought it," she wrote, "a choice regaile, and of which luckily the Doctr is very fond ...which often makes up the greatest part of our supper." Needing utensils of her own, she sent to Carr End for a small clay bakestone since "they make the sweetest Bread," and asked for a bag of oatmeal to be dispatched, preferably by sea as the carriage by land amounted to several times the value of the meal itself.

Ann was naturally uncertain of her position in her brother's home, and particularly of its permanence, during this early period of her life in London but within five years it is evident that she was fully established as the mistress of the household. She sought to render her brother any service she could "unless," she wrote, "a better helpmeet were provided and then in proportion as my brother's advantage were likely to be increased and established." But she added, one suspects with some relief, "at present no proper object (as he thinks) rises to his view." Her confidence grew as it became apparent that "no proper object" would ever materialise. The doctor's work made it difficult for him to consider marriage. He was regularly seeing patients from 9 in the morning until 9 at night, returning home every day exhausted from his labours. He became increasingly dependent on his sister who was continually thankful that "Brother considering his thin Habite Bears continual fatigue of Body, and anxcious care of mind for those under his care and atendance...in general enjoys a better state of health than could be expected." At the same time he for his part was very solicitous for his sister's welfare. He even suggested that she spend more money on her clothes, thinking her "peniuerious or supersticious or both" for wearing a dress "as plain as when in the country."

The growing relationship that developed between the doctor and his sister, and their closeness at this time with the family at Carr End, is illustrated by Ann's correspondence. It also provides evidence that she wrote as she spoke, with a north country accent. Papers she always spelt "pappers," and when questioning whether any of the doctor's old clothes would be useful for the children, Alexander was asked "to give me whint." The old clothes were sent in a trunk. "The Doctr," she wrote, "was so kind as to give me credit of it, but if I furnished it, thou knows by what benevolence." The trunk contained a book for each of the children and some old shirts "which the doctor bantered me a good deal about as not worth sending but I knew by experience would be acceptable." Then there was a yard of fine cloth, a gown of "best silk camblet" for Alexander's wife, several cannisters of tea and one pound of chocolate. The doctor said that she had "stript him to the skin" but it clearly gave him satisfaction to part with what his sister thought would be serviceable.

The close relationship with Alexander did not last through life, as later events will show, but both the doctor and his sister retained for their brother Samuel an affection and religious regard that endured until his death in 1772. Samuel had been an unusually errant member of the family as a young man. He had, he said, "drunk up iniquity as an ox drinketh up water." His father, a Quaker preacher who made three ministering visits to Friends in American colonies, told him on the eve of his departure for his last visit to America in 1736, "And now, son Samuel, farewell! – and unless it be as a changed man, I cannot say that I ever wish to see thee again." Samuel, however, underwent a deep religious awakening during his father's absence and in 1738 he married Susanna Croudson, a ministering Friend 15 years his senior. They lived in Warrington where he set up a shopkeeping business, and he soon became a preacher with an unusual gift for stirring the souls of his fellow men.

In the summer of 1754 Samuel felt moved to emulate his father and make a visit to the Quaker settlements in the American colonies. Alexander travelled to say goodbye to him at the general meeting at Marsdenheight "which," he wrote in his diary, "is this year held a week sooner than usual that Samll might attend before he go abroad."[10] Samuel left Warrington on 2 August, travelled as far as Leek in Staffordshire with his wife and other Friends, and was then greeted at St Albans by his sister Ann, who joined him for the last stage into London. At his brother's house he met John Churchman, an American Friend from East Nottingham in Pennsylvania who had been on a religious visit to England, Ireland, and Holland since 1750. Churchman was to be his companion across the sea. Four days later Ann accompanied the two Friends to Gravesend where they went on board the *Caroline*, Stephen Mesnard commanding, and on 10 August, Ann wrote, "the wind being pretty fair," she saw them on board for the last time "and in the space of an hour they were wafted out of our sight." The pilot left them the following day, bearing a letter from Samuel for the London household to tell them that all was well. But it was a particularly trying time for Samuel's companion, John Churchman, who wrote to Ann that "we lay in the Downs until 3rd day ye 13th of ye 8th mo the wind being contrary and therefore did not go thro' ye Chanel until ye 18th, during which time," he told Ann after he reached his home in Pennsylvania, "that grievous lax continued on me, which was very wearing and before ye Disorder left me I had a sore fit of ye piles which continued near 2 weeks."[11]

During the next two years the doctor and his sister were kept constantly in touch with Samuel Fothergill's arduous journey through the colonies. October 1754 found him in Philadelphia complaining that "the greatest inconvenience I find is the number of mosquitos, a little venomous fly, that have within these few nights severely handled me, and so swelled my hands as to render it not easy to write." Another letter followed in November describing his plans to visit Virginia, and then in December he wrote from Curles-upon-James' River to reassure them that "my health is preserved to my admiration." He wrote too that 16 English bodies had been found murdered by Indians in the back parts of South Carolina, a foretaste of horrors to come. By April 1755 he was back in Philadelphia having paid a general visit to Friends in Maryland, Virginia, North and South Carolina, and some of the remoter parts of Pennsylvania. He had already covered a total distance of 4000 miles. In June he was in Newport, Rhode Island, and from Nantucket on 28 June he wrote to Ann that he was awaiting a boat to take him to Martha's Vineyard. Alas his loyal horse was dead. "He travelled 150 miles with me without having so much as a quartern of English oats; I was obliged to beg a little Indian bread for my own support, for none I could buy, and I divided it honestly between him and myself."

Two months later he wrote from Boston to describe his meeting in Faneuil Hall where 2000 people heard him preach, and where, he told his brother and sister, "Truth was as a canopy over the meeting." In the same letter he reported the ignominious news of General Braddock's total defeat "with the loss of about 700 men killed, himself and sixty officers amongst them." From East Nottingham, home of John Churchman, he told Ann in October that he had now travelled 6200 miles. It was hard work. He had returned from a yearly meeting in Maryland with John Churchman. They had found the work laborious and some of the older people were "not only dry, but very dry." In November he was in Philadelphia again, alarmed by an earthquake and disturbed by the distracted state of the province whose outer settlements were in a state of turmoil after the defeat of Braddock at Fort Duquesne. By the spring of 1756 he had "the first perception of approaching liberty to revisit his native land," and Ann was able to look forward to seeing him again. John Churchman wrote to her, telling her of the value of her brother's visit and how "if he has not much increased in words and fine eloquence, I am sensible he has improved in the rest of his ministry...Dear Nancy," he went on, "thy countenance is as familiar to me this hour as it was when I enjoyed that quiet rest at your house...there are few Friends in England that I more remember than you."[12]

Samuel had a last meeting in Philadelphia where his warnings of trials and tribulations to come, delivered to a large audience two years before "when not so much as a handsbreadth of cloud appeared over our land," were seen to have been prophetic. Friends' minds "were seized with awful dread," wondering whether this last warning was like that of Jeremiah before the destruction of Jerusalem. It was a period of agonising choice for Friends in Philadelphia, particularly those who sat in the provincial assembly, whether to accept the implications of war or to hold to their pacifist principles. The Fothergills were influential in shaping opinion. Dr Fothergill, correspondent of the London yearly meeting with the Pennsylvania Quakers, wrote from London urging and encouraging their pacificism, and in Philadelphia Samuel told them, "If the potsherds of the earth clash together, let them clash."

The preacher was now tired. He had travelled, according to his journal, 8765 miles, and on 5 June 1756 he embarked on the *Charming Polly*, reaching Dublin just over a month later. There he was held up by contrary winds for two weeks, but he arrived home by the end of July, accompanied by Catherine Payton, long to be his associate in his ministry and a close friend of the doctor and his sister. They were able to write from London on 2 August to Israel Pemberton in Philadelphia with the news of Samuel's return.

During his absence, life for the London household had become increasingly hectic. The doctor was now one of London's most successful physicians and so busy that he increasingly left his correspondence with his brother to Ann. He wrote briefly to Samuel, in March 1757, of "having mounted not less than fifty single pairs of stairs today." There were visits from the family and from many others. His sister was now his trusted confidante, his friend and supporter in all that he did; they understood each other and their lives had grown together. "We are in a sort of publick station," he wrote, "the objects of numerous applications of very different natures." One such application, in July 1757, was Franklin's first visit to the Fothergill household when he arrived in London to represent the affairs of the Pennsylvania assembly.[13] It was a meeting of friends since the doctor and Franklin already knew each other by correspondence; their friendship, which grew warmer through the years, was to continue until the doctor's death in 1780.

The Fothergills were also increasingly prosperous. The doctor's practice had grown, and in a letter to Alexander he was able to report that he was helping Ann by investing £200 for her with an India captain, the interest being 24% over 20 months. But their numerous activities meant a great deal of work for Ann. She wrote despairingly of the excessive demands made upon her, "By one means or another it becomes more and more difficult and allmost impossible to find one uninterupted qurter of an hour." In August 1757 the doctor decided to take a brief respite in Scarborough, leaving Ann in London. It was an experimental holiday. Ann reported that he had been little wanted in his absence and he, exhausted by his labours, felt he had done himself some justice.

There were, however, those who thought that the doctor's motives were less than altruistic. James Jenkins remembered Dr Fothergill at one time as "an obsequious guinea-collecting doctor," although it was not an opinion in which he persisted.[14] Some of his friends, however, were concerned at his prosperity and Samuel wrote to Ann:

Do my dear Sister endeavour to persuade him he cannot be justified in destroying himself however laudable the motive. He and thyself have often told me so and I firmly believe it – & I hope to practice agreeable to that belief – I believe his motives are good, but some envious tongues are ready to say the desire of accumulating abundance is the cause of subjecting himself to so much fatigue. But this from those who don't know him.[15]

Perhaps it was the increasingly frenetic activity of the Gracechurch Street household that led the doctor and his sister to look for a more peaceful environment outside London. In 1762 Ann had been with her brother for nearly 13 years and her domestic responsibilities were now about to increase. The doctor, keen to develop his botanical interests, had apparently kept a garden and house at Lambeth but he now bought from Admiral Elliot a property at Upton in Essex where he was to create a botanical garden unrivalled in Europe for its collections of American plants. So March 1763 found Ann busy packing up at Lambeth and irritated at not being able to move into the new country house. "The person my brother brought Upton of," she wrote, "and paid him above 6 months ago & since which time he has no right to be there but of suffrance, is so ungenerious not to say very unjust as to keep possession yet, his family in the House, his Cattle in the fields picking up every blade of grass as it rises and we obliged to accomodate our servants and our goods as we can."

Ann was constantly jealous of her brother's welfare. In the same letter, written to Samuel, she describes how the doctor is in bed with a fever. Ann is distressed that he will insist on getting up to have his bed made, a liberty, she wrote, that he would never have allowed a patient. Furthermore, she was concerned that he would admit many of his patients' apothecaries to his room "to consult with him and charge his mind with care and solicitude for many others when he needs to be exempted from all but his own." But he recovered and soon Ann could write to their brother Samuel that "the smelts they came very fresh and regaled several besides ourselves."

The house that Ann was to create at Upton was described by an American who made a visit there the year after the doctor bought it. "The house is old," she wrote, "the rooms very large and most genteely furnished...very pretty tapestry and the utmost neatness and order...and attention in the servants beyond what I almost ever met with." The doctor and his sister, the writer went on, do not admit "of that mechanical politeness that shews itself in external forms, yet they excel in the kind attention they give to the wants of others. The garden, full of flowering shrubs and a variety of hedges, was a most pleasing spot."[16]

The property at Upton, although excellent for his horticultural activities, was too near London to allow the peace and relaxation that the doctor needed. Within two years he was looking for another country retreat, farther from the demands of his patients in the metropolis and near to his brother Samuel and his other relations at Warrington in Lancashire. Ann wrote to Alexander about the plan, in which they had enlisted Samuel's help, "It was Bro: Drs desire and request that it might be kept as private as possible, that a large circle might not be apprized of it and accordingly prepared to frequent the place allso."

Brother Samuel had unfortunately mentioned the plan very freely and others had proposed visits to the new retreat, "which is not the thing he need leave home in pursuit of," wrote Ann.[17] They finally took a lease on Lea Hall, a small country house near Middlewich in Cheshire, 150 miles from London, and within easy reach of Warrington. It was a square built house, of the Queen Anne period, standing on its own in a small walled garden, about two miles outside the town. It was possible to walk out on the roof and view the surrounding landscape, which was flat and quite unlike the hills and valleys of Wensleydale. The rooms were beautifully panelled and there was a fine staircase. A later owner commented on the excellence of the cellars which had three large pillars in the centre. For the remaining years of their life together the doctor and his sister Ann spent two months every summer in this comfortable rural retreat, assured for a little while of relief from the fatigue of life in London and able "to recover the power of recollection" as the doctor put it.

Despite the appearance of severity that the Fothergill household gave to the outside world, it is interesting that the doctor and his sister were not teetotallers. For their first visit to Lea Hall in the summer of 1765 Samuel was asked to procure for them brandy, a fine mountain white wine, and six gallons of red port, with which to stock their cellars. "A rough good-bodied wine I like best," the doctor wrote. Furniture and other possessions were dispatched from London to Liverpool by sea and some of the servants were sent on ahead. Then, in that summer of the Stamp Act crisis, the doctor and his sister set off in their coach on the journey to Lea Hall, taking with them, as they so often did, an American visitor. This year it was Elizabeth Graeme of Philadelphia, who was to meet at Lea Hall her fellow American the Reverend Richard Peters and go on with him to Scotland. It may well have been these American visitors who gave the doctor the sort of detailed knowledge of American affairs that he needed for the pro-

American pamphlet that he was preparing, *Considerations relative to the North American Colonies*.[18] A preliminary draft was soon sent to his friend the Earl of Dartmouth, Secretary of State for the American Colonies, and the pamphlet was published anonymously later in the year.

Two years later the doctor and his sister decided to move from the house in Gracechurch Street where they had lived together for nearly 20 years. They chose a house in Harpur Street, Bloomsbury, just to the north of Red Lion Square, at that time a newly developing area of the city. The front door led into a hall with a window on the left and there was a fine curved staircase leading to the first floor where there were two good drawing rooms. At the back, a large dining room occupied the entire rear ground floor, with an alcove between Ionic pillars and a high, exquisitely carved chimney piece.[19] It was to this house and its domestic problems that Ann came in 1767. Silver was bought and no doubt many other things besides.[20] Everything was at first new and strange, she wrote in October soon after her return from their summer recess at Lea Hall. "All busy," she told brother Samuel, "nothing finished...we share our house and is long like to do so with different classes of workmen, joiners, carpenters, painters, plumbers, smiths &c &c, which makes a busy dissipating scene." She wisely decided to defer "pappering" until the summer. There was a major advantage in the move. Her brother was to "reserve the afternoons more to himself to be at liberty to attend the meetings for business which he has done more since we came here than he was allowed to do for years befor." The doctor was now 55 years old. He hoped gradually to lessen both his business and his other encumbrances. It seems to have been a vain hope. Ann wrote that her brother was "as busy as usual – much abroad and Ingaged when at home." She herself was content with the move. She found that she could walk from the new house to attend Gracechurch Street meeting "with allacrity." At the same time she revealed to her brother Samuel something of her inward calmness of spirit when she told him that she even found it possible "to be in solitude in the streets of London."

An intimate account of the family at Harpur Street at this

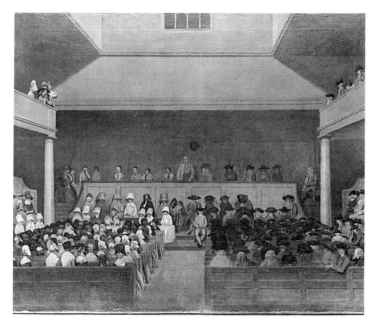

9 Friends' meeting, Gracechurch Street, about 1770. The figure in the
light suit to the right by the pillar is said to be Dr John Fothergill
(Library Committee of the Religious Society of Friends, London)

time is given by the London diary of Betty Fothergill, who
came along with her two sisters Ann and Molly to stay for the
winter of 1769–70.[21] Their father Joseph, the doctor's
brother, had died in 1761 and they were escorted from
Warrington by their Uncle Samuel and his companion,
Catherine Payton. Betty was an attractive young woman of
17, just engaged to Alexander Chorley who patiently waited
for her in Lancashire. They left Warrington on 19 October
1769 and travelled in a postchaise. On 21 October Betty
reported that "London from an eminence nr. Highgate presented itself to our view covered with a thick pall of smoke."
They soon arrived in Harpur Street "which we found
perfectly still and very unlike the idea I had formed of the
hurry and bustle of London." They were greeted by their

aunt but it was evening before she saw her uncle doctor "who received me with that cheerful benignity which is his peculiar characteristic." His niece always found him agreeable, perhaps because, as Ann put it, "My brother loves to Gratifye rather than restrict young persons of our sex in what seems not quite improper."

It was the only time in their lives that the doctor and his sister were able to play the part of parents to their nieces, and this period was acutely observed by the young Betty. There were many domestic chores to be carried out in the household over which Ann Fothergill so capably presided. Sometimes they stayed quietly at home, as on the day when the formidable Catherine Payton was "too much indisposed with the toothache to venture out." The old aunt ensured that her nieces saw as much of London as any visitor would today. They witnessed the revels to celebrate John Wilkes's release from the King's Bench Prison, saw "that pompous trifle the Lord Mayor's show," watched the King and Queen on their way to the House of Lords, and were taken for walks not only in the genteel streets near their home where the Duke of Bedford and the Spanish ambassador lived, but also "thro' the filthy walks of Fleet market & some other places I had not been in before."

At the beginning of November they went down with their aunt to Upton. Betty on this first visit waxed rhapsodic:

When we arrived at the little door that leads into the garden a different scene opened upon our view – the winter was not the time for viewing it to advantage yet it appeared delightful from the agreeable and judicious manner its walks and shrubbery were laid out. Everything around displays the good taste of the owner, who excels not more in this art as in almost every other – At the end of a broad gravel walk, which goes up from the Door stands the house which tho it is not Elegant is perfectly near and genteel. Adjoining to one end is the large greenhouse – separated from one of the front Parlors by a wall in which there is a glass door. So in this room you may sit and bid the Storms of winter defiance, whilst the three senses of feeling seeing and smelling are gratifyd to the Utmost, the first by the warmth communicated from a good fire, the second by a view of oranges myrtles and every other curious delightful shrub that feast the eye with the blossoming appearance of a perpetual spring – and the third with the fragrandt odours arising from this Eden. Here are also several hot houses full of the most scarce and curious plants... If any person who may happen to read this has any inclination to become a Poet, I would advise them to repair to Upton as soon as the pleasant Month of May comes and there seat themselves under the extensive branches of an old oak tree that grows on the bank of a Canal.

But it was not always so idyllic. She went again just after Christmas and this changeable young woman recorded that her spirits were "allways uncommon low after visiting Upton."

At home the girls helped to entertain the stream of visitors who came to the doctor's house. Many were members of the prosperous Quaker families who lived in the neighbourhood. Others included young physicians enjoying her uncle's patronage. John Coakley Lettsom, Dr Fothergill's biographer and his successor in practice, was a constant visitor, taking the girls on visits to the British Museum or simply staying for tea. Born in the West Indies, he had come to England when he was 6 years old and Samuel Fothergill had become his guardian. It was Samuel who had recommended him to his doctor brother; he was therefore almost one of the family. For a little while he and Betty became a little too close and Ann Fothergill seems to have reminded her niece of her obligations to her fiancé in the north. After a visit with her aunt, Uncle Samuel, and sister Molly to the Museum in late November, Betty recorded that:

I had a good deal of conversation with my Aunt upon various subjects but particularly upon one... which I was surprised to see her so well acquainted with. It convinced me of her penetration and that her eye pierces deeper than many people imagine... for the sake of the person concerned I could wish it not to have seen quite so far.

Two days later Ann accompanied Samuel as far as Barnet on his way back to Warrington where no doubt he reported on the state of affairs at Harpur Street to Alexander Chorley, who wisely made an early visit to London to make sure of his future wife.

When Ann returned from Barnet the following day, she found John Ellis at breakfast, a visitor whom Betty found "a very humorous comical old gentleman." Perhaps he had come to study the corals and shells in the doctor's cabinets, for several of the corals in the Hunterian collections in Glasgow belonged to Fothergill and were used and illustrated by Ellis in his *Natural History of Many Curious and Uncommon Zoophytes*.[22] On 10 January 1770 Betty spent a quiet day at home. Her aunt, who was sitting beside her, was writing to brother Samuel now at home in Warrington. Ann's letter was a gossipy account of the affairs of the family. Molly had been "much indisposed for about 2 weeks" and was causing her aunt some concern. Nanny seemed well and Betty, wrote Ann, "we think looks full as well as when she came & seems easy and satisfied with her present situation," but she added cautiously, "for the time being." Her doctor brother, however, she lamented, "sustaines a situation much like the continued hurry of a whirlwind."

One day Dr Lettsom brought his friend Dr Bostock from Liverpool to breakfast, a young man whose intelligence made an impression on Betty. He was to be one of the first physicians at the Liverpool Infirmary. It was this same Bostock, an advocate of republican principles, who had first convinced Benjamin Rush when they were students together in Edinburgh, of the absurdity of kings and of hereditary power. Betty recorded on 10 March 1770: "He appears to be a very sensible agreeable little man, and if nature has not been very liberal with regard to the height of his person, she has perhaps made amends by the extent of his mind."

Other distinguished visitors included the famous surgeon from St Bartholomew's Hospital, Percival Pott, and on 18 May a more celebrated visitor called. Betty, who was "obliged to attend to the vulgar task of getting up Linnen," was greatly distressed at being unable to meet him. The visitor was Benjamin Franklin, and so, for the sake of some ironing, we are denied an account of the famous philosopher from the pen of this lively young woman.

Franklin was a not infrequent visitor at the Harpur Street house. No doubt he was offered the rough good bodied port that the doctor liked best. What went with it can only be a matter of surmise, but a tantalising glimpse of what it might have been is given by a small handwritten book dating from 1727 which is preserved by a Fothergill descendant now living in New Jersey.[23] The book, most of which is in Ann Fothergill's characteristic handwriting, is her recipe book. The earliest recipe, on how "To Pott Beef," although started in her own writing, is continued in the hand of her brother Alexander, and so may date as far back as her life at Carr End. Then there is a recipe from a friend in Manchester on how to make an almond pudding – dated 1749, just before her arrival in London. Others were clearly from contemporary recipe books. "To stew Carp," for example, is taken from F Chambertin, 1752, and must have been copied in her early years in the metropolis. Her "Whipt Sillybable" would do for anyone today:

Take a pint of Thick Creame two spoonfulls of white wine the Juse of a Lemmon and the Rinde grated as much sugar as will make it sweet put altogether into a bason & whiske it all one way till its very thick then fill your glasses.

There were also instructions of how to stew pigeons or to "Boyl elles," to "Dress Scotch Scollops" or to "Make new ale drink old." There were blackberry, elderberry, or raisin wines and there was an excellent recipe for Mead. "Biskits" were made as follows:

Take 8 Eggs beat them with half ye white put in one pound of sugar and a pound of flour mix ym well then have the papers Buttered lett ym be double. Straw them with fine sugar and some Carraways then on long Sticks & put them in the Oven again to drye.

The last recipe in the book is dated 1773 and is for a mundane universal sauce. From the evidence of this book, however, it is clear that the Fothergills entertained their guests well; one is tempted to surmise that some of these recipes were fed to Benjamin Franklin.

For Dr Fothergill, closely concerned in the affairs of the American colonies, the years leading up to the revolution of 1776 were full of concern and foreboding. Indirect evidence suggests that Ann shared the doctor's fears as well as his pro-American opinions. But domestic chores and family problems demanded her constant attention. From 1770 onwards her beloved brother Samuel was constantly ailing. After his return from London at the beginning of the year, he was unwell for six weeks. In February 1771 it was Ann's turn to be unwell, with an attack of rheumatism "accute in my left side." Nevertheless, she was able to make some purchases in town for her uncle and for Betty, now married to Alexander Chorley. She described her shopping expedition:

I have procured and it is sent away today near as I can China to thy order. S Tittley's[24] is the same of what thou saw on the Table tho' of 40 setts in 8 or 9 months only 3 or 4 now remains so much have they been approved at the price which is (£)3:3:0 – perhaps Betty Chorley will not quite approve of hers. If not I shall be glad to take them for our owne use if she will give them Houseroom till we come to Lea Hall. She will think the Coffee cups rather too small. So did I but in this Article there is no Choice, tis the only dozen of nankeen Coffee Cups I ever saw to be sold apart, for 6 in a compleat sett is the common allowance, none to spare. The price of this Dozen is (£)1:1:0 – 6 of the same Sort was sold in another shop for (£)0:18:0. I could have no other choice of either Slop Bason or Sugar dish Nankeen but this – nor them without the addition of the plates all which cost (£)1:11:0. I had the choice of 2 potts: the form of the other pleased me Better, it would not poure well. I will answer for this in that respect: or take any or all again if she dont like them the price of 6s – a Box (£)0:1:6 – the whole charge for which I have the Bill is £5:2:6.

Molly was now about to be married to Robert Watson of Waterford in Ireland and Ann wrote to explain that her doctor brother was prepared to send £100 for the couple "which they might put to what use they please," but he balked at meeting her removal expenses to her new home. By July Ann was writing of Samuel's "painful Indisposition," which persisted into November. And the doctor also was unwell. He had been, wrote Ann, "poorly and drooping" ever since their return from their summer retreat at Lea Hall, and now he was "as thin and languid as I ever saw him go about." It was scarcely surprising. The doctor was engaged at this time in an unfortunate dispute with a Dr Leeds who had been awarded damages against him by a majority of a group of five Quaker arbitrators who judged that he had unjustly criticised Leeds. The affair had occupied Dr Fothergill's attention throughout his summer holiday at Lea Hall and during the long winter. It was not until May 1772 that Lord Chief Justice Mansfield at the Court of King's Bench set the award aside as "partial and therefore corrupt and unjust."[19] With Samuel slowly deteriorating in Warrington and all the worry and concern created by the Leeds affair, it was a sad winter for Ann. In early 1772 she made a brief visit to her dying brother and in March she wrote to him with the chilling news that the doctor "thought an advancing dropsey inevitable and that thy constitution is so impaired as not to admitt the usual remedys...and with great concern both then and repeatedly since has expressed himself with anxiety and without hope." Samuel, undismayed, replied to Ann, "I continue too bulky, tho' something diminished, yesterday morning my belly ached violently, a sensation I endeavoured to allay by scratching, & by some means tap'd myself of a full half-pint of water. Which I hope was of use, & is proof the water is not died in my Bowells."[25]

On 27 May, just over two weeks before his death, she wrote again to tell him that "I have often remembered thee on my pillow. In such a Dispossion as that I could offer myself in thy stead if provedance would accept so mean an offering." Samuel died, greatly mourned, on 15 June 1772.

There were further family problems to come. During the 1760s there had been some hints of a cooling of the relationship that had existed between the Harpur Street household and Alexander Fothergill at Carr End. The doctor and his sister had made a visit there on their way home in 1763 from a holiday in Scarborough, in the days before they had taken on Lea Hall. But Ann had written to Alexander in 1765 that "I think we ought not to become nearly indifferent to each other unless some just occasion is given." During the Leeds affair, however, Alexander, with the legal training that he put to good use in his native valley, had proved particularly valuable to Dr Fothergill. The doctor, writing from Lea Hall in the summer of 1771, had asked him to go to Edinburgh to obtain affidavits essential to his cause. Fothergill's London lawyer, Charlton Palmer, wrote to say that "the notes on this case seem to have been drawn by an able lawyer, and if they are your Brother's I should not have been afraid of trusting him with the Edinboro' business without any other agent whatsoever."

But Alexander was becoming increasingly involved in debt. In 1762 he had mortgaged part of the family property to Thomas Simpson of Richmond, Yorkshire, for £400. Then in 1773 he had obtained £600 from a Richard Seymour of Aldburgh, near Richmond, on the remainder of the property. The Carr End farm was therefore mortgaged to the hilt. At the same time Alexander's behaviour was increasingly criticised by his fellow Quakers in Wensleydale. Complaints had been made at the preparative meeting for Wensleydale in 1771.[26] On 4 September three Friends were asked by the meeting to speak to Alexander Fothergill, James Wetherall, and John Thwait "requesting better conduct for the future by living a more selfe denying life." A month later it was recorded that, although James Wetherall and John Thwait had undertaken "that they will behave more orderly for the future," Alexander had still not been spoken to. Three months after this, Alexander was in London but his brother and sister were seeing little of him, at least on his own. Ann wrote to Samuel:

Brother Alexander is yet in Town. He and our relations in Gr – ch street are pretty well, we see him sometimes to Breakfast, when we are liable to have promiscuse company, or 1st day evenings when his familys are with him, that we have not had an opportunity of privat conversation on his owne affairs. We have Invited him to Lodge a few nights with us But he declines it aledging that his Children are then most at Liberty from Busines for a little Conversation, &c he seems not in haste to return Home. He says nothing when he intends it. I believe he is In qrters agreeable to him at J Freemans and amuses himself by attending the parliament House to hear their debaits, But I dont hear he has any Business.[27]

By 1774 Alexander could avoid his accusers no longer. For 20 years he had had the unenviable task of acting as surveyor for the turnpike road that climbed over the hill from Wensleydale, across Cam and down to Ingleton and Lancaster, one of the loneliest and most desolate roads in England, and he was now charged by the turnpike trustees with misappropriation of funds. At the same time, as he recorded in his diary for 26

February, two Friends approached him after a meeting and accused him of "disorderly conduct, principally as to women...with having two bastard children at Richmond & others elsewhere, and some other general charges of that sort." Alexander protested his innocence, admitting only that he might have been "imprudent in being at times occasionally in company with persons not well accounted of." The news obviously reached London for on 29 September he recorded that "Dear Brother Doctr Fothergill having desired me to meet him at Knaresbro' tomorrow afternoon I set out this evening to Middleham to Shorten next day's work." The erring Alexander's diary for the next two days records the affecting family reunion:

30th Sepr – I went by Rippon. Thence to Scotton, where I went to see Friends Burying Ground belonging Knairsbro: Meeting where my Worthy Father's Body was interred the year 1744. Thence to Knairsbro' where I met with Dr. Brother & Sister alighted a little before I got there. We spent the evening together in which both Brother and Sister manifested the highest & strongest Brotherly Concern affection and regard to and for me, in persuading advising & intreating for my good and true interest and this in the most tender and affectionate manner, Not opbraidingly, and went then to sleep – A little whereof fell to my share: as I wanted much to drink in and receive their advice, and that I may retain it and profitt by it.
First Octobr. I was up Early. Brother & Sister came down at 8. We breakfasted together & spent some time in conversation, then they got a Chaise and came with me to Scotton. I conducted them to the Burying Ground, and as near as I could remember to Dear Father's Grave where we stood in silent contemplation about 15 minutes...Bro and Sister tenderly repeated their former advice which was strengthened by our present Situation, and here we took an affectionate leave of each other. They returned to their coach to set out for London, and I came homewards. But so buryd in thought that I miss the way and I believe I made 10 into 15 or 16 miles to Rippon and got but to Middleham being a Rainy Dark evening.[28]

Alexander subsequently confessed to the preparative meeting of Wensleydale and the monthly meeting of Richmond that "There came up Briars and Thorns and the spirit of the World prevailed in too many instances (tho' not so many as were unjustly charged) a disorderly and very blameable conduct gave my friends just cause to testify against me as was done."[29] The sympathetic encouragement that the doctor and his sister gave to their brother illustrates the spirit of forgiveness with which these quiet Quakers approached the frailty of their fellows. It was not always so. Ann's views of sexual nonconformity were naturally conservative. In February 1771 she had told Samuel of the death of John Williams (John Hill's son in law), leaving "a sorrowfull young widow and childe." Next year, however, she had written sadly:

I am just returned from Bush Hill where I have been this afternoon to pay a visit of condolence to that worthy pair John Hill and his wife who are in great distress for a Beloved Daughters Samefull misconduct unsuspected by them or I believe any of her friends; the widow Williams whose Husband thou visited near his end about 15 months ago, and for whom she seemed unfegnidly to greve much is about 5 months gone with Childe By her Shopman and they were privetly married 3 weeks a goe.

The doctor and his sister returned from Lea Hall in 1774 to a winter of toil for Dr Fothergill. He had important literary commitments and was carrying out clinical studies for the medical society which he had founded. His efforts during that winter as a peacemaker between Franklin and the British government have already been described. By the following summer he was exhausted. On 20 July 1775 rumours of a bloody battle near Boston were circulating in London, confirmed by General Gage's own account of the Battle of Bunker Hill which was published on 25 July.[30] The doctor and his sister went to Lea Hall almost with a sense of relief and Ann could write to her niece that "my brother is better than might be expected after 10 months unremitting and most ardious Labour that he himself acknowledges he ever passed through." For Ann the change to life in the country was "allmost to the extreame, from comparatively a whirl-wind to a calme." She herself had not been well and she too required the respite. She had a "rheumatick fever" with pain in her ankles, spreading to above the knees, but mercifully she was able to report, "the pain has mostly been remote from the vitals." This letter was written to her niece Sally Hird, now living in Leeds, Yorkshire. Sally was the second daughter of her brother Joseph and elder sister of the three nieces who had stayed in London for the winter of 1769–1770. She had been married to Abraham Tetley but was left a widow soon after the death of her Uncle Samuel in 1772. It had in fact been Sally who had nursed the dying Samuel, and her "kind, affectionate, constant attention" to him had particularly endeared her to the doctor and his sister. She was now married again, to Dr William Hird, a prominent physician in Leeds. In December the doctor and his sister were back at full pace in London and Ann was asked to write to her niece Sally again, this time to ask her doctor husband to send his observations on "A Disorder like a Bad Cold" which had prevailed both in London and in other places. It was the first time in her correspondence that he appears to have asked her to help him with his medical affairs.

During 1776 her ill health persisted. Her brother reported that, although they had had a favourable summer in Cheshire, she had had more entertaining than she would have liked. She had also accompanied him in Yorkshire as one of a committee appointed by the yearly meeting to make a general visit to meetings throughout the country. "Our return to town was to her anxious and affecting. I perceived a weakness in her voice and a kind of flutter that was unusual to her." And so he arranged for her to go to a south coast resort, to Deal in Kent, where she had friends and where she could stay with a small family. "Her disease was labour, and the cure must be rest... We are now likely to be separated longer than we have been these twenty years or near it," he added sadly to Sally Hird.

They were now aging. In 1777 he was 65 and she nearly 60. Then she had an accident to her leg. It appears to have been a fracture, for her brother told her it was the "era for broken shins," but by December she was happily restored and could "walk about my usual occasions without pain." She was writing to her niece in Leeds in the same way that she had to Alexander and his young family nearly 30 years before. "About 10 days since a Box was sent to you containing Sundreys" and "by the time this reaches thee I hope a Barril of oysters may have arrived for you."

The journey to Lea Hall in July 1778 was eventful. Their cousin, Benjamin Waterhouse, then a medical student at Edinburgh and future professor of medicine at Harvard, was to spend the holiday with them. As he had been two summers in London, Ann thought the country air would do him good, particularly as there seemed no way in which he could get back to his native Rhode Island at that time. It had been a remarkably hot, dry summer. Ann told her niece "horses from the violent heat and suffocation of dust dropped down dead on the road in their harness." Ben Waterhouse went on ahead with the coach to take a look at St Albans and the next day, 20 July, he was to go to Hockliffe, 37 miles from London, where the doctor and his sister would meet him. On the way the advance party met a dreadful storm of thunder and lightning, with hail "as large as any of them ever saw." The doctor's party did not get away from Harpur Street until after 8 30 in the morning, but it was fine when they set out. Ann's account of the journey gives us the flavour of travel 200 years ago as well as describing the storm:

Just before we got up Highgate Hill a moderate shower fall, just sufficient to lay the Dust and render traviling pleasant. At Barnet we Chainged horses – during that little time (which was about 10 o'clock) we were surrounded with Black darkness indeed, and several loud Claps of thunder and very strong flashes of lightning. But little more rain than to lay the dust – traveling with great expedition with 4 horses prevented us hearing so much of the thunder But I could perceive it allmost continual – at Albans we stopt to Breakfast during which time a heavy shower fel But was over by the time we were ready to set out and we had little more rain till we came to Dunstable Hill where it came very heavy indeed. But we soon were at our Inn where we and our advance party were mutually pleased to meet again and see each other safe and well – about 4 o'clock we set out and had a fine evening to Stoney Stratford.

She described their preservation on that stormy day with gratitude since "many Both men and women and Cattle lost their lives with In and around London (as we have since been informed)." Benjamin Waterhouse, whose constitution Ann found "allways puney," enjoyed the later part of the journey to Lea Hall, particularly the "Diversified prospects and large extent of well cultivated country." It was a busy summer, with more visitors than they cared for, but they returned to London refreshed.

That winter, however, it was the doctor who fell seriously ill. In November he had an attack of prostatic obstruction, mercifully relieved by his friend the surgeon Percival Pott. Sally Hird, the young daughter of Dr Hird by his first marriage, came to stay at Harpur Street and give her help; and the doctor recovered – so much so that by February 1779 Ann was reporting that he "is Imbarked as much as ever from Early till very late as usual. Sometime Home to a hasty dinner Betwixt 4 and 5 o'clock & out again till 9 or near 10 at night and some days without any dinner out as late – and of consequence up writing till betwixt 11 and 12." It was no way for an elderly and infirm physician to take care of himself.

There had been other problems. Alexander Fothergill had to make repayments of his loans and in November, during the doctor's illness, he had written: "By the last 1st day's post we received from Son Thomas the distressing account of thy sudain and dangerous illness with which thou was visited... and tho' reading and writing may be too troublesom in thy present poor state yet 'tis my duty to write..." and he recorded how he had received the bank bills for £400 to pay off the legatees of Thomas Simpson, to whom he had mortgaged part of the Carr End property in 1762.[31] But there were further difficulties ahead. The first part of the mortgage was now paid off, but there remained the £600 which was owed to Richard Seymour. Concerned lest the illness prove fatal, Alexander was pressing the doctor for further help. On 2 January, when the doctor was still incapacitated, Alexander wrote again. He himself had been unwell, as well as his wife: "I as well as dr sister and thyself have had a rap at the Door of my old house on earth... but necessity seems to require that I remind thee that the £600 must or is promised to be paid... on the 2d day of next month."[32]

By 4 February the doctor had arranged with Charlton Palmer to send a further £600 to pay off the remainder of the mortgage, but it is not surprising that an uncharacteristic and querulous note had crept into his writing. "The losses, the expenses I have had were it only for thy own family, (and I do not mean this by way of reflection) are such as would have afforded me, with what little I have remaining, some tolerable provision against old age."[33] But Carr End now effectively belonged to the doctor.

During the summer of 1779 it was Ann's turn to be ill. A Friend, missing her presence at the monthly meeting, discovered that she was unwell and wrote encouragingly: "Remember the very hairs of your head are all number'd – not a Sparrow can fall to the ground without your heavenly Father's knowledge and the blessed Lip of Truth has said you are of more value than many Sparrows."[3]

She had had a recurrence of her rheumatism and the doctor insisted that she spend a period at the spa at Buxton. She stayed less than two weeks but to her surprise her brother spent the whole time with her, "a long time for my brother to devote to me." The next summer was to be their last holiday at Lea Hall together. The journey north was hectic as always. At every stop there was a press of apothecaries with their patients "that put him allmost out of patience." But it was a quiet and satisfying holiday with visits from their nieces and young families. "A peaceful pleasing retreat to me it is," Ann wrote, "I often walk the garding alone whilst my brother is writing or otherwise engaged – and say in my Heart what more could we ask for."

Their journey back to London took them to Ackworth, the famous Quaker school which the doctor had played a major part in founding during the previous two years. Ann wrote that "we scarce ever had a more satisfactory journey Home – the roads were generally good, the wether most favourable." They were welcomed home by their "family," their servants, and although it was past 6 o'clock the doctor set off at once to pay several visits. If Ann had had any premonition of her brother's impending death during her solitary walks in the garden at Lea Hall, she showed no sign of it in her letters that autumn. But in December 1780 the doctor had a further attack of prostatic obstruction which even the skill of Percival Pott could not relieve. David Barclay, living in nearby Red Lion Square, wrote on 15 December to

Dr Hird and his wife that "altho I have no commission from thy worthy Uncle Dr Fothergill, I could not with satisfaction longer defer informing Thee and they valuable wife that my dear Friend is very much indisposed." The following day he told Dr Hird that "Your Aunt is preserved much in the calmness, & sustains this shock with fortitude & resolution – she joins in affectionate regard." Ann did not desire their presence "under a roof where there is nothing but distress." She had her niece Alice Chorley with her and the doctor too did not want to cause his relations pain by seeing him in his present afflicted situation. The end came, a merciful release, on the day after Christmas.[34] The doctor was to be buried at Winchmore Hill, a burial ground described by a Quaker diarist as the "Westminster Abbey of the Friends of Middlesex where our Kings, Statemen and Poets repose."[14] It was in the country, 10 miles north of Harpur Street, and there was an ancient meeting house. On 5 January more than 70 coaches followed the doctor through Islington and on to his last resting place. It was a long day for the mourners and for the devoted Ann, alone with her grief.

Dr William Cuming, her brother's friend from student days in Edinburgh, now practising in Dorchester, knew something of the extent of her loss and understood her relationship with her brother. "Your loss," he wrote on 10 January, "it must be confessed is incomparably the greatest; but you are by no means the only sufferer – all his friends, his acquaintance, the publick – all partake of it and share with you."[35] Sir George Savile, member of Parliament for York and leader of the Yorkshire Association which was actively lobbying in opposition to the American war, called to present his compliments. There was now the problem of the estate. Upton had to be sold, as well as the house in Harpur Street. She felt it "irksome to leave the house desolate and without inhabitant." By April 1781 she was arranging with a "gentleman of the name of Leigh of York Street" to sell her brother's books by auction. The sale, by Leigh and Sotheby, lasted eight days. There was also the "family" to be cared for. It was not easy to get them new employment. By April she reported that "Thos Greenfield not yet got a place nor Joseph Imploy."

Soon, however, she had moved into a smaller house, No 68 Great Russell Street, just opposite the British Museum and off Bloomsbury Square. In the summer of 1782 she went to bathe in the sea at Brighthelmstone for a few weeks, since she felt "several weakening complaints increasing upon me." Despite these symptoms, she was to live on for another 20 years. Brother Alexander, now over 70, had also been in town but, although she greeted him cordially, she told her niece Sally Hird, "thou will believe the remembrance of the disimilarity Could not add to my Comfort." Alexander may well have been in London to see his sister about the mortgages on Carr End. In his will, Dr Fothergill had desired "my Sister Ann Fothergill to take up and pay off my brother Alexander Fothergill the Mortgage on his estates and to pay him any money that shall be remaining of the sum of one thousand eight hundred pounds after discharging such mortgages and all costs and Charges attending the transfer thereof." Now, in November 1782, Ann arranged that the mortgage be transferred to Alexander's eldest son William and to John Chorley, his son in law. Alexander returned to Carr End which he no longer owned, and spent his last years there. He died in 1788 at the age of 79.

Through these last years Ann's nieces came to stay with her. By now she was an old lady living with the past, but still concerned for her brother's memory and reputation, as evidenced by her firm letter in 1783 to Baron Dimsdale, the inoculator of the Empress Catherine of Russia and her family, setting to rights his recollection of the events leading to his selection for that important undertaking. She followed her brother's custom of befriending and helping young physicians in London. Robert Willan, a young Yorkshireman who had been encouraged by Dr Fothergill, "experienced much active friendship from Mrs Fothergill, the doctor's surviving sister" in setting up in practice in London in 1783 (see Chapter 7).

For the rest of her life Ann remained kind and benevolent and she was much given, it was said, to hospitality. Twice a week she had a dinner provided for strangers who attended Westminster meeting. In 1790 she was one of the subscribers to the new meeting house at Winchmore Hill where her brother was buried, and it was there that she too was interred after her death in 1802 at the age of 84. In that quiet graveyard she lies beside the brother whom she loved.

The deep and satisfying relationship that developed between brother and sister was the basis of a partnership which was of inestimable importance to Dr Fothergill in a life which was spent, according to Franklin, "always projecting something for the Good of his Country and of Mankind in General, and putting others who had it in their Power what was out of his own Reach, but whatever was within it he took care to do himself." Ann always knew how much she owed to her brother, how much her life had been shaped by him. She may not always have appreciated how much she came to mean to him. Although gratified by his support during her illness in 1779, she seems to have been genuinely surprised that he spent 12 whole days with her at Buxton. By then, however, he had been signing many of his letters J and A Fothergill for years. There is little doubt that she was closer to him, and dearer, than he would ever himself have been able to say. Ann became, during her life with him, a figure of significance in her own right. She was one of the few British housewives who had the privilege of entertaining, at her house in Harpur Street, two men who subsequently signed the Declaration of Independence, both of whom remembered her well. In later life, Ann may have appeared a trifle formidable, but like so many members of the Society of Friends she had a warm and compassionate heart. Her letters, despite an endearing idiosyncracy of spelling, reflect the sturdy independence of spirit of the north country non-conformist. Her independence of mind since early life is best illustrated by the inscription on the front of her little recipe book. Above, in the beautiful eighteenth century copperplate of a 15 year old, is written "John Fothergill;" beside, another hand has put "not his book." Beneath, that same hand, in firm thick handwriting, has penned the words "Ann Fothergill, Her Book."

NOTES

1 Corner GW. *The autobiography of Benjamin Rush*. Princeton: Princeton University Press, 1948: 45–46.

2 Larabee, LW. *The Papers of Benjamin Franklin*. Vol. 10. New Haven and London: Yale University Press, 1966: 172.

3 MS autograph letter, Sarah Shewell to Ann Fothergill, 9 July 1779. Portfolio 22:21. Library of the Society of Friends, London.

4 Crosfield G. *Memoirs of the life and gospel labours of Samuel Fothergill*. Liverpool: D Marples and London: Charles Gilpin, 1843: 229. The letters of Samuel Fothergill quoted in this chapter are derived from Crosfield unless otherwise stated.

5 Corner BC, Booth CC. *Chain of friendship. Letters of Dr Fothergill*. Cambridge, Massachusetts: Harvard University Press, 1971: 132. Dr Fothergill's letters quoted in this chapter are from this source unless otherwise stated.

6 Ann Fothergill's letters are preserved in the collections at the Library of the Society of Friends, London. Her letters quoted in this chapter are taken from these collections.

7 MS autograph letter, Joseph Fothergill to Alexander Fothergill, 19 January 1748. Library of the Society of Friends, London.

8 Fothergill J. *An account of the sore throat attended with ulcers*. London: L Davis, 1748. Six editions of the work were published during Fothergill's lifetime.

9 Hartley M, Ingilby J. *Life and traditions in the Yorkshire dales*. London: JM Dent and Sons, 1968: 27–8.

10 MS diary of Alexander Fothergill, 27 July 1754. North Yorkshire County Library, Northallerton, Yorkshire.

11 MS autograph letter, John Churchman to Ann Fothergill, 15 10 mo, 1754. Portfolio 21:29. Library of the Society of Friends, London.

12 MS autograph letter, John Churchman to Ann Fothergill, 23 5 mo, 1765. Portfolio 21:28. Library of the Society of Friends, London.

13 Van Doren C, ed. *Benjamin Franklin's autobiographical writings*. London: Cresset Press, 1946:786.

14 Typescript copy of original MS, James Jenkins, The Records and Recollections of James Jenkins from 1761 to 1821, pp 24; 385. Library of the Society of Friends, London.

15 MS autograph letter, Samuel Fothergill to Ann Fothergill, 3 May 1760. Portfolio 22:20. Library of the Society of Friends, London.

16 Extract "from EG's journal, 1764," in Milcah Martha Moore's commonplace book. In the possession of Miss Sara G Smith, Philadelphia.

17 Typescript copy made by R Hingston Fox of letter from Ann Fothergill to Alexander Fothergill, 14th 5 mo, 1756. Portfolio 38:84. Library of the Society of Friends, London.

18 Fothergill J. *Considerations relative to the North American colonies*. London: Henry Kent, 1765. (Published anonymously.)

19 Fox RH. *Dr John Fothergill and his friends*. London: Longmans, Green: 1919.

20 Some of Dr Fothergill's silver cutlery, still preserved, bears the hallmark 1767.

21 MS autograph diary of Betty Fothergill. Library of the Society of Friends, London.

22 Solander D. *Natural history of many curious and uncommon zoophytes, collected from various parts of the globe by the late John Ellis, Esq, FRS. Systematically arranged and described by the late Daniel Solander MD FRS.* London: Benjamin White and Peter Elmsly, 1786.

23 MS recipe book in handwriting of Ann Fothergill, inscribed "Ann Fothergill, Her Book." In the possession of Mrs Winifred Fothergill Quinlan, Townbank, New Jersey.

24 "S Tittley" refers to Sally Tetley, second daughter of Joseph Fothergill, then married to Abraham Tetley but soon to be widowed.

25 MS autograph letter, Samuel Fothergill to Ann Fothergill 27th 4 mo, 1772. Portfolio 22:24. Library of the Society of Friends, London.

26 MS records of preparative meeting for Wensleydale. North Yorkshire County Library, Northallerton, Yorkshire.

27 Alexander Fothergill's daughter Ann was married to James Freeman of Gracechurch Street, where Alexander was lodging.

28 MS diary of Alexander Fothergill. Entries for 29, 30 September, and 1 October, 1774. North Yorkshire County Library, Northallerton, Yorkshire.

29 MS autograph document by Alexander Fothergill to Richmond monthly meeting. Library of the Society of Friends, London.

30 Ketchum RM. *The battle for Bunker Hill*. London: Cresset Press, 1962: 161.

31 MS autograph letter, Alexander Fothergill to Dr John Fothergill, undated. Portfolio 38:111. Library of the Society of Friends, London.

32 MS autograph letter, Alexander Fothergill to Dr John Fothergill, 2nd 1st mo, 1779. Portfolio 38:111. Library of the Society of Friends, London.

33 MS autograph letter, J Fothergill to Alexander Fothergill, undated. Portfolio 38:111. Library of the Society of Friends, London.

34 MS autograph letters, David Barclay to Dr William Hird, 15–24th 12 mo, 1780. Portfolio 21:99–106. Library of the Society of Friends, London.

35 Lettsom JC. *The works of John Fothergill MD...with some account of his life*. London: C Dilly, 1784.

149

7 The Willans of Marthwaite

In the spring of 1812, the year of Napoleon's ill fated venture into Russia, Richard Willan, a gentleman farmer in Yorkshire, received a letter from Madeira.[1] The letter, dated 14 April, came by Penzance and Kendal, and it took four weeks to reach its destination at The Hill, in Marthwaite near Sedbergh, where Richard lived. It related the sad news of the death of his younger brother, Robert Willan, whose pioneer work on dermatology was widely acclaimed and who is remembered as the founder of British dermatology.

The country home of the Willans in Marthwaite is today very much as it was in the eighteenth century. From the upper part of Wensleydale you can look westwards and upwards towards the Westmorland border, near which Robert Willan was born, and see the deep valleys, the broad hillsides, the crags, moors, and grey stone walls of that lovely land. If you then go up to the head of Wensleydale, to the watershed of the Pennines, you come to the top of a narrow valley, Garsdale, which leads down on the western side to Sedbergh, the small market town with a famous grammar school founded in 1525. At Sedbergh itself, at the end of this valley, there is the eighteenth century schoolhouse, now the school library, where Willan, like John Fothergill, was a pupil. The door through which Robert Willan hurried as a boy has the date 1716 above it and there is also the motto of the school *Dura virum nutrix*. In Willan's time this was the best school in the north and there he became an accomplished classical scholar.

Adapted from the *British Journal of Dermatology* 1968; **80**: 459–86, and from *Medical History* 1981; **25**: 181–96.

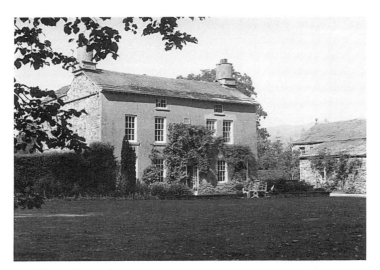

10   The Hill, Marthwaite

From Sedbergh, if you travel south west on the Kirkby Lonsdale road, you come after three miles or so to the Willan home. You see The Hill first from the road, a fairly typical dales farmhouse of the early eighteenth century, at the end of an avenue of gracious trees. The date stone over the door bears the inscription R.W. 1712 – Robert Willan's grand-father. On one of the barns, now sadly derelict, there was also a date stone with R. and A.W. (for his parents Robert and Ann Willan) and 1748 carved upon it.

Robert Willan, the dermatologist, was the youngest child of the sixth generation of Willans known to have lived in Marthwaite since the middle of the seventeenth century. The Willans were Quakers. The first Willan of Marthwaite identi-fiable in the Quaker records seems to have been Anthony who died in 1670.[2] His son, Richard, married Alice Croft of nearby Killington in 1659, and he died at The Hill in 1706. His will indicates that he was not a wealthy man, his major legacy, to his wife, being only £5.[3] It was his second son, Robert Willan (1663–1737), who created the fortunes of the Willan family. He played an active part in the affairs of the Society of Friends at Sedbergh throughout his life, attending

151

meetings at the old meeting house at Briggflatts near Sedbergh. The building dates from 1675 and retains to this day the quiet simplicity of eighteenth century Quakerism. This Robert Willan once recorded how, "I had the advantage beyond many of Education under the care of Believing Parents and Masters for my furtherance in ye Knowledge and Life thereof and for my preservation therein in my young years..." Despite these advantages, he was during those early years not immune from the world's temptations, as the following account of the results of a late seventeenth century debauch will show. In a testimony to his monthly meeting on 27 September 1691, when he was 28 years old, he confessed to having been "prevailed upon to take more strong drink than was good or convenient for me" and he went on to describe how

coming from Lancaster having there taken too much strong Liquor and in my coming homewards wth another man being full of strong drink and riding fast I fell from my mare and being parted she run away homewards. And the man Rode after her and I followed after in my boots expecting to have met him coming back with the Mare, but she having taken another way I missed them and so came home on foote in ye night. Then the man finding the Mare, and wanting me, Occasioned a great Noise and Blunder in the Country and put People in strange thoughts what was become of me. And all this work and Stirr I do sincerely acknowledge was occasion'd only thorow taking over much strong drink before we came out...[4]

It was a problem that was to occasion difficulties for a later generation of the family.

Robert Willan was married in 1692 to Mary Birkett, daughter of Miles Birkett of Hartmell, and their first child, Richard, was born the following year. Soon afterwards they appear to have moved to Hewthwaite in the valley of Dent, some five miles from the family home at The Hill. Two more sons were to be born to Robert Willan while he lived in Dent. According to Norman Penney's *The First Publishers of Truth*, the Quakers of Dent had no meeting house until 1700 and they therefore gathered for worship in each other's houses, including "Robert Willan's house at East Banke in Dent".[5] The house still has old oak panelling but it has been extensively altered since the seventeenth century and only the remnants of what must have been stone mullioned windows can now be seen.

Dentdale starts as a narrow valley running south from the town of Sedbergh, widening out after several miles to form a broad valley around the town of Dent. Hewthwaite, on the east side of the valley, is halfway between Sedbergh and Dent town. In the seventeenth century it was a pastoral community of "statesmen," men who owned their small ancestral homes and who kept flocks of sheep on their hill pastures. For centuries wool was the staple product of the Yorkshire dales so it is not surprising that knitting should have become a major industry in those valleys in the years before the Industrial Revolution. In the seventeenth and eighteenth centuries – until knee breeches were superseded by long trousers – Dent was famous for the manufacture and export of knitted stockings, and the Dent knitters were immortalised by Robert Southey as the "Terrible knitters e' Dent," the word terrible being used in its dialect sense of great. Adam Sedgwick, born in Dent and later Woodwardian professor of geology in the University of Cambridge, recorded during the nineteenth century memories of the great days of knitting in his native valley. He wrote that some of the more enterprising of the statesmen of Dent became middlemen, acting between the village manufacturers and consumers, sometimes riding up to London "to deal personally with the merchants of Cheapside, and to keep alive the current of rural industry."[6] Robert Willan appears to have been one of these successful eighteenth century hosiers. We can imagine the trains of packhorses filing down the narrow lane from Hewthwaite to the valley below, see the milkmaids knitting as they drove the cattle to their fields, and remember the "sittings" at which the country people met together in the winter evenings to knit "with a speed that cheated the eye", while they listened to readings from Defoe or Bunyan.[7]

The stocking trade brought prosperity to Robert Willan, for by 1700 he was able to move to Castley, a larger and more impressive house just to the north of Sedbergh. The house, now called Castlehow, is little changed today from its appearance in the early eighteenth century. It has the original stone mullioned windows, and a carved date stone above the door carries the initials R. and M. W., for Robert and Mary, his wife, with the date 1701 beneath. Inside, the house is panelled in oak and there is a fine staircase in the Jacobean style. Beside the fireplace in the main downstairs room there is an oak cupboard with a decorated door and the same initials and date carved upon it.

Their next son, Robert, was born at the end of 1700 (old style), followed by Alice and Elizabeth at two year intervals, both births being recorded as at Castley. Two years later, in 1706, Richard Willan, father of Robert the hosier, died at his home at The Hill. The inventory of his goods and effects serves to illustrate his interests, the modest extent of his property, and the changes that were to occur in the fortunes of the family within one generation. Richard was evidently a farmer, for beasts and horses amounted to £44 10s 0d out of the total inventory which was valued at just over £93. His "money in his purse," apparel, and riding saddle accounted for £6 and there were silver spoons worth £2 10s 0d and a clock at £1. He felt no need to leave any of his property to his son Robert living in some style at Castley, but there were five shillings for his 13 year old grandson Richard and the residue went to his son Edward, who was named as his executor.

Robert and Mary Willan were to have two more children at Castley, but then as so often happened in that century, disaster struck. In 1710, shortly after the birth of their last child, Mary Willan died, soon to be followed by the infant named after her.

By then, Richard, the eldest son, was 17 years old and he no doubt joined his father in his business. Two years later the house at The Hill was either renovated or rebuilt and a date stone with the initial RW 1712 was set into the lintel above the door, the single initials being those of Richard, still a bachelor. It seems likely that Richard moved to The Hill at this time; perhaps significantly it was the year of his father's remarriage, to Alice Burgess of Chester. Richard himself was married in 1716 to Hannah Wardell, but within five years she too was dead, leaving him in 1721 with his two young sons, Robert, the father of the dermatologist, and Lancelot. A

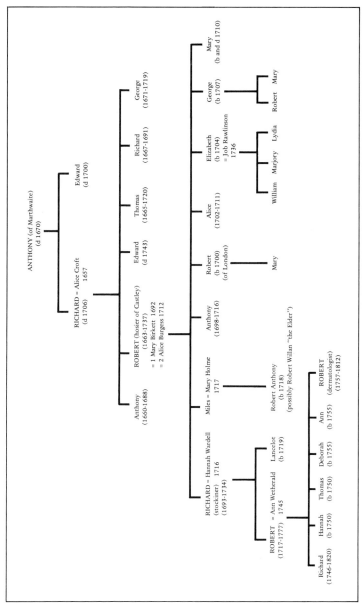

The Willan family

friend from Kendal, Alice Cragg, brought them up; Richard Willan in his will made her a legacy "in regard to her consideration for my children in their infancie."[8]

By this time, Robert Willan of Castley, the patriarch of the family, had lost three other children. Alice died in 1711 at the age of 9, Anthony at 18 in the year of his elder brother Richard's marriage, Miles in 1720 at the age of 25. Miles, who was named after his maternal grandfather, Miles Birkett, had married a non-Quaker, Mary Holme, in 1717. No doubt it was a grief to his father, so long a pillar of the Sedbergh Friends' meeting, when the monthly meeting recorded its testimony against Miles for being "married by a Priest with a Woman of another persuasion."[9] Their only son was born the following year and was baptised Robert Anthony in Sedbergh church in July 1718.[10] It was only two years later that Miles Willan himself died, possibly suddenly since he left no will. Mary Willan made over her interest in her husband's estate to her wealthy father in law. Perhaps it was as well; the assets were valued at £49 13s od but there were debts of £132 "upon speciality."[11]

By now Robert Willan was aging. Increasingly during the ensuing years he seems to have made his business over to his son Richard living at The Hill. Richard seems not to have enjoyed robust health. He made his first will in 1727, adding a codicil in 1734, five days before his premature death, at the age of 41, on 14 April. Richard was, by dales standards, a relatively wealthy man. His inventory, which describes him as a "Stockiner," amounted to a total of £1225 10s od. Of this, £300 was accounted for by "stock in trade, stockins and other Debts," and there was £663 owing to the deceased on securities. "Plaite" alone was worth £50, and his "purse and apparel" were valued at £55. Richard appointed his father Robert, uncle Edward, and two friends as executors and trustees. He left the major part of his property to his elder son, Robert, to be held in trust until he attained the age of 21. The sum of £500 was to go to his second son, Lancelot, His Wardell brothers in law were asked to supervise the boys' education. If, however, both the sons were to die before reaching the age of 21 the property was to go to his younger brother, Robert Willan, whom he described as "of London," and there were also to be appropriate legacies to his nephew Robert Anthony, to his niece Mary, and to his younger brother George. The fourth day of September, 1734, must have been a sad day for the grieving father when he put his signature, along with his fellow executors, to the obligation to "truly execute and perform the last Will and Testament" of his eldest son.

By then over 70, Robert Willan lived on at Castley for another three years. In 1736 he had the pleasure of seeing his only surviving daughter Elizabeth married at the age of 32 to Job Rawlinson of Graythwaite Hall in Lancashire. It was an excellent marriage, for the Rawlinsons were established iron-masters with furnaces and forges in Lancashire, West-morland, and as far afield as Invergarry in Scotland. They were closely connected with other Quaker families such as the Fords, Crosfields, and Backhouses in those early years of the Industrial Revolution in England.[13] Ironically it was this revolution that was to end the stocking trade that had sustained so many in the dales of northwest Yorkshire for so long.

Robert Willan died in November 1737 at the age of 74. Many of his immediate family had already predeceased him. His eldest brother, Anthony, had died young; his younger brother, Richard, died in Barbados at the age of 24, and his youngest brother, George, who had moved to London and possibly acted as his factor, died in Aldgate in 1719 leaving three daughters. His brother Thomas, who also left three daughters, died in Kendal a year later. Robert Willan was not the last of his own generation to die, for his brother Edward survived him for seven years. Nevertheless, for many Sed-bergh Quakers the death of Robert Willan must have been like the end of an era.

Robert Willan's bequests to his children indicate the extent to which he had already helped them in their affairs. Robert "of London" received only £10, his father "having given to him largely heretofore," and George owed his father more than £400 at the time of his death, much of which sum was bequeathed to him. Elizabeth Rawlinson, however, was to have Castley and its land, and to her husband, Job, Robert Willan left his silver tobacco box. Castley is said later to have become an academy. The Hewthwaite property in Dent was sold by the executors to pay other legacies and expenses. Robert's grandchildren all received sums of money, the largest share going to Robert Anthony who was to inherit £150 when he reached the age of 21 in 1739 and in addition got the "screwtore that stands in the parlour." He also left property at Briggflatts to his grandson Robert who the following year, at 21 years old, was to inherit the property at The Hill under the terms of his father Richard's will.[14]

No details are available of the subsequent lives of any of the grandchildren of Robert Willan, with the exception of his grandson Robert. Robert Anthony, in particular, does not appear in the records of the Sedbergh meetings of the Friends, and when his mother died in 1744 there is no mention of him in her will.[15]

Robert Willan, inheritor of The Hill, married Ann Wetherald in 1745 and took her to live with him at the family home in Marthwaite. Here their six children were born between 1746 and 1757, the last being the dermatologist. Robert Willan put a date stone on a building at The Hill in 1748 with the initials of himself and his wife. He did not remain a lifelong Quaker, for he seems to have shared his grandfather's early difficulty with strong drink. In 1758 his monthly meeting drew up a paper of their disunity with him on account of his "drinking to excess and breaking word."[16]

There is little doubt that this Robert Willan, the father of the dermatologist, became a medical practitioner in the Sedbergh district. He enjoyed, according to his son's biographer, "an extensive medical reputation and practice." At the time of his marriage the Friends record him as Robert Willan MD, but there is considerable doubt as to whether he ever had a university degree. When he died in 1777 he was described as a "man-midwife," and it seems more likely that he was one of those country practitioners who received an early training apprenticed to an apothecary but did not proceed to a university degree. It would have been open to him as a Quaker to attend the medical school in Edinburgh, but there is no evidence that he ever did so. A Robert Willan appears in Alexander Monro's list of students in Edinburgh for the years 1739, 1740, and 1743, and this Robert Willan graduated MD in 1745.[17] While it is possible that there were two Robert Willans at Edinburgh between 1739 and 1745, there was only one who graduated MD and he can be positively identified as a bachelor who, having gone from Edinburgh to practice in Scarborough, emigrated to Pennsylvania in 1748. He was the author while in Scarborough of a book on *The King's Evil*.[18] The origins of this Robert Willan MD, described by Munk as Robert Willan "the Elder",[19] are not established with certainty, but from the facts of his life it is likely that he was a member of the Willan family of Marthwaite. He may well have been Robert Anthony Willan, the son of Miles Willan and the grandson of Robert of Castley, under whose will he would have benefited at precisely the time that he started as a medical student.

Robert Willan, the future dermatologist, was born at The Hill in 1757. He was educated at Sedbergh School where he became an accomplished classical scholar, even, according to the school register "surpassing his master, Dr Bateman, in knowledge of Greek."[20] He then went to Edinburgh and in the summer of 1780 graduated MD at the age of 23. Soon afterwards he travelled to London. There John Fothergill, then aged 68, offered him assistance and urged him to settle in the capital.[21] The young Willan would have done this but his plans were thwarted by the unfortunate death of Dr Fothergill in December of the same year. Almost at the same time news came of the death of an elderly relative, Dr Trotter of Darlington, with whom it had been suggested Willan should work. Willan therefore decided to take advantage of this opening and he travelled northwards again early in 1781 to start practice at Darlington, only 40 miles or so from his home near Sedbergh.

While he was in Darlington Willan became interested in mineral waters, like so many of his contemporaries. Near Darlington there was a small village called Croft, with a spring producing "a fine clear sparkling water: smelling strongly of sulphur," and the custom was to drink between four and nine pints of it, which must have made the dressing room provided by the thoughtful owner of the spa very necessary. Willan at this early stage of his career was certainly no revolutionary and he had a conventional belief in the curative powers of mineral waters. Dedicating his *Observations on the sulphur-water at Croft near Darlington* to Sir Joseph Banks he wrote, "As nature has consulted the convenience and necessity of human life in dispensing everywhere with liberal hand, the simple element of water, so hath she provided an alleviation of human misery, by impregnating, in particular situations, that element with principles which are found extremely useful in the cure of disease."[22] He went on, as was the custom of physicians of the time, to recommend the waters of Croft spa for all manner of ailments including discharges, chronic weakness, gravel, rickets, inflammation of the eyes, and so on. Already at this early stage of his career, however, his practice may have stimulated an interest in skin disease for he gives a fairly extensive list of disorders of the skin in which the spa water was helpful. He was also curious about the high incidence of skin disease, asking "Why are the nations of the North, and especially this kingdom, more liable to cutaneous affections?" – a question which occupied him for the remainder of his working life.

In 1782, after less than two years in Darlington, Robert Willan returned to London, where he was befriended and much helped by Dr Fothergill's sister and companion Ann who was then living alone in the city. The following year, 1783, Willan was appointed physician to the new public dispensary in Carey Street, where he was to work for the next 20 years. It must have been at this stage that he began his systematic studies of diseases of the skin, which were no doubt common disorders among the London poor who flocked to the public dispensary for his advice, and the next seven years must have been the busiest and most exciting of his life. Although he was working as a general physician it was during this period that he prepared his classification and description of cutaneous diseases, and in 1790 his work was presented to the Medical Society of London.[23] It was this that won him the Fothergillian medal of the society.

Despite his success Willan was not well known at this early stage of his career – he was still only 33 – and many of his friends now advised him to publish his work. It was a massive undertaking, entailing the reproduction of a large number of drawings and paintings of skin disorders, and it was probably difficult for Willan to find a publisher at once. The first part of the work, including Willan's classification of papulae, appeared in 1798 and was at once translated into German, an edition appearing in Breslau in 1799. Further parts of the work were issued in 1801, and 1805 (rashes) and the fourth part – the remainder of the rashes and the bullae, including an amended edition of the previous three parts – was published as volume I of Willan's *Cutaneous Disorders* in 1808.[24] This work, although incomplete, was a remarkable achievement. The descriptions and classifications of skin diesease introduced rational thinking into a disorganised subject and they justifiably established Willan's scientific reputation; in effect, he achieved for dermatology what Linnaeus had done for botany. At the same time his clinical skill was being increasingly recognised, and his practice became so busy that by 1803 he had to resign from the Carey Street dispensary. The governors recognised his 20 years of service by presenting him with a fine piece of plate, now in the possession of Sedbergh School.

Something is known of Willan's method of practice. Bateman, his biographer, admirer, and pupil, tells us that he was "a close and faithful observer of disease," but an indifferent therapeutist.[25] A few of Willan's letters survive and there is one in the Wellcome collection which illustrates that physicians must have got into the habit of sending him drawings of skin diseases that puzzled them, and Willan would then reply. The letter is to Lettsom.

As far as I can judge by your drawing which is on a reduced scale, the complaint is the Lichenose eruption succeeding in some persons to the use of Mercury either internally or externally. You will know from the particulars of ye case whether the appearance was referable to that cause. I have sent a drawing (nat^l size) by way of comparison. Yours truly, R Willan.[26]

He also advised his brother Richard, living at the family

home at The Hill, on the problems of his health, and another letter reveals his therapeutic approach to have been entirely conventional for his time. "This humid season is not very good for you," he wrote to Richard Willan,

and generally it conduces to form the scorbutic disposition in the body. Your medicine should be as beneficial as the Cheltenham water. There is no great probability of its being purgative; I wished Mr Dawson or Wallis to regulate the proportion of the Cheltenham or Epsom Salt in it so that it might prove sufficiently laxative to prevent the necessity of taking sulphur or any further medicine at the same time.[27] I wish the remedy to clear off gently the inflammation of the stomach and bowels which has been so troublesome. It is often succeeded by the impetiginous or scorbutic eruptions or this may sometimes stand in place of it, and of the gout, which is another of its attendants. The milk of sulphur is particularly useful in that form of scurvy...

How beneficial this advice was to Richard Willan is not recorded. His brother went on to give an interesting description of the torment of toothache and the courage of a child faced with the horror of a dental extraction over 150 years ago. "The little boy," he wrote, "after considerable suffering from a fungus at the root of one of the grinder teeth, got perfectly well. He went firmly and steadily to have the tooth drawn when his cold and y[e] inflammation got better, and he never winced in the operation. He had not fully recovered his bloom and good looks till Christmas: but now he is growing rapidly, has spread out and is quite muscular, taking constant and violent exercise in all forms..."[28] Willan's proud description of this episode was pardonable for the "little boy" was his own son. He describes this incident further in another letter, and goes on to praise the intellectual abilities of his boy. "His progress in literature has been retarded for the present tho' his capabilities are great and his memory strong. He can repeat verbatim little poems which strike his fancy, when they have been read to him 3 or 4 times in a good accent. We propose to follow your idea of giving him correct French pronunciation while the organs are flexible..." The family bond between Robert Willan and his brother Richard was obviously a close one. Another letter refers to financial transactions between them, and there is also an amusing reference to the problems of transportation.[29] Willan, the classical scholar, evidently called his horses by classical names. "My old horse Achilles is well-nigh demolished," he told his brother, "and young Telemachus seems very thin & tottering. I want two more but am fearful, as it wd more than double the heavy tax on us already; and the price of oats is here so enormous, the stable would become more expensive than our kitchen." He wrote with all the forthright directness of a dalesman.

All successful physicians have to advise others less fortunate in their careers. Another letter, preserved at the Library of the Society of Friends in London, illustrates how Willan reacted when consulted by Dr Rutter of Liverpool about a medical man who practice was seriously threatened by his ill health and who was considering a move to the south. "My dear Friend," he wrote, "it seems proper to answer thy letter with which I am favoured immediately..." and he went on to describe the situation in the area suggested by Rutter on the outskirts of London.

Tottenham which is now extended to Edmonton makes a large village, but is well cultivated by med¹ practitioners: Holt a surgeon is situated at one end of it, Maule at the other. Neither of these has so much business in the place as Hammond who lives at Edmonton. His brothers partake of it, one of whom is settled at Enfield, the other still nearer at Southgate. A gentleman well recommended to our friends, who form a large society at Tottenham, wᵈ get some business amongst them, but perhaps of no great extent. I do not at present know of any certain vacancy in the neighbourhood: a clear one indeed seldom occurs, as surgeons always dispose of whatever business they can transfer for a consideration in money, with regard to which much fraud is practised...[30]

In later life Willan's practice was predominantly in dermatology, but he was a man of very much wider interests both professionally and in the use of his scanty leisure time. He wrote on vaccination, smallpox and its history, recorded unusual and informative cases of all sorts, was interested in hygiene and public health, the cure of alcoholism, and chlorosis; and he joined Lettsom and a group of other eminent London physicians in planning a fever hospital, following the precepts which had been laid down in Chester by his fellow dalesman, Dr John Haygarth, whose work on the prevention of contagious fevers by segregation was increasingly accepted internationally at that time. Robert Willan was also an antiquary and historian. He wrote, among other things, a *History of the Ministry of Jesus Christ* – a compendium of the narratives of the four gospels, with notes. This was first published in 1782, and a further edition came out in 1803, his collaborator M Willan probably being his wife.[31][32] Another interesting work was *A list of the Ancient Words at present used in the Mountainous District of the West Riding of Yorkshire*. In this work he enlisted the aid of his brother Richard in Yorkshire and wrote to him giving a list of "old words wch I remember at school, and wch are antient Anglo Saxon," asking Richard to add what he could.[33] He included words such as "beck" (brook), "dub" (pool), "fettle" (mend), "laith" (a barn), "lake" (to idle), and "tarn," all of which are familiar words today, but "brant," "cowp," "mappen," "roggle," and "wrydden" will be lost on all but the expert. He also commented on the courting customs of the people of the dales, describing how after "strong ale and strong punch, besides kissing and romping...the rustic nymph is finally conducted by her partner of the dance to her father's house, which both enter without noise, and seated on the antique lang settle, prolong conversation in gentle whispers, till the first streaks of dawn admonish the youth to retire." He compares such practices favourably with the enormities committed at similar festivities in the Metropolis.[34]

Willan married relatively late in life, in 1800, when he was 43, and he had one son, the little boy whose dental problems he so vividly described. His wife Mary was not a member of the Society of Friends. She was the widow of a Dr Scott. The Willans lived in some style in Bloomsbury Square. The minutes of the Carey Street dispensary dated 20 May 1800 record that the governors voted that plate to the value of 50 guineas be presented to Dr Willan on the occasion of his recent marriage.[35] The Royal College of Physicians of London possesses two miniature portraits of Robert Willan and his wife and an indifferent oil painting whose artist is unknown. These were presented by Miss MEC Howell, great granddaughter of the dermatologist.[36] There is another portrait of Willan, on loan from the governors of Sedbergh School, which hangs outside the Willan Room at the college.

Willan's contemporaries liked him as a person and had the highest regard for his abilities. Bateman described how "in his intercourse with his professional brethren, he was liberal and independent, and extremely tender of giving offence."[25] At his death the *Gentleman's Magazine* recorded that "in addition to his great merits as a physician, and as an accurate and classical writer, he was one of the most amiable of men, a sincere friend, a good husband and an affectionate father. He was in truth, a model of the perfect human character; a benevolent and skilful Physician, a correct and sound philosopher, and a truly virtuous man."[37]

Willan died in 1812, at the early age of 54, before he had had time to complete the second volume of his work. This was to include pustulae, vesicles, tubercles, and maculae and it was not until five years after his death that it was published by his friend and pupil Dr Bateman.[38] It is usually said that his death was due to tuberculosis. This diagnosis, however, is unsatisfactory. It is true that in the spring of 1811 he suddenly expectorated some blood whilst helping a patient, but this symptom was accompanied by breathlessness which became more marked in the next few weeks, so much so that he could not lie flat in bed at night. At the same time his pulse was noted to be irregular. Since he also developed oedema of the feet and ultimately a severe anasarca, it seems more likely that his condition was due to cardiac failure. In September 1811, on the assumption that he was becoming phthisical, his friends persuaded him to go to Madeira. He left with his friend Ashby Smith on 10 October and must have had a miserable passage for he was 53 days at sea, detained by foul winds in the Downs and at Portsmouth, and during this time he developed severe ascites. But he arrived in Madeira safe and sound on 1 December, and by the following February felt so much better that he contemplated a return to England. This, however, was only a temporary respite; his dropsy returned and he died, in Madeira, on 7 April 1812.

His last days are graphically described by his friend Ashby

Smith, who wrote from Madeira on 14 April to inform Willan's brother, at home at The Hill. "His decay," wrote Ashby Smith to Richard Willan, "was gradual and unattended by pain – he was not at all confined to his bed, and retained to the last his cheerfulness, serenity and self possession – he had the most perfect knowledge of his impending dissolution, and with his usual acumen, traced and remarked on each progressive symptom; till within 3 hr. of its taking place, it has never been my lot to witness a deathbed scene attended with so much resignation, confidence and peace." The funeral took place the day afterwards, Robert Willan having sensibly "given particular instruction that his remains should not be removed to England for interment."[1] His gravestone is preserved in an old cemetery wall in Madeira and reads "Sacred to the Memory of Robert Willan., M.D., F.R.S. &c of London who died on this Island 7th April 1812 aged 53 years."[39]

It is difficult to make accurate diagnoses at such a distance of time and without pathological information, but it seems likely that Willan suffered from cardiac failure, possibly due to rheumatic heart disease, which itself might have been associated with that damp farmhouse in the north country where he lived as a boy. Whatever it was that took him to his Maker, as he lay dying in distant Madeira he must have remembered that old grey house in Yorkshire, the green fields around it, and the beauty of the sunlight on the hills and valleys of his native land.

Today only date stones remain on the houses near Sedbergh where the Willan family lived for so long. Richard, who received the news of his famous brother's death in Madeira in 1812, had inherited the property at The Hill from his father in 1777. He parted company with the Friends in 1788, and they recorded how "Richard Willan acknowledged the kindness of Friends but there did not appear any desire in him of returning to our Society again and having joined himself to the established religion of this Nation, we do not look upon him as a member of our Society."[40]

Long after his death in 1820 at the age of 74, Richard Willan was remembered by Adam Sedgwick who described him as "a thorough Dalesman...a lively cheerful man with a love for classical learning..." Unlike his father, he was a man of temperate habits – "no small praise", wrote Sedgwick, "during those days of deep potations among the Country Squires of the North of England."[6] He taught Adam Sedgwick how to fish, and shot grouse enthusiastically on the moors around Dent. Sedgwick's recollections of Richard Willan were written when he was over 80, and it is perhaps not surprising that the old man's memories of the admired friend of his youth may not have been entirely accurate. He recorded that Richard Willan had fought as a volunteer at the battle on the Heights of Abraham, an unlikely story since in 1759 Richard would have been scarcely 13 years old.

According to Sedgwick, Richard Willan retained "his pleasant bright address even to old age." Until weighed down by infirmity, he was "always a welcome guest at the whist table of an evening party at Sedbergh, or at a graver meeting of the intellectual men from the neighbouring Dales." When he died he was buried in Sedbergh churchyard by a priest who was a lifelong friend, and his tombstone stands against the north wall of the church. He was the last of the Willans of Marthwaite.

NOTES

1 MS autograph letter, Ashby Smith to Richard Willan Esq, Maderia, 14 April 1812. Medical Society of London.
2 The Willan genealogy has been derived from the records of the Society of Friends and from wills of several generations of the Willan family.
3 MS will and inventory of Richard Willan, 1706. Lancashire Record Office.
4 Minute books of Sedbergh monthly meeting, 19th 7th mo 1691. County Record Office, Kendal, Cumbria.
5 Penney N. The first publishers of truth. London: Headley Bros, 1907.
6 Sedgwick A. Supplement to the memorial to the trustees of the Cowgill chapel. Cambridge: Cambridge University Press, 1870: 62–4; 212–3.
7 Hartley M, Igilby J. The old hand-knitters of the dales. Clapham: Dalesman Publishing, 1951.
8 MS will of Richard Willan. Lancashire Record Office.

9 Minute books of Sedbergh monthly meeting, 4 November 1717. County Record Office, Kendal, Cumbria.

10 Parish records, Sedbergh Parish Church, kindly provided by the Reverend A Rogers.

11 MS inventory of goods and chattels of Myles Willan, 1720. Lancashire Record Office.

12 MS inventory of goods and chattels of Richard Willan, stockiner, 1734. Lancashire Record Office.

13 Raistrick A. *Quakers in science and industry*. London: Bannisdale Press, 1950: 102.

14 MS will and inventory of Robert Willan, hosier of Castley, 1737. Lancashire Record Office.

15 MS will and inventory of Mary Willan, 1744. Lancashire Record Office.

16 Minute books of Sedbergh monthly meeting, 6th and 7th mo 1758. County Record Office, Kendal, Cumbria.

17 Monro A, *primus*. List of students. Edinburgh University Library.

18 Willan R, Sr. *An essay on the king's evil*. London: M Cooper, 1746.

19 Munk W. *Roll of the Royal College of Physicians of London*. Vol 2. London: Royal College of Physicians, 1878: 350.

20 *Sedbergh School register, 1546–1909*. Leeds; Richard Jackson, 1909: 198.

21 Lane JE. Robert Willan. *Archs Dermatol* 1926; 13: 737–60.

22 Willan R, Jr. *Observations on the sulphur-water at Croft near Darlington*. London: J Johnson and W Brown, 1782.

23 MacCormac H. At the public dispensary with Willan and Bateman. *Br J Dermatol* 1933; 45: 385–95.

24 Beswick TSL. Robert Willan: the solution of a ninety year old mystery. *J Hist Med* 1957; 12: 349–65.

25 Bateman T. Biographical memoir of the late Dr Willan. *Edin Med Surg J* 1812; 8: 502.

26 MS autograph letter, Robert Willan to Dr Lettsom, 12 January 1810. Wellcome Institute Library, Euston Road, London.

27 John Dawson was the mathematical genius who had taught Robert Willan (see Chapter 8).

28 MS autograph letter, Robert Willan to Richard Willan, undated. Library of the Medical Society of London.

29 MS autograph letter, Robert Willan to Richard Willan, 24 February 1805. Library of the Royal College of Physicians of London.

30 MS autograph letter, Robert Willan to Dr Rutter, undated. Library of the Society of Friends, London.

31 Willan R. *The history of the ministry of Jesus Christ, combined from the narrations of the four evangelists*. London: James Phillips and W Brown 1782.

32 Willan R, Willan M. *The united gospel: or ministry of our lord and saviour Jesus Christ, combined from the narrations of the four evangelists*. London: W Phillips, 1803.

33 MS autograph letter, Robert Willan to Richard Willan, undated. Library of the Medical Society of London.

34 Willan R. A list of the ancient words at present used in the mountainous district of the West Riding of Yorkshire. In: *Archaelogia or Miscellaneous tracts relating to Antiquity*. Vol 17. London: Society of Antiquaries of London, 1814: 138.

35 These minutes are preserved in the Library of the Royal College of Physicians of London and have been analysed by MacCormac (see note 23).

36 Lane JE. Portraits of Robert Willan. *Arch Dermatol* 1929; **20**: 54–8.

37 *Gentleman's Magazine* 1812; **82**: 545.

38 Bateman T. *Delineations of cutaneous diseases exhibiting the characteristic appearance of the principal genera and species comprised in the classification of the late Dr Willan: and completing the series of engravings begun by that author*. London: Longman, Hurst, Rees, Orme, and Brown, 1817.

39 Willan was in fact 54 when he died, not 53 as the gravestone states.

40 Minute books of Sedbergh monthly meeting, 29th 7th mo. 1788. County Record Office, Kendal, Cumbria.

8 A rural genius

The men from the Yorkshire dales whom we remember today often made their fame and fortune in cities far from their birthplace, or even in islands overseas. There were also, however, those who stayed at home, farming in fair weather and foul, and living out their lives in the relative obscurity of town or village in the shelter of those northern valleys.

This chapter describes a humble son of one of the Yorkshire dales, a man who had no formal education and who was virtually self taught. Yet he became a country practitioner who knew and tutored some of his most distinguished compatriots. He worked for most of his long life in the valley of his birth, but he was also a remarkable mathematical genius with a well deserved national reputation, and this brought to him as pupils at his modest home at Sedbergh 12 men who were to become senior wranglers at the University of Cambridge.[1]

John Dawson was born at Raygill Farm in Garsdale in 1734. His father, William Dawson, was a "statesman" earning at that time not more than £10 or £12 in a year. Dawson's birthplace is little altered by the passage of nearly 250 years, and the valley of Garsdale, never penetrated by railway or bus route, scarcely visited by tourists even today, is serene and untroubled by the passing centuries. Inside the house the present occupants preserve a carved cupboard door on which can be read the initials JD 1667, inscribed by an earlier member of the Dawson family.

Paper read to the Osler Club, 11 June 1970. *British Medical Journal* 1970; iv: 171–3.

Until he was over 20 years old John Dawson worked as a shepherd on the hills. High on the moor above his home there is a stone called Dawson's Rock where, according to local tradition, young Dawson sat and worked out a system of conic sections entirely for himself. His family's limited resources made formal education unavailable to him, and according to one account Dawson educated himself by begging or borrowing books and doing a little teaching. As early as 1756, however, when he was 22, his reputation as a rural intellect began to be known locally, and in the summer of that year three young men about to enter the University of Cambridge went to read with him. The first was John Haygarth, born in Garsdale at nearby Swarthgill and a pupil at Sedbergh School.[2] Haygarth was then 16 years old and was later to become internationally famous for his work on the epidemiology of infectious disease. The second was a young man called Sedgwick, who became vicar of Dent and the father of Adam Sedgwick, professor of geology at Cambridge. The third became an obscure clergyman in Leicestershire. Sedgwick, according to his son, spoke of this Garsdale summer with Dawson in 1756 as one of great happiness and profit.

Soon after this, Dawson was taken on as an assistant by a Mr Bracken of Lancaster, a well known country surgeon and apothecary with an extensive practice. Here Dawson, too old to be a regular apprentice, learned the rudiments of the profession that was to be his livelihood. Later he set up as a surgeon and apothecary at Sedbergh, the market town at the foot of his native valley and some five miles from his birthplace.

He lived at first a life that was abstemious in the extreme, his purpose being to save up enough money to travel to Edinburgh for further medical study. At the end of that first year, with £100 of hard earned money stitched into the lining of his waistcoat, he set off on foot for the Scottish capital, where he attended classes in medicine. There he lived in conditions of the sternest self denial until his funds ran out, and he then walked back to Sedbergh. His popularity in his native dales was such that work flowed to him and he was continuously sought locally. Within another two years he had saved up £300, and with this sum stitched in small parcels of gold in his waistcoat he travelled to London, mostly on foot, although he is said to have done part of the journey by stage wagon, the mode of transport of the poor. London, however, was more expensive than Edinburgh, and he could not live as quietly as he had there, for in London his mathematical abilities were beginning to be recognised. He got through a course of medical and surgical lectures, obtained some sort of a diploma, and then went back to his home at Sedbergh. For the next 20 or 30 years he earned his living as a practitioner in that town, attending the sick, helping the dying, delivering women in childbirth, occupying himself with the manifold duties of the dedicated country doctor. He married Ann Thirlbeck in 1767, when he was 33, and the ceremony was conducted by Dr Bateman, then headmaster of Sedbergh School and Robert Willan's classical teacher. Dawson and his wife had one daughter.

We know little of his method of practice. But Robert Willan, a pupil of Dawson's before he went to Edinburgh University, refers to him in a letter to his brother Richard, living at the family home near Sedbergh, whom Dawson was evidently attending.[3] Sedgwick, vicar at nearby Dent, called him in 1785 to deliver his wife of their son, Adam, and John Haygarth, Sedgwick's fellow pupil with Dawson in 1756, gives a case report received from Dawson in 1780 in one of his books on smallpox.[4] By now Haygarth was at Chester, developing his plans for exterminating casual smallpox from Great Britain and advising the introduction of general inoculation. It was just a few years before Jenner's discovery. Dawson describes the death from confluent smallpox of a young man called John Airey in a fetid upstairs room in a back street at Sedbergh. His report describes the preventive measures that he took and shows how, despite the fact that many were susceptible, no one else in the town contracted the disease. This is interesting, since it shows that Dawson at that time was following the rules laid down by Haygarth, his fellow dalesman, for the treatment and prevention of infectious fevers. These were the rules that Haygarth later

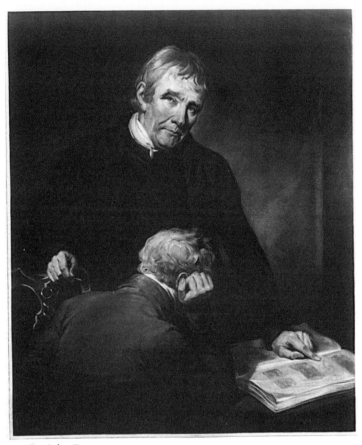

11   Dr John Dawson
(Royal College of Physicians of London)

published as his famous *Letter to Dr Percival on the Prevention of Infectious Fevers*, rules of isolation, cleanliness, and ventilation which have persisted to this day.[5]

In 1790 Dawson relinquished his practice as an apothecary but he lived on until 1820, dying a venerable intellectual ruin at the advanced age of 86. He was known, revered, and respected in his native valleys as the local medical practitioner. But it is not for this that he is remembered, but for his mathematics, which won him renown as a remarkable and influential tutor. In many ways it is through his pupils that we know him today.

How Dawson developed his mathematical abilities is not known. He published relatively little, but engaged in controversy with William Emerson, who refused to accept some of Thomas Simpson's work pointing out a slip by Newton in the problem of precession. Dawson's independent analysis supported Simpson. In 1769 Dawson, the country practitioner, wrote an anonymous pamphlet in reply to a geometrical essay by Mathew Stewart, professor of mathematics at the University of Edinburgh. Stewart had tried to calculate the distance of the sun from the earth using the theory of gravity, attempting to determine the extent to which the orbit of the moon around the earth is disturbed by gravitational pull in different positions. In his pamphlet Dawson pointed out that the only really effective way of calculating the sun's distance was by a careful observation of the transit of Venus,[6] and it was to do this that James Cook, another Yorkshireman, sailed to Tahiti in that year on his first voyage of exploration. Dawson was proved right in this controversy, and this brought him the friendship and esteem of a wide group of philosophers of the time. He was visited at Sedbergh by the Edinburgh mathematician John Playfair, by Lord Webb Seymour, and later by Lord Brougham. His other publications included an analysis of the work of the Reverend C Wildbore, who had sought to describe the velocities of water issuing from a vessel in motion. Dawson was also interested in theology, and in 1781 published a tract attacking Joseph Priestley's doctrine of philosophical necessity.

Dawson's reputation as a mathematical teacher and his method of teaching have been well described by Adam Sedgwick, who was his pupil in 1804, and who must be considered one of Dawson's most brilliant pupils. It was with Sedgwick, then professor at Cambridge, that Charles Darwin in the summer of 1831 spent several weeks studying rock formations in Wales and making a geological map of the country. In fact on his return home from this trip on 29 August he was greeted with the letter from George Peacock offering him the post of naturalist on the *Beagle*. Darwin once described Sedgwick as a "talking giant," and when he got to Ascension Island on his way home from his epic voyage he related how the news that Sedgwick had said that "Charles Darwin should take a place amongst the leading scientific men" fired him with enthusiasm for geology. "After reading this letter," wrote Darwin, "I clambered over the mountains with a bounding step and made the volcanic rocks resound under my geological hammer."[7]

According to Sedgwick, Dawson took students during the summer vacations, and after giving up his practice in 1790 he devoted himself entirely to mathematical teaching. He charged five shillings a week for instruction and would teach for as long as his pupils would learn. His pupils seem to have come from far and wide. Dr Butler, later headmaster of Harrow, was his pupil in 1792. In a letter he describes his journey from the south and how he paid one and sixpence a week for an excellent room at the best hotel in town, the King's Arms. Breakfast was twopence, and dinner for tenpence a day was "a leg of mutton and potatoes both hot; ham and tongue, gooseberry tarts, cheese, butter and bread; pretty well for tenpence." Between 1781 and 1794 Dawson had eight senior wranglers among his pupils, and the senior wranglers for 1797, 1798, 1800, and 1807 were all Dawson's men. One of these was James Inman, another Garsdale man, afterwards mathematical professor at the Royal Naval College and the author of Inman's tables. In addition to these men, Dawson's pupils included John Haygarth and Robert Willan, to whom reference has been made, George Birkbeck of Settle, the founder of Mechanics' Institutes, and Adam Sedgwick. Such a galaxy of intellectual talent is a remarkable tribute to the abilities of this extraordinary country practitioner.

Whether Dawson was ever on the staff of Sedbergh School as a regular teacher is uncertain. A fair number of Sedbergh boys may well have benefited from his instruction, though only three of his senior wranglers were Sedberghians. He certainly had close links with the school, for the school history records how Dawson wrote a memorandum describing the problems of Dr Bateman, the headmaster who had officiated at his wedding. "People here," wrote Dawson, "have made free with him. He has twice been pulled by the nose, besides being very rudely teated in other ways." Such was the lot of the eighteenth century schoolmaster.

In these days, when mathematics are vital for the analysis of the results of clinical investigation, it is interesting to look back and examine whether Dawson's mathematical abilities were ever applied to the medicine that he practised. We have no record of whether this was so, but his pupil and neighbour from Garsdale, John Haygarth, certainly made use of his ingenuity. In his *Inquiry into How to Prevent the Small Pox*, published when he was working at Chester, Haygarth records how "It occurred to me that it might be computed arithmetically by the doctrine of chances...if one, two or three persons were exposed to the variolous infection, what degree of probability there was that one or more of these would catch the distemper."[8] Dawson calculated the odds for Haygarth on the assumption that one person in 20 might be not liable to smallpox. So that if a single child in a family escapes the disorder then the likelihood that he was never exposed is probable in a degree of 19 to 1. If two in a family escape the probability is 400 to 1, and if three escape then the odds are above 8000 to 1. Later on, when Haygarth had come to believe that it would be possible to exterminate smallpox in the community, Dawson calculated for him the increase in population that might result. This was done on the assumption that either 30 000 or 35 000 people might survive annually if the disease were eradicated.[4]

One of the surviving portraits of Dawson shows him sitting on a rock with the old Sedbergh schoolhouse, now the school library, in the background. Adam Sedgwick has left us a delightful description of his admired teacher. "Simple in manner," he wrote, "cheerful and mirthful in temper, with a dress approaching that of the higher class of venerable old Quakers of the Dales, without any stiffness or affectation of superiority, yet did he bear at first sight a very commanding presence...His powerful, projecting forehead and well-chiselled features told of much thought, and might have implied severity had not a soft radiant benevolence played over his fine old face..."[9]

Dawson died on 19 September 1820 and he was buried at Sedbergh. Some years later his former pupils erected a monument to his memory in the church. There the fine black marble bust of John Dawson can be seen today. The inscription was written by John Bell of Trinity, distinguished leader in the Chancery Bar and senior wrangler in 1786, and it reads "In memory of John Dawson of Sedbergh...Distinguished by his profound knowledge of mathematics, beloved for his amiable simplicity of character, and revered for his exemplary discharge of every moral and religious duty."

That simple character, John Dawson, perhaps would not have wished that he should be remembered today by the publication of an account of his life. But it serves to illustrate how this remarkable man achieved serenity in the obscurity of medical practice and in the study of mathematics in a remote valley of the Yorkshire dales.

NOTES

1 Clark JW, Hughes T McK. *The life and letters of the Reverend Adam Sedgwick*. Cambridge: Cambridge University Press, 1890: 60–70.
2 Elliott J. A medical pioneer: John Haygarth of Chester. *Br Med J* 1913; i: 235–41.
3 MS autograph letter, Robert Willan to Richard Willan, undated. Library of the Medical Society of London. (See also Chapter 7.)
4 Haygarth J. *A sketch of a plan to exterminate the casual small pox from Great Britain and to introduce general inoculation*. London: J Johnson, 1793: 193; 205.
5 Haygarth J. *A letter to Dr Percival on the prevention of infectious fevers*. Bath: R Cruttwell, 1801.
6 Dawson J. *Four propositions showing not only that the distance of the sun as attempted to be determined from the theory of gravity by a late author is upon his own principles erroneous but also that it is more probable this capital question can never be satisfactorily answered by any calculus of this kind*. Newcastle: J White and T Saint, 1769.
7 Moorhead A. *Darwin and the Beagle*. London: Hamish Hamilton, 1969.
8 Haygarth J. *An inquiry into how to prevent the small pox*. London: J Johnson, 1784.
9 Sedgwick A. *Supplement to the memorial to the trustees of the Cowgill chapel*. Cambridge: Cambridge University Press, 1870: 49.

9 The conquest of smallpox

The origins of smallpox are shrouded in mystery. Smallpox virus has uniquely afflicted man and it presumably first emerged as a viral mutation during or after the neolithic revolution, when the introduction of new methods of agriculture and the herding of cattle led to the creation of the earliest civilised communities. There are those who believe that the skin rash of the mummy of Rameses V of Egypt, who died in the twelfth century BC, was due to smallpox. If this were so it is curious that there is no clear description of the disease either in the Biblical record, or in the Hippocratic writings, or in any of the medical texts of the Roman era. In fact it seems likely that smallpox had its origins in the orient. It appears to have been present in India since the earliest times. It was known in China in the Tcheou dynasty, about 1100 BC, when the name for the malady was "tai-tou." Smallpox was later recorded in Arabia in the sixth century at the siege of Mecca and it seems likely that the disease was brought into Europe through Spain, following its conquest by the Moors in 710. Nevertheless, there is also evidence that the disease was already present in Europe at an earlier date. Gregory of Tours gives a description of the condition in France in the sixth century and an epidemic is referred to by Marius, Bishop of Avenche in AD 570. It was he who first used the term "Variola." The first clear description of the disease, however, was written by the great Arabic physician Rhazes, who worked in Baghdad and who died about AD 930.[1]

The Jenner lecture given at St George's Hospital Medical School, 7 March 1985. *Quarterly Journal of Medicine* 1985; 57: 811–23.

It was an ubiquitous disorder that respected no one and afflicted virtually all susceptible individuals at some stage of their lives. Variola major had a high mortality, particularly among children, with case fatality rates of as much as 20 or 40%. There was, however, another minor form of the disease, with a far lower mortality. Those who survived were often severely disfigured, and sometimes alopecic, and the eyes were not infrequently affected so that smallpox was an important cause of blindness from corneal scarring. Three of the early Arab caliphs were apparently pitted with smallpox and two had a white spot in each of their eyes. As with other infectious diseases, smallpox was often spread by travellers. The Spaniards took smallpox with them to the West Indies in 1507 and to Mexico in 1520 resulting in devastating epidemics which decimated the native Indian population. It has been stated that the phenomenal success of a few conquistadores in defeating the Aztec and Inca kingdoms may have been in large part due to an epidemic of smallpox in the New World, which is thought to have caused more than three and a half million deaths within a few years.[2] There is also some evidence to suggest that hostile Indians were sometimes deliberately exposed to the disease for the purpose of causing epidemics, a practice which was not restricted to the American continent during the colonial era.

From the sixteenth to the eighteenth centuries smallpox was the most devastating disease in the Western world. It destroyed dynasties, decimated armies and broke hearts. Lord Macaulay in a famous passage described the disease in the seventeenth century as "the most terrible of the ministers of death...smallpox was always present filling the church-yards with corpses...and making the eyes and cheeks of the betrothed maiden objects of horror to the lover." Queen Elizabeth suffered from it, became bald as a result of her illness and throughout her life was concerned about the disfiguring marks on her face. The brother of King Charles II died from a malignant attack soon after the royal family returned to London after the Restoration in 1660. Queen Mary II, wife of William of Orange, died of the disease in London in 1694, and the Duke of Gloucester, only surviving

child of Queen Anne, died of smallpox in 1700. This precipitated a constitutional crisis which resulted in the Act of
Settlement ensuring the Protestant Hanoverian succcession
after her death and it also established that no King or Queen
of England could leave the country without permission.
Hence the accession of George I and the Hanoverian dynasty
were due to smallpox. The Emperor Joseph of Austria
succumbed to a severe attack in 1717, and in 1774 Louis XV
was at the Trianon, favourite retreat of his mistress, la
Marquise de Pompadour, when by candlelight the early
lesions of smallpox were first noted on his skin. His death
from the disease soon afterwards at Versailles was made
known to a waiting world when the candle which had been
kept burning in a window of his room was extinguished.
George Washington was fortunate in surviving an attack
during his visit to Barbados in 1751, developing an immunity
which protected him during that winter which "tried men's
souls" at Valley Forge in 1777, when smallpox broke out in
the American revolutionary army.

It is not surprising that from the earliest times there should
have been attempts to control, or treat, so dread a disease,
however unavailing the methods used. In India there was a
centuries old custom of propitiating Shitala Mata, the Hindu
goddess of smallpox. Traditionally she is represented as
riding on a donkey with a basketful of grain upon her head.
In one hand she has a pitcher of water and in the other a
broom. The belief has been that when she shakes her head she
spills the grain and each grain turns into a smallpox pustule.
The victim survived if she cleaned the spilt grain with water,
but did not if she used only the dry broom.[3] Belief in such
superstition may seem naive today but it was unquestionably
less harmful to the patient than the murderous regimens of
bleeding and purging to which English physicians for
centuries condemned their unfortunate patients.

The first protective measure to emerge was the technique
of inoculation, inducing a mild and usually non-fatal attack
of the disease. Material was taken from a smallpox vesicle
and inoculated into the skin. Some days later a mild rash,
with relatively few pustules, would develop around the site of

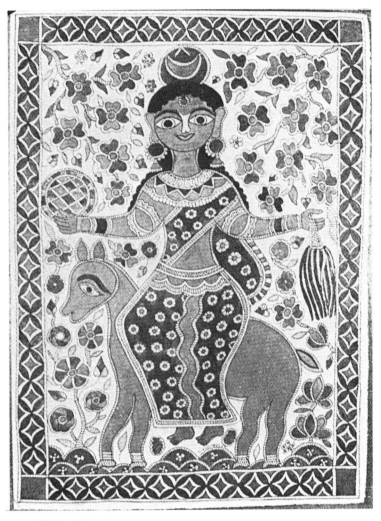

12   Shitala Mata

inoculation and thereafter the individual usually had a lifelong protection. The origins of the practice are lost in
antiquity. It appears to have been part of folk medicine in
Europe as early as the seventeenth century for there are
reports that "buying the smallpox," in which smallpox scabs

were rubbed into the skin, was a common practice in Wales, Poland, and southern Italy. It is also evident that African folk medicine knew of the efficacy of inoculation since the Reverend Cotton Mather of Boston, notorious for his part in the witchcraft trials of Salem, learnt of the practice from his African slave Onisemus in 1716, and Cadwallader Colden recorded the use of inoculation among his slaves in a communication to a society of physicians in London in 1753. The practice may well have originally developed in China, and a report to the Royal Society in London in 1700 described the Chinese method of inoculation against smallpox by inserting crust material into the nostrils of the individual.[4]

In England the deaths of Queen Mary and of the son and heir of Queen Anne made a deep impression in court circles and among men of learning. There was therefore considerable interest in the practice of inoculation when reports of its use in Turkey first reached London during the second decade of the eighteenth century. Edward Tarry was practising medicine in the Levant in 1706 and when he returned to Enfield in 1712 he claimed to have seen 4000 inoculated. There were discussions on the practice of inoculation at the Royal Society during the next two years but it was the account sent from Turkey by the Italian physician Dr Emanuel Timoni in 1714 that commanded the most attention.[5] His paper was read to the Royal Society on 3 June. The Royal Society continued to seek information from physicians in Turkey as a result of Timoni's report. Further interest was created by the return to London in 1716 of the two sons of the secretary to the British ambassador in Turkey, both of whom had been safely inoculated. In July of that year Cotton Mather wrote to the Royal Society from Boston with the information on inoculation obtained from his African slave and asked why the practice had not been tried in England. Despite the interest created by these events nothing active was done by any fellow of the Royal Society, nor did any member of the medical profession have the courage to recommend inoculation in this country. The effective introduction of the practice into Britain was due not to the efforts of a conservative medical profession but to the energy and enthusiasm of a young society belle and lady of letters whose own beauty had been ravished by an attack of smallpox despite the ministrations of the most distinguished members of the Royal College of Physicians of London. As a result she was to hate and mistrust the orthodox medical profession until her dying day.

Lady Mary Wortley Montagu was born in 1695, the daughter of Henry Pierrepoint, Lord Kingston, a member of the famous Kit Cat Club whose members included the architect Vanbrugh, the Dukes of Marlborough and New-castle, Addison, Steele, Congreve, and the physician and poet Samuel Garth.[6] According to her granddaughter, Lady Louisa Stuart, Lady Mary had been brought to the club as a child by her father, and passed from lap to distinguished lap before being toasted as their beauty of the year by the members, a day that she would never forget. As a young woman she was a close friend of Alexander Pope, a friendship sadly to end in recrimination. He mocked her as "Sappho at her toilet's greasy task" in his *Epistle on the Characters of Women* and he may have had her in mind when he wrote that "every woman is at heart a rake." Lady Mary herself wrote satirical poetry which achieved a certain contemporary fame. She married Henry Wortley Montagu, younger son of the Earl of Sandwich, in 1712, and in 1715 suffered the severe attack of smallpox which seriously afflicted her good looks. She was attended by Dr Hans Sloane, as he then was, and her father's friend of the Kit Cat Club, Sir Samuel Garth, known as much for his poetry as for his medical skills. Lady Mary's disillusion with her medical advisers was expressed in the verses she wrote after her recovery. Garth, she wrote, was

Known

By his red cloak and his superior frown,
And why, he cried, this grief and this despair?
You shall again be well, again be fair:
Believe my oath; (with that an oath he swore),
False was his oath; my beauty is no more.

She recovered, however, with the loss of her eyelashes, and a year later, her husband was appointed British ambassador to Turkey. She immediately became interested in the technique of variolation to prevent smallpox and within a few weeks of her arrival there, in the spring of 1717, she wrote her famous letter to Sarah Chiswell describing, not entirely accurately, the practice of inoculation as carried out in Constantinople. In 1718, with the help of Charles Maitland, surgeon to the embassy, she had her son safely inoculated. The boy developed about 100 crusts in all, but they all fell off "without leaving any one mark or impress behind them."

Lady Mary left Constantinople in 1718 and returned to England, where in the spring of 1721 an epidemic of smallpox raged in London with a high mortality in children. She now had her daughter inoculated, again by Maitland, and she invited three learned physicians of the Royal College of Physicians of London, one of them Sir Hans Sloane, to visit the young lady. There may have been an element of vindictiveness in this last invitation, since she so well remembered Sir Hans's visit to her when she lay ill with smallpox "masked o'er and trembling at the sight of day." Sir Hans, she had written

> came, my fortune to deplore,
> (A golden-headed cane well carved he bore)
> Cordials, he cried, my spirits must restore:
> Beauty is fled and spirit is no more.

It was an experience she intended that her own children should never suffer.

Sir Hans Sloane seems at this time, nevertheless, to have been unconvinced about the virtues of the procedure and it was probably Princess Caroline, the Princess of Wales, and possibly Lady Mary herself who played an influential role in arranging for the so called Newgate experiments to be carried out. The Princess's daughter had recently had smallpox and she was anxious that her other children be inoculated. Before this was done inoculation was successfully carried out by Maitland on six Newgate felons who were pardoned for their participation in this experiment, and soon afterwards the royal children were themselves inoculated. It was perhaps natural that women, who will risk much in the search for beauty, as well as for their children, should have been the prime movers in introducing inoculation in Britain.

With royal patronage the practice became fashionable and throughout the latter half of the eighteenth century inoculation was the method of prevention universally adopted. James Jurin, secretary to the Royal Society and later physician to Guy's Hospital, played a leading role in obtaining statistical evidence on the efficacy of inoculation, and the physician Richard Mead became an important early supporter of the practice.[7] There was at first considerable controversy over the best method of inoculation. There was also the disadvantage that there was a distinct mortality, which led to considerable opposition. The practice lost ground during the 1730s and before 1740 inoculation was practised only on an insignificant scale. Contemporary hesitation by medical men to recommend inoculation was clearly stated by Dr William Hillary, in his book *A Rational and Mechanical Essay on the Small Pox*, which was published in 1735.[8] By 1750, however, the practice was gaining ground and a London physician, writing to a brother who had just lost his eldest son from smallpox, strongly recommended inoculation for his remaining children and told him that it was "an operation easy to be performed." He went on to describe how a common sewing thread should be pulled through a ripe pock, dried, and then put into a dry vial or little box. When needed, an eighth of an inch or so of thread was cut off, and this was laid on an area of skin that had been scratched with the point of a needle. A plaster was applied and the whole was done.[9] It was not, however, until the Suttons introduced their improved method of inoculation in the 1760s that the practice became widely popular.[10] Other practitioners of inoculation included Dr Thomas Dimsdale, who travelled to Russia in 1768 at the request of Catherine the Great, whom he inoculated together with her son.[11] Dimsdale was rewarded with £10000 and Catherine created him a Baron of the Empire. In the second half of the eighteenth century increasing numbers of individuals were inoculated throughout England, and general inoculations were introduced in a number of towns throughout the kingdom. In the American colonies, Benjamin Franklin had been an early supporter of innoculation, particularly after the death of his 4 year old son in 1736. It is a feature of the heartbreak caused by smallpox that even in old age this unsentimental old philosopher grieved for his boy "of whom," he wrote, "I could never think without a sigh."[12] He, therefore, had a particular personal reason for publishing an account of the success of inoculation in America in 1759, together with "Plain Instructions by which any person may be enabled to perform the operation" – instructions which were written in plain English, easy for a layman to understand, by Samuel Johnson's admired physician, Dr William Heberden.[13] The results of these efforts appear to have been a significant reduction in the smallpox mortality during the eighteenth century, the figures for Boston, Massachusetts, for example, falling from 175 deaths from smallpox per 1000 population in 1677–8 to 10 per 1000, or even less, during 1778 and 1792.[14]

One of the factors contributing to the dilatoriness of the orthodox medical profession of the day in recognising the value of inoculation in preventing smallpox may have been their conception of the mode of propagation of contagious distempers. For more than a century the ideas of Thomas Sydenham had prevailed and his theories had been accepted without hesitation by later writers. Sydenham held that the epidemic propagation of contagious disease was to be attributed to the inherent constitution of the individual as well as to a "peculiar occult constitution of the air." This view was reflected by Richard Mead in his discourse concerning pestilential contagion, published in 1720, in which he wrote that "when the constitution of the air happens to favour infection it rages with great violence." As a young man, Sir Hans Sloane had been recommended as a pupil to Sydenham and he was imbued with the same ideas.

The idea that the spread of infectious disease was due to atmospheric miasmata was not really challenged until John Haygarth, working as a physician in Chester in the late eighteenth century, began to "ascertain by clinical observations according to what law the variolous infection is propagated." Haygarth was refreshingly blunt in his condemnation of Sydenham's ideas. "While such an opinion prevails," he wrote, "the wildest visionary can never entertain a hope to retard the progress of this malady [smallpox] except by prayer and the merciful interposition of Providence." He soon established to his own satisfaction that a patient with smallpox was infectious but only to a distance of a very few feet. Immediate contact was not always the usual transfer and he concluded that the air could transmit infection. These conclusions led him in 1778 to propose the formation of a Smallpox Society in Chester which would have as its purpose the promotion of inoculation for the effective prevention of smallpox, together with a strict policy of isolation. A general inoculation was to be carried out every two years and in the intervals rules for prevention were introduced. These rules contained useful advice on cleanliness but the most significant was the effective isolation of the patient.[15] It was Haygarth who first recognised the importance of isolation in the control of epidemics and in 1783 he introduced separate fever wards at the Chester Hospital, the first example of the use of isolation in the control of infectious fevers in hospital.[16]

In the story of the conquest of smallpox, Haygarth's long forgotten contribution has been largely overshadowed by Jenner's discovery of vaccination at the end of the eighteenth century, yet Haygarth had the vision to see that it should be possible to eradicate smallpox completely. He recognised that any attempt to exterminate, or even to limit it, might be thought "too visionary or chimerical to deserve any serious attention," an interesting forewarning of the misgivings expressed by many when the World Health Organisation embarked on its eradication programme. Yet as early as 1778, the year after smallpox had raged among the troops of Washington's army at Valley Forge, he had submitted a plan for exterminating smallpox in Great Britain to his friend and fellow dalesman, the London physician Dr John Fothergill. Fothergill had always been interested in smallpox; it was he who recommended his fellow Quaker Dr Thomas Dimsdale to Catherine the Great's ambassador in London.

Haygarth subsequently published his *Sketch of a plan to exterminate the casual smallpox from Great Britain and to introduce General Inoculation* in 1793.[17] Haygarth's plan was ambitious and far ahead of its time. He proposed a nationwide policy of inoculation which would be reinforced by legal authority, with directors, inspectors, rewards, and punishments. In particular he favoured the enactment of a law to reward the observation of his rules of prevention, which had proved so successful in Chester. Transgression was to be punished by a fine and, if unable to pay, the offender was to be publicly exposed in the nearest market town with a label on his breast saying "Behold a villain who has wilfully and wickedly spread the smallpox." He recognised that his plan might be dismissed as too visionary, and that it might be seen as either "an extravagant and dangerous innovation," or as "an invasion of personal liberty." He was anxious to encourage a dispassionate and considered debate of his proposals and earnestly entreated his readers not to dismiss his ideas out of hand. He also included the calculations made by his old mathematical teacher, John Dawson of Sedbergh, on the increase that might be expected to occur in the population of Great Britain were smallpox to be eradicated. It is interesting to speculate what might have happened if vaccination had not been discovered by Jenner within five years of the publication of Haygarth's book.

The conquest of smallpox owes a great deal to folk medicine and to the beliefs of country people. As has been shown, inoculation which was essential in paving the way for the discovery of vaccination, emerged from the practices of the unorthodox. Vaccination also had its roots in folk medicine. As with so many discoveries, claims for priority are often advanced by others after the fruits of a new idea have already become apparent. Although Jenner's book on the "Variolae vaccinae" was not published until 1798, there is evidence that individuals had occasionally inoculated cowpox as a means of preventing smallpox. Benjamin Jesty, a farmer who lived near Yeovil in Somerset, vaccinated his wife and two sons with cowpox material in 1774, the year of the death of Louis XV, but the same two sons were inoculated in the traditional manner 15 years later, which does little to strengthen the view that cowpox was thought universally to be protective.[4] There is no evidence that Jenner knew of Jesty's activities and it is to Jenner alone, as Parliament was later to recognise, that the credit for introducing vaccination belongs.

Edward Jenner was born in May 1749 in Berkeley near Bristol, the son of a country parson.[18] He was first apprenticed to a surgeon apothecary in Sodbury and then came to London in 1770. He was registered as a surgical pupil of Mr Hunter's at St George's Hospital in October of that year. At the hospital he would have undertaken the usual tasks of a student, attending at operations and helping with dressings. But Jenner was also a resident at John Hunter's house in Jermyn Street and was a pupil at the Hunters' famous anatomy school in Windmill Street. It was here that he first met Joseph Banks, future president of the Royal Society. In 1771 Lieutenant James Cook had returned to England in the *Endeavour*, after his first voyage during which he had explored the whole coast of both islands of New Zealand and the eastern seaboard of Australia. Joseph Banks, who had ample private means, had been the naturalist on the *Endeavour* and he had returned laden with South Sea trophies. He now needed help with arranging the extensive collection of specimens that he had made during the voyage. It was Hunter who suggested that his pupil Edward Jenner should be employed to sort out the material and mount and classify the various specimens. Banks was so impressed with the young Jenner's work that he offered him the post of botanist on the *Resolution*, then being prepared for Cook's remarkable second voyage; Zoffany was to have been the artist. None of this came to pass for Cook to his relief sailed without Joseph Banks; and Jenner, unhappy in London, returned to his native Gloucestershire. Here he worked as a country surgeon but indulged his love of natural history. He corresponded faithfully with his old teacher John Hunter who ensured his election as a fellow of the Royal Society in 1788. His first degree of MD was obtained from the University of St Andrews in 1792, a simple matter requiring only a fee and a recommendation, but he was now a physician and could be addressed as doctor.

Jenner as a country practitioner undertook the task of inoculation for his patients. He had always been interested in smallpox and before he went to London, when he was an apprentice in Sodbury, he had been intrigued by the chance remark of a dairy maid that an attack of cowpox might prevent smallpox; but the subject apparently never formed part of his correspondence with John Hunter, though he may have discussed cowpox with his friends in London during a visit in 1788. It was in fact an epidemic of smallpox in his native Gloucestershire in 1778 after his return from London that stimulated his further interest, because he found that there were individuals who were utterly resistant to all his attempts to inoculate them with smallpox. He noted that these were patients who had contracted cowpox previously. For some years Jenner was concerned with defining the different pustular diseases of the udders of the cow as well as studying the condition of grease in horses. John Haygarth, hearing of his efforts, wrote from Chester in 1794 to Jenner's ecclesiastical friend Dr Worthington, "I hope no reliance will be placed upon vulgar stories, the author should admit nothing but what has been proved by his own personal observation, both in the brute and human species." It was an interesting echo of John Hunter's famous advice not to speculate, but to experiment.

Two years later Jenner first successfully demonstrated that the boy James Phipps, inoculated in the arm with cowpox obtained from the hand of a milkmaid, Sarah Nelmes, could not then receive smallpox by inoculation. Sarah's cowpox was contracted from the cow "Blossom" whose hide is preserved in the library of St George's Hospital. Jenner sent his account of this experiment to his friend Everard Home, John Hunter's brother in law, for submission to the Royal Society. Home thought the account curious, but quite naturally he was not satisfied with a single case only, or with the apparent paradox, pointed out by Jenner, that an individual might have cowpox twice. If 20 or 30 children were inoculated with the cowpox and afterwards with the smallpox without contracting it he might be led to change his opinion. At present, however, he told Sir Joseph Banks in a letter preserved in the library of the Royal Botanic Gardens in Kew, "I want faith."[19]

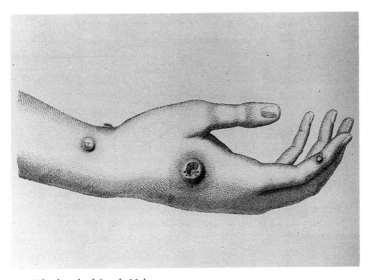

13 The hand of Sarah Nelmes
(Royal College of Physicians of London)

Banks quite reasonably returned Jenner's paper on the grounds that the technique of vaccination had not been satisfactorily validated and he did not refer the paper to the committee responsible for the publication of the *Philosophical Transactions*. It was for this reason that the Royal Society did not publish this epoch making discovery by one of its most distinguished fellows (see Chapter 1). Jenner did not in fact write up his findings until two years later, when, after further experiments, he published the *Inquiry into the causes and effects of Variolae Vaccinae* – literally, smallpox of the cow – as a book dedicated to his friend and collaborator, Dr Caleb Hillier Parry.[20]

Jenner's discovery, as with so many others that have benefited mankind, was not greeted with wholehearted and general enthusiasm at once. But there were some who were immediately impressed, among them the London physician and pupil of John Fothergill, John Coakley Lettsom. Lettsom was one of Jenner's earliest supporters and he at once sent a copy of the *Variolae Vaccinae* to Fothergill's cousin in

Boston, Benjamin Waterhouse, whom he had known as a student in London. Dr Henry Cline was the first to use Jenner's vaccine in the capital city and Dr William Woodville and Dr George Pearson, who had obtained cowpox material from a dairy in Gray's Inn Lane, were later responsible for carrying out numerous vaccinations in the metropolis.[4]

Although Woodville and Pearson found reason to disagree with Jenner on a variety of matters, their extensive experience effectively confirmed his observations and led to widespread acceptance of the procedure.[21] In 1803 Lettsom ensured that Jenner was awarded the Fothergillian medal of the Medical Society of London, and his portrait was added to the famous painting of the members of that society receiving the title deeds of their house from Lettsom. By 1806 even the conservative Royal College of Physicians of London, which never admitted Jenner – an unlettered surgeon unversed in the ancients – to their membership, had produced a report supporting vaccination. But there were others who considered the practice to be contrary to the will of God. Some said that smallpox was sent to chasten the population. Birch suggested that smallpox was "a merciful provision on the part of Providence to lessen the burthen of a poor man's family" and Rowley, a learned member of the University of Oxford, argued that it was "impious and profane to wrest out of the hands of the Almighty the Divine dispensation of Providence," a view which that blunt Yorkshireman John Haygarth would have fiercely disputed.

On the Continent, however, where inoculation had never enjoyed the support it received in England, the practice of vaccination spread rapidly. By 1799 vaccinations had been carried out in Hanover and Vienna and by a year later in Greece, Turkey, and as far afield as India and Ceylon. In 1800, despite the Napoleonic wars, France sent observers to England and Woodville took vaccine to Paris. By 1805, the year of Trafalgar, Napoleon had ordered the vaccination of all troops who had not had smallpox.

Although at that time nothing could travel faster than a horse on land or than the vagaries of the wind would drive a sailing ship at sea, it was remarkable how the extensive correspondence of the intimate world of medical savants ensured that they kept abreast of the latest developments. In the United States, Waterhouse had published news of Jenner's discovery in the Boston newspapers in 1799 as soon as he received his copy of Jenner's *Inquiry* from Lettsom. A year later he obtained lymph from his old friend John Haygarth, then removed from Chester to Bath, where he was living in some style at No 15, The Royal Crescent. Haygarth, for whom Waterhouse had obtained the honorary degree of MD at Harvard in 1794, was an enthusiastic supporter of Jenner and the first vaccine institution in England was founded in Bath, the home of Caleb Hillier Parry, the physician to whom Jenner had dedicated his work in 1798.

On 8 July 1800 Waterhouse vaccinated his son and soon afterwards six members of his household. He then asked Dr Aspen Wall, of the Inoculation Hospital in Brookline, to inoculate them with smallpox. None responded. Waterhouse, therefore, deserves considerable credit, firstly for having acted upon Jenner's experiments, then for having repeated them, and finally for having shown clearly to himself and to his fellow citizens that vaccination could successfully protect against smallpox. There were problems over the supply of lymph in New England at this early stage, with Waterhouse initially seeking to maintain a monopoly. He soon realised the error of his ways, however, and from 1801 a universal supply was assured. In later years Oliver Wendell Holmes was to remember being vaccinated as a child sitting on the knee of the aging Benjamin Waterhouse.

Jenner, however, made one major error in his assessment of the value of vaccination. To the day that he died from a cerebral haemorrhage in 1823 – the year of the foundation of the *Lancet* – he believed that a single vaccination would prevent smallpox. As Everard Home had pointed out in 1796 in his review of Jenner's first paper offered to the Royal Society, cowpox could occur more than once, suggesting that immunity might not be lifelong. But it was not until a significant number of cases of smallpox had occurred in vaccinated individuals that it was realised that repeated vaccination was necessary.

The government's actions on vaccination began with the awards to Jenner by Parliament of £10000 in 1802 and of a further £20000 in 1806. The remainder of the nineteenth century was taken up with legislation. The first Vaccination Act, which empowered guardians and overseers of parishes in England and Wales to contract with registered medical practitioners to perform vaccinations, was passed in 1840. The eighth section of this Act proposed by Thomas Wakley, the founder and editor of the *Lancet*, who was now a member of Parliament, made the old practice of inoculation illegal. Other Acts followed, all encouraging compulsory vaccination of infants, but vaccination was never universal and at the end of the century a conscientious objection clause was introduced, which effectively reduced the number of the population vaccinated. Smallpox was therefore never eradicated, and although it became rare in Britain it continued to occur right up to the era of the eradication programme of the World Health Organisation (WHO). There was smallpox in London in 1927, in Bilston in 1947, and further outbreaks occurred in Glasgow in 1950, in Brighton in 1950-1, and in the industrial Pennines in 1953.[4]

Who it was who first conceived the idea that smallpox really could be totally eradicated is uncertain. Jenner, writing of vaccination in 1801, considered that "the annihilation of the smallpox the most dreadful scourge of the human species must be the result of this practice,"[22] yet it was to be 177 years before this dream came true. One of the first initiatives was taken by the Pan-American Health Organisation in 1950. Stimulated by its director, the organisation resolved to eradicate smallpox from the Americas. By 1958 considerable progress had been made, but there was still smallpox in Brazil, Colombia, Peru, and Ecuador. At the same time the new communist regime of Mao Tse Tung, with its commitment to the welfare of the people of China, embarked on a mass vaccination campaign which was launched in 1950. With excellent organisation and widespread community cooperation the programme was entirely successful and by 1960 endemic smallpox had been eradicated from China, the last case occurring in the southern province of Yunnan. Since then there have been no imported cases.

There had been a number of tentative initiatives at the WHO during the same period but the commitment of the organisation to total eradication began in 1958, when Professor Victor Zhdanov, Vice Minister of Health in the Soviet Union, proposed to the World Health Assembly that the global eradication of smallpox should be undertaken. At first the programme entailed worldwide mass vaccination programmes aiming at 80% of the population. This was an enormous task and in those early years it was all too apparent that it was not succeeding. An expert committee called together by WHO in 1964 recommended that the target should be increased to 100% of the population, manifestly an impossible undertaking. In 1966 the World Health Assembly made a last effort to rescue the programme which was in obvious danger of total collapse. A large sum ($2·5 million) was voted for smallpox eradication, an important proportion of the assembly's budget. At that time there were still 34 countries in which smallpox was endemic so the budget, on average, represented no more that $75 000 per country. It had to be admitted that only the most visionary among the delegates really believed that eradication was feasible.[23]

There were, however, a number of technical advances in smallpox control that were vital in ensuring the final successful outcome.[24] The first was the development of effective heat stable vaccines. The original fluid lymph could not be maintained in the environment of developing countries where the absence of electricity or effective refrigeration made preservation impossible. Between 1948 and 1953 however, LH Collier, working at the Lister Institute in London, had succeeded in developing a stable freeze dried vaccine for use in tropical countries.[25] In 1969 Arita and Henderson, who were the leading spirits in the World Health Organisation's eradication programme, convened a meeting at which a step by step manual describing the method of manufacturing sufficient freeze dried vaccine was produced. At first it was estimated that 250 million doses would be required yearly and the Soviet Union was one of the major contributors of vaccine during those early years. As a result of the initiatives of the WHO, however, 80% of the vaccine required by the eradication programmme was being produced in the developing countries themselves by 1973. The vaccine was stable in tropical climates and would last for at least a month. It was also of standardised efficacy.

The second technical advance was the invention by Wyeth Laboratories of the bifurcated needle.[26] Effectively it was a sewing needle with the end cut off at the eyed end. Between the tines of the needle just sufficient vaccine could be held in solution to ensure a satisfactory vaccination. Wyeth generously waived all the royalties on this invention. Soon afterwards WHO workers in Pakistan invented a needle holder, which would hold both sterilised and used needles, so that the trained vaccinator simply required a quantity of needles, access to boiling water for sterilization, and a supply of freeze dried vaccine for a month's effective work in the field. It was also shown that cleaning the skin with spirit simply rearranged the bacteria on the surface and was therefore unnecessary. All that was needed was to clear away any excessive dirt.

The eradication programmes in different countries began between 1967 and 1969, and by 1971 all were in operation. The intention was to achieve 100% nationwide vaccination, but it soon became clear that there was a simpler way forward. It was shown in Nigeria that a sensitive system for the detection of cases and the subsequent containment of outbreaks by vaccination was an effective method of smallpox control in a developing country. This method was called "surveillance-containment" and it was clearly more practicable than the target of 100% vaccination in all countries.

The progress of the programme now became impressive. In much of Africa and South America smallpox was eradicated and by 1970 the number of countries where it was endemic had fallen to 17. By 1973 smallpox was confined to the Indian subcontinent, Ethiopia, and Botswana. Eradication in India proved a particular problem. The Indian programme had been first launched in 1962 with mass vaccination of the population as its aim. But by 1967 it was clear that it was far from achieving its objective, particularly in the northern states. There were also objections to vaccination on religious grounds, few Hindus wishing to use something which came originally from a cow, an animal sacred to them. Yet gradually prejudice and superstition were broken down and in 1973 Indian health workers, funded jointly by the Indian government, WHO, and the Swedish International Development Authority, mounted an ambitious new programme of search and containment. At first it seemed that smallpox was increasing, but this was in fact due to the increased accuracy of case reporting. In January 1975, operation Target Zero was launched. By the end of the programme it was envisaged that 120000 health workers would have visited more than 100 million households. Rewards, increasing to as much as a 1000 rupees as the disease finally came under control, were given for case reporting and on 24 May 1975 Saiban Bibi, a woman of 30 living on a railway platform in Assam, became India's last known smallpox victim. It was a formidable achievement which was due in great part to the dedication of Indian health workers. The last case in Pakistan had been in October 1974 in Naipur, and on 16 October 1975 a three year old girl, Rahima Banu of Bangladesh, was the last victim of smallpox in Asia, its ancient homeland.

Only Ethiopia and Somalia remained, but here there were special difficulties. Constant civil war, guerrilla activity, and attacks upon WHO personnel hampered the eradication programme. The identification of the disease among rapidly mobile nomads was to prove a particular challenge. Furthermore, the disease was of a mild type with a low mortality and morbidity, so that sufferers were able to continue their daily affairs, thereby spreading the disease. It was to the credit of the intrepid national and WHO staff and to volunteers from the United States, Japan, and Austria that smallpox was finally conquered in this part of the world. Ali Maalin, a 23 year old cook in Merka, Somalia, was the last person to suffer from a natural infection of the disease that had plagued mankind for at least 3 millenia.[23] But it was not quite the end. In Birmingham in 1978 two cases of smallpox occurred as a result of the escape of virus from a laboratory that was carrying out important work for the World Health Organisation. It was a sad and tragic postscript to a uniquely remarkable achievement.[27]

Since then, no further case of smallpox has occurred anywhere in the world and in 1980 the 33rd World Health Assembly solemnly made the following declaration: "that the world and all its peoples have won freedom from smallpox which was the most devastating disease sweeping through many countries since earliest times, leaving death, blindness and disfigurement in its wake and which, only a decade ago, was rampant in Africa, Asia and South America." At the same time Professor Frank Fenner, the Australian chairman of the Global Commission for the Certification of Smallpox Eradication presented the official certificate of eradication to the president of the assembly who was in no sense exaggerating when he described this achievement as unique in the history of mankind.[28]

It may be questioned why supplies of smallpox virus are still maintained anywhere in the world today and why the WHO continued to support work on smallpox and related viruses after the disease had been effectively eradicated. The very good reason lies in the desire to establish that smallpox has truly been eradicated and that there can be no animal reservoir for a virus related to smallpox which might by mutation become pathogenic to man. A pox virus of monkeys was first isolated in the laboratory in 1958, but it was not until the eradication programme was well under way that monkeypox was first discovered in man in the Basankusu district of Zaire in 1970. Between then and 1979, 47 patients with monkeypox were described; cases were detected in Zaire, Liberia, Nigeria, Ivory Coast, and Sierra Leone and this distribution coincides with the tropical rain forest areas of Central and West Africa. Most cases occur in children under the age of 10. In only four cases has there been evidence of person to person spread. Nevertheless, it is an unpleasant disorder with a significant mortality.

Other animal pox viruses which persist include cowpox,

tanapox, ratpox, racoonpox and camelpox, this last being recognised in Iran in the early 1970s and in Somalia between 1977 and 1979. The World Health Organisation has continued to encourage research into methods of identifying the different pox viruses, and it was to this work that the Birmingham laboratory was making important contributions. The genomic structure of the different pox viruses must be clearly established and so it is essential to prepare appropriate DNA maps of all orthopox viruses including variola and monkeypox viruses. Currently, no known orthopox virus has shown a DNA pattern with a potential for mutation to a variola like pattern in a one or two step process, but it is vital to ensure that no such virus emerges. For these reasons the World Health Organisation continues still to support two collaborating centres both of which hold smallpox virus under conditions of very strict containment. They also maintain a large stock of preserved vaccine just in case vaccination might ever again be required.

Surveillance has continued in the period after eradication. Between 1978 and 1982, 176 rumours of cases of possible smallpox were investigated by the World Health Organisation in 60 different countries. With the exception of the Birmingham cases in 1978, all were false alarms, the vast majority being cases of chickenpox or other skin diseases. The position with regard to monkeypox is being kept under specially close surveillance.

Can we, therefore, regard the threat of smallpox as being completely eliminated? There appear to be no hidden loci of the disease in isolated or remote communities anywhere in the globe today. A recent article in the *Lancet* has questioned whether archaeologists interested in tombs or ancient graveyards might be at risk, but this seems a most unlikely hazard since all the evidence suggests that the virus is unlikely to have remained viable. Whether the same argument applies to bodies of individuals dying of smallpox and buried under freezing conditions, as in the arctic, seems less certain. The use of smallpox virus for biological warfare or for an act of terrorism is, one supposes, remotely possible, but seems extremely unlikely. All the evidence in fact indicates that the disease has been removed from the globe and that man will not again suffer its horrors.

The conquest of smallpox is a truly remarkable story which owes so much to so many. It had its origins in folk medicine, was made possible by science and technology, and was effectively achieved by the global partnership of men and women of many nations with a wide spectrum of political, social, and religious views. It has been a miraculous achievement that owes nothing to providence and represents an example of what can be achieved by the unity of the human will.

NOTES

1 Dixon CW. *Smallpox*. London: J and A Churchill, 1962.
2 Benenson AS. Smallpox. *In*: Evans SC, ed; *Viral infections in humans: epidemiology and control*. London: John Wiley, 1976: 428–55.
3 Anonymous. Reaching target zero. *WHO Chronicle* 1979; 33: 359–63.
4 Dixon CW. *Smallpox*. London: J and A Churchill, 1962: 217; 270; 265–7; 308–449.
5 Timoni E. An account or history of the procuring the smallpox by incision, or inoculation; as it has for some time been practised at Constantinople. *Phil Trans R Soc Lond* 1714–16; 29: 72–82.
6 Halsband R. *The life of Lady Mary Wortley Montagu*. London: Oxford University Press, 1956.
7 Jurin J. *An account of the success of inoculating the smallpox for the year 1724*. London: J Peele, 1725.
8 Hillary W. *A rational and mechanical essay on the smallpox*. London: G Strachan, 1735.
9 Corner BC, Booth CC. *Chain of friendship. Letters of Dr John Fothergill 1735–1780*. Cambridge, Massachusetts: Harvard University Press, 1971.
10 Sutton, D. *The inoculator or Suttonian system of inoculation fully set forth in a plain and familiar manner*. London: T Gilbert and C Dilly, 1796.
11 Fox RH. *Dr Fothergill and his friends*. London: Longmans, Green, 1919: 79–98.
12 Van Doren C, ed Benjamin Franklin's *Autobiographical writings*. London: Cresset Press, 1946: 38.
13 Pepper W. *The medical side of Benjamin Franklin*. New York City: Argosy-Antiquaria, 1970.

14 Razzell PE. *Smallpox in the 18th century*. London: Caliban Books, 1980.

15 Haygarth J. *An inquiry into how to prevent the small pox*. London: J Johnson, 1784.

16 Elliot J. A medical pioneer: John Haygarth of Chester. *Br Med J* 1913; iv: 235–241.

17 Haygarth J. *A sketch of a plan to exterminate the casual smallpox from Great Britain and to introduce general inoculation*. London: J Johnson. 1793.

18 Fisk D. *Dr Jenner of Berkeley*. London: Heinemann, 1959.

19 MS autograph letter, E Home to Sir Joseph Banks, 21 April 1797. Banks MSS, Library of the Royal Botanic Gardens, Kew.

20 Jenner E. *An inquiry into the cause and effects of the variolae vaccinae*. London: Sampson Low, 1798.

21 Behbehani AM. The smallpox story: life and death of an old disease. *Microbiol Rev* 1983; **47**: 455–509.

22 Jenner E. *Origin of the vaccine inoculation*. London: DN Shury, 1801.

23 Henderson DA. The deliberate extinction of a species. *Proc Am Phil Soc* 1980; **126**: 461–471.

24 Arita I. How technology contributed to the success of global smallpox eradication. *WHO Chronicle* 1980; **34**: 175–7.

25 Collier LH. Appropriate technology in the development of freeze dried smallpox vaccine. *WHO Chronicle* 1980; **34**: 178–9.

26 Rubin BA. A note on the development of the bifurcated needle for smallpox vaccination. *WHO Chronicle* 1980; **34**: 180–1.

27 Department of Health and Social Security. *Report of the investigation into the cause of the 1978 Birmingham smallpox occurrence*. London: HMSO, 1980. (Shooter report.)

28 Decisions of the World Health Assembly. *WHO Chronicle* 1980; **34**: 258–63.

10 The development of medical journals in Britain

The Renaissance of learning was closely associated with the development of the new technology that led to the development of printing and the publication of books. During the scientific revolution that followed the Renaissance in Europe it was initially in published books that the new breed of scientists brought their work before the public, and for the most part they published in Latin, the lingua franca of their time. In England, however, it was some time before medical matters were published even as books, particularly if their authors were promulgating ideas which challenged contemporary thought. In 1628, for example, William Harvey published *De Motu Cordis* in Leyden and Frankfurt in Latin, no suitable vehicle for publication being available to him in England. The increase in publication that occurred during the century and a half that followed Harvey's death in 1657, however, brought an increasing amount of medical material before the public, and by the end of the eighteenth century Latin had been virtually replaced by English as the language of medical communication.

The story of the publication of medical journals reflects the history of both medical practice and science. Medical papers were first published, usually in Latin, in the proceedings of learned societies, and societies subsequently emerged which were specifically devoted to medical subjects. Medical journals also became a vehicle for the expression of dissent and for the

Based on the Hastings memorial lecture delivered on 7 July 1982 at BMA House to celebrate the 150th anniversary of the British Medical Association, and on the Bishop memorial lecture of the Library Association for 1981.

publication of medicopolitical ideas. During the first half of the nineteenth century, for example, both the *Lancet* and the predecessors of the *British Medical Journal* played leading roles in the reform movement that led to the Medical Act of 1858. Since that time journals have increasingly reflected scientific advances and the development of specialisation, so that the modern era has been associated particularly with the development of the specialist journal. It is only recently that the increasing subjugation of health to politics has again encouraged the appearance of a style of radical medico-political journalism associated with a previous era.

The first journal in which medical men chose to publish was the *Philosophical Transactions* of the Royal Society. The Royal Society, founded in 1660 by Charles II, began the publication of the *Philosophical Transactions* in 1665 and in its pages one can read Newton's *Principia* as well as the works of those Oxford physiologists who followed Harvey at the end of the seventeenth century. During the first half of the eighteenth century many medical men communicated their work to the Royal Society, still frequently in Latin. Some of the clinical contributions of that era are in fact of the most appalling banality, particularly when compared with the papers published alongside them. In 1720, for example, Edmund Halley published a distinguished communication on the magnitude of Sirius,[1] and in the same volume there is an affidavit sworn before a magistrate in Scotland to the effect that a boy had lived for three years without food,[2] a publication that does little credit to a society whose motto is *Nullius in Verba*.

By the middle of the eighteenth century there was general dissatisfaction with the decline of scientific activity within the Royal Society and it was the Earl of Macclesfield, future president and a mathematician and astronomer of distinction, who persuaded his colleagues to set up a committee to review all papers before publication in an attempt to improve the quality of the *Philosophical Transactions*. The Royal Society therefore first introduced the concept of refereeing. Significantly, there was a medical member of the committee, William Heberden. The Royal Society owes to Heberden's influence the general improvement in the standard of medical and biological papers that were published in the second half of the eighteenth century, which include much of John Hunter's most important work (see Chapter 1).

In Edinburgh in 1731 the first medical journal in Britain appeared. The Edinburgh medical school had been founded in 1726 by that distinguished group of young professors who were trained by Boerhaave in Leyden. Edinburgh practised the same freedom from religious sectarianism and bigotry that had been a feature both of Harvey's alma mater at Padua and of Leyden. Edinburgh was therefore a haven for the nonconformist. It was the medical men associated with the new medical school who first published the *Medical Essays and Observations* in Edinburgh. Appropriately, they dedicated their new journal to the Royal Society.

By the middle of the eighteenth century an appreciable number of graduates of the Edinburgh medical school were practising successfully in London, many of them licentiates of the London College of Physicians by examination. Because they were not graduates of Oxford and Cambridge, however, they were debarred from the fellowship of the Royal College of Physicians, a matter which led first to disgruntled murmurings and later to open rebellion.[3]

It was this group of disaffected Scottish graduates, Dr William Hunter, Sir William Watson, and Dr John Fothergill among them, who founded the first society of physicians in London, thus providing an alternative forum for medical discussion in the capital to the Royal Society and the Royal College of Physicians. In 1752, the same year that the Royal Society reformed its practices, the Society of Physicians began to publish a selection of the papers read before it. Six volumes, entitled the *Medical Observations and Inquiries*, were issued between 1757 and 1784. A member wrote later that this small society had "communicated more useful knowledge to the world than the College has done in their corporate capacity since the time of their first foundation" – perhaps something of an exaggeration.

In 1767, however, stung to action by the activities of their rebel licentiates, William Heberden and his friend Sir George

Baker persuaded the Royal College of Physicians to publish their own *Medical Transactions*. Heberden's influence can be discerned in the preface to the first volume, which demonstrates his adherence to Newtonian prinicples. "The experience of many ages," he wrote, "hath more than sufficiently shown that mere abstract reasonings have tended very little to the promotion of natural knowledge. By laying these aside and attending carefully to what nature hath either by chance or upon experiment offered to our observation, a greater progress hath been made in this part of Philosophy, since the beginning of the last century, than had been till that time from the days of Aristotle." The *Medical Transactions* provided a useful forum for the publication of medical papers but it was unfortunate for the college that the Scottish licentiates refused to submit papers in protest against their continued exclusion from the fellowship.

The Medical Society of London was founded in 1773 by another Quaker physician, who was a protégé of John Fothergill and a graduate of the University of Edinburgh: John Coakley Lettsom. This society not only provided a forum for scientific discussion but was also a meeting place for physicians, surgeons, and apothecaries – a unitarian concept of the medical profession far ahead of its time. It, too, published its proceedings, and if one excludes the *Philosophical Transactions* this is the only medical journal of the eighteenth century in this country that survives to this day.

It is interesting to examine the extent to which medical journals had replaced books as a vehicle for publishing original work by the end of the eighteenth century. At that time much medical work was still being published in books despite the emergence of the published volumes of proceedings. The major discoveries of the Age of Reason were the belated recognition by the Royal Navy that scurvy could be prevented, the introduction of digitalis by Withering, the description of angina pectoris and its association with heart disease by Heberden and Fothergill, the replacement of inoculation for smallpox by vaccination, and the discovery of the new gases, among which nitrous oxide was to be the most medically significant. Lind and Withering both published their work as books, as did most of the discoverers of the new gases, including Humphrey Davy. Heberden described angina pectoris at a meeting of the Royal College of Physicians in July 1769 and then published his observations in the newly founded *Medical Transactions* in 1772. Fothergill, who first recognised the relationship between angina pectoris and coronary heart disease, described his observations in the *Medical Observations and Inquiries* that he himself had founded.[4] Jenner, after his unsuccessful attempt to have his work on vaccination published by the Royal Society, reported it in his famous book.

The first half of the nineteenth century was associated with the movement for reform. Reform in England, however, was not limited to political matters but was felt across the whole spectrum of the nation's life, and there was nothing in that era more in need of reform than medicine and the medical profession. Apart from Edinburgh, there was no satisfactory system of university education in medicine. There was a multiplicity of schools in the metropolis, where nepotism was rife. There were private schools such as the Clutterbuck school in Aldersgate and the Windmill Street school, which had been founded in the previous century by the Hunters. The privileged royal colleges wielded enormous power and both surgeons and apothecaries licensed their own practitioners. There was also tension between the provinces and the metropolis. In this environment Thomas Wakley founded the *Lancet*, a radical journal whose carefully chosen name implied its future function of incising "the abscess on the medical body politic."[5]

Thomas Wakley passed the examination of the Royal College of Surgeons in 1817, at the age of 22.[6] He married well and settled down to practise as a surgeon in Argyll Street. Here he might have had a successful if undistinguished professional career had it not been for the events of 1820. In January of that year the old mad King died. The following month a group of radical desperadoes, intent on murdering the Prime Minister and his entire cabinet, were apprehended. The five ringleaders of what came to be known as the Cato Street Conspiracy were duly hanged on May Day 1820 outside

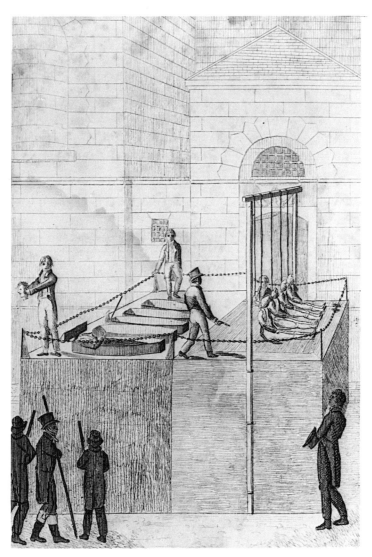

14 The execution of the Cato Street conspirators. (The assistant
    executioner can be seen exhibiting the severed head of the chief
    conspirator, Arthur Littlewood, to the crowd in Newgate Street)
    (Museum of London)

Newgate Prison. As their bodies were cut down, a figure dressed in sailor's clothes and with face masked appeared on the scaffold and skilfully decapitated the corpses. Obviously an expert, he was in fact Tom Parker, anatomy assistant at St Thomas's. Rumour put it about, however, that the masked man had been a surgeon from Argyll Street, and the only surgeon living there was Wakley. In August a gang of men supposedly sympathetic to the Cato Street conspirators burst in on Wakley, assaulted him, and burnt his house to the ground. Subsequently the unfortunate Wakley was accused of having been his own arsonist to obtain the insurance, a calumny he successfully contested in court with the insurance company, but he had lost his house and his practice, a disaster to a young man within six months of his marriage.

It was at this time that Wakley met William Cobbett, the radical reforming journalist, then editor of the *Weekly Political Register* and the *Evening Post*. Cobbett had exhumed the bones of Tom Paine and preserved them in his home. He had had some experience of attacking the medical establishment during an earlier part of his life in the United States. In his periodical *The Rush Light* he had for two years "flung the worst abuse that any honest physician had to bear" at Dr Benjamin Rush of Philadelphia, violently attacking the murderous regimen of bleeding and purging for which he was famous.[7] Cobbett, like Wakley, believed himself to be a target of the Cato Street conspirators' friends and this was the bond that brought the two men together. Cobbett, as ardent a supporter of political reform as Wakley was to be for the reform of the medical profession, played an important role in encouraging Wakley to take up radical medical journalism.

The year 1823 was recorded by Smart in his *Economic Annals* as "a quietly prosperous year," and was memorable to Harriet Martineau as the year in which Birkbeck founded the London Mechanics' Institute, the starting point for the Mechanics' Institute movement in England.[8] But for medicine, the truly momentous event was the publication of the *Lancet*, which first appeared on 5 October, a Sunday. The objectives of the *Lancet* were clearly set out in the opening issue. Most importantly, it was to publish for the first time the lectures of the distinguished men who taught in the London medical schools. There was also to be medical and surgical intelligence, to encourage the publication of case reports. Finally, there were to be non-medical topics, including comments on the current political scene and drama and chess – interests of the editor – but these did not last long. It was the decision to publish the lectures of the London teachers that at once brought Wakley into conflict with the profession, and particularly with the surgeons and their college, since it threatened both their power and their pocket.

Although Astley Cooper did not object to his lectures being published anonymously, Abernethy, senior surgeon at St Bartholomew's, applied to the Court of Chancery for an injunction against publication on the grounds that it infringed copyright. His lectures were published by Wakley so accurately that they included all his well known nautical expletives. Abernethy lost his case, and Wakley, who had retained the future Lord Brougham as his counsel, at once found his position greatly strengthened. The circulation of the *Lancet* increased and at the same time the venomous nature of Wakley's attacks against nepotism and privilege continued. There were repeated lawsuits, nine in all in a six year period, with results which were overall favourable to Wakley.

During the years that preceded the Medical Act of 1858 the *Lancet* poured out a stream of malevolence and vitriol against the Royal College of Physicians, the Royal College of Surgeons of London, and the Worshipful Company of Apothecaries, who were castigated as "the old hags of Rhubarb Hall." Not unnaturally, Wakley was subjected to equal abuse. The *Medical Gazette*, founded by Brodie and Abernethy, described unhappily how a set of literary plunderers had "broken on the peace and quiet of our profession."

Charles Hastings, founder of the British Medical Association, was an almost exact contemporary of Thomas Wakley.[9] Born in 1794 in Ludlow, he graduated MD in Edinburgh in 1818. He was then elected as physician to the Worcester Infirmary and within six weeks was involved like Wakley in controversy, for he charged the junior surgeon,

Thomas Stephenson, with professional misconduct. The character of Hastings, however, was in striking contrast to that of Wakley. He worked diligently throughout his life as a respected physician in Worcester, and it was through the institutions that he created and the committees that he served that he influenced the cause of medical reform, to which he was no less dedicated than Wakley. More successful than Wakley in the corridors of power, he was a conventional figure who began his public career as an officer of the local Worcestershire Medical and Surgical Society. When he died in 1867 he had played the major role in founding the British Medical Association, had been knighted, and had become the most respected medical man in the kingdom. The *Lancet*, at the time of his death, graciously commented that he was an amiable physician "who has rendered good service to his profession and has never, so far as we know, made himself an enemy."

Hastings's first venture into medical journalism was in 1828 when he persuaded his fellow members of the Worcestershire Medical Society to launch the *Midland Medical and Surgical Reporter*. It was specifically aimed at providing a forum for the publication of medical reports from the provinces, as at that time medical journals were confined to London, Edinburgh, and Dublin. In 1829 Sir Henry Halford, the president of the Royal College of Physicians, known as the "eel backed baronet" by virtue of his courtly manners, wrote to congratulate the Society of Physicians and the Medical Practitioners in the Midland Counties on their endeavours and did them the honour of asking permission to join their society.

Meanwhile, in the metropolis there had been attempts to form a Metropolitan Society of General Practitioners of Medicine, as well as a movement towards a national College of Medicine, supported by Wakley. Hastings was aware of these developments and in 1832 – appropriately the year when the great Reform Bill was passed enthusiastically by the House of Commons, but reluctantly by a House of Lords threatened with the creation by the monarch of an excess of radical peers – he decided in consultation with Edward

Barlow of Bath and other colleagues to form the Provincial Medical Association. The provincial practitioners considered that they could make a contribution to medical science just as significant if not greater than that of their colleagues in the metropolitan hospitals. Haygarth in Chester, Percival in Manchester, and Withering in Birmingham had all been provincial practitioners. In Hastings's own city of Worcester, Dr Wall had made important contributions to medicine as well as to porcelain. In addition they had the shining example of Edward Jenner, a country surgeon who had made the most important discovery of the age.

At the same time the publisher of the *Midland Reporter* was going into liquidation, and it was for these reasons that its successor became the *Transactions of the Provincial Medical Association*, which continued until 1853. Meanwhile, after considerable thought and with Hastings's active support, the association decided to establish a regular weekly journal and in 1840 they founded the *Provincial Medical and Surgical Journal*, later to become the *British Medical Journal*. The association and the *Journal* were almost immediately successful for they sought to cater for medical practitioners throughout the country and bring together physicians, surgeons, and apothecaries under one umbrella. It was not all plain sailing, however, for it took some years before the various regions of the provinces were united. Wakley, who was not always a supporter of Hastings, was soon writing that the association should become the British Medical Association.

By the early 1850s the movement for a national association had become almost irresistable, particularly in the metropolitan countries. Sir Charles Hastings, who had been knighted in 1850, was initially uncertain of the need for change as he felt there might be a lessening of the esprit de corps in the provinces. But he withdrew his objections, and at a momentous meeting in Dee's Hotel in Birmingham in 1855 the decision was taken that gave birth to the British Medical Association, the creation of Charles Hastings, which has now served a united profession for 150 years.

In 1853 the *Provincial Medical and Surgical Journal* amalgamated with the *London Journal of Medicine* to become the *Association Medical Journal*. In 1857, following the foundation of the British Medical Association, it became the *British Medical Journal* that we know today. During the remainder of the nineteenth century, the *Lancet* and the *British Medical Journal* were the leading medical publications in Britain and in 1881 the *British Medical Journal* had the privilege of publishing the proceedings of the great International Congress of Medicine in London presided over by Sir James Paget, at which both Lister and Virchow were present. The Prince of Wales and the future Kaiser were also there.

The later years of the nineteenth century and the first decades of the twentieth were associated with the development of journals which reflected the new scientific discoveries in physiology and medicine, the cellular pathology of Virchow and Rokitansky, and the bacterial origin of disease. The *Journal of Physiology*, for example, was founded in London in 1878 and the *Journal of Pathology and Bacteriology*, forerunner of the present *Journal of Pathology*, in 1892. The *Quarterly Journal of Medicine* continues to be the official publication of the Association of Physicians of Great Britain and Ireland and was first published in 1907; the *British Journal of Surgery* first appeared in 1913.

In the history of the United Kingdom the effects of having an empire were an important influence on the mother country. Physicians and surgeons followed trade and the flag to far flung corners of the globe. William Hillary had published his book on the *Diseases of the West India Islands* in London in 1759 (see Chapter 3). By the end of the nineteenth century there were to be journals reflecting the discoveries of Manson, Ross, and others. The *Journal of Tropical Medicine and Hygiene* first appeared in 1898, and the *Transactions of the Society for Tropical Medicine and Hygiene* (later to be *Royal*) have been published since 1907. Sir James Mackenzie founded the journal *Heart* in the following year as a reflection of his own scientific interests, and he appointed the future Sir Thomas Lewis as its first editor, at the tender age of 27. Lewis, however, in later life was more interested in the general than the specific and he changed its name in 1931 to *Clinical Science*; the journal continues with this name despite a brief flirtation with molecular medicine.

It might be assumed that the general journals would feel threatened by the modern development of the specialist journal. It is therefore all the more to the credit of the *British Medical Journal* that this journal has played a generous and pioneering role in encouraging specialist journals, usually in association with the relevant society or association. The first of these, the *Archives of Disease in Childhood* and the *Journal of Neurology and Psychopathology*, were founded in 1926, late in Dawson Williams's time as editor. There are now 13 specialist journals, as well as six professional and scientific publications published by the *British Medical Journal* on an agency basis. Other general journals, such as the *Journal of Physiology*, have successfully resisted the fragmentation that has afflicted both medicine and pathology in the modern era. The *Quarterly Journal of Medicine*, with a declining circulation, has been less successful; its preservation of archaic editorial practices, until very recently, has probably reflected the conservatism of its parent body.

The development of what has come to be known as the "throwaway journal" is a feature of recent years which may perhaps owe something to the increasing interplay between politics and health that followed the foundation of the National Health Service in 1948. One of the best known was *World Medicine*, whose style of radical journalism on subjects such as the reconstitution of the General Medical Council or the alleged skeletons in the cupboards at the Royal Society of Medicine was reminiscent of Thomas Wakley. It also published material that produced from many established figures of the profession a chorus of orchestrated outrage similar to that provoked by Wakley in his prime. The significance to the story of medical publishing of *World Medicine* and its contemporaries remains to be assessed by historians. It is well to remember, however, that for many established members of a conservative profession in the 1820s the *Lancet* was a throwaway journal too.

Medical journalism has been of vital importance for the diffusion of knowledge and of new ideas in this country. The story of medical journals and the characters of the men who made them is as fascinating as any other aspect of medical history. For many the contemporary scene may seem staid and conservative by comparison with previous eras. There is, however, one lesson that can be learnt: nothing great was ever achieved unless by a radical.

NOTES

1 Halley E. Some remarks on a late essay of Mr Cassini, wherein he proposed to find, by observation, the parallax and magnitude of Sirius. *Philos Trans* 1720; **31**: 28–30.
2 Blair P. A copy of an affidavit made in Scotland concerning a boy's living a considerable time without food. *Philos Trans* 1720; **31**: 28–30.
3 Stevenson LG. The siege of Warwick Lane. *J Hist Med Allied Sci* 1952; **8**: 105–22.
4 Corner BC, Booth, CC. *Chain of friendship. Letters of Dr Fothergill 1735–1780*. Cambridge, Massachusetts: Harvard University Press, 1971.
5 Frogatt P. *The Lancet*: Wakley's instrument for medical education reform. *J Soc Occup Med* 1979; **29**: 45–53.
6 Sprigge SS. *The life and times of Thomas Wakley*. London: Longmans, Green, 1897.
7 Corner GW. *The autobiography of Benjamin Rush*. Princeton: Princeton University Press, 1948.
8 Kelly T. *George Birkbeck, pioneer of adult education*. Liverpool: Liverpool University Press, 1957.
9 McMenemy WH. *The life and times of Sir Charles Hastings*. Edinburgh and London: Livingstone, 1959.

11 Technology and medicine

Technology is as old as man. As Benjamin Franklin aptly remarked, man has always been a tool making animal, and it was his capacity to make tools that led to the development of crafts such as carpentry, building, metal smelting, weaponry, leather tanning, weaving, and so on. From these crafts there emerged through the centuries the technology that has become one of the four environments within which man lives, the others being the cosmic, the natural, and the social.

Science, however, has a different tradition and is a more recent development in man's history. It belonged originally to mathematics and astronomy or to the aristocratic speculative philosophy of the Greeks and Romans, and became the experimental science we know today only after the Renaissance. For the ensuing centuries, science and technology were largely divorced from each other, pursuing different paths, not only as a result of class division but also because initially the work of the scientist in his laboratory had little relevance to that of workers, craftsmen, and metal founders who were developing their own technology. It was not until after the Industrial Revolution that science and technology came together and that technology became more firmly based on science. Von Liebig, for example, was the father of organic chemistry and it was his basic scientific discoveries that were to lead to the development of the first synthetic fertilisers; and Faraday's work was the scientific basis upon which Edison and Swan developed the technology of the electric light bulb.

From the *Proceedings of the Royal Society of London* (Series B) 1985; **224**: 267–85.

Medicine and medical technology have evolved in a similar way. As with many of man's other practical activities, medicine first developed as a craft and from ancient times technology has, therefore, been an essential part of its practice. One of the earliest of medical technologies was applied to the treatment of broken limbs: the splinting of the legs of Egyptian mummies is a prehistoric example which serves to emphasise that medical technology has always been with us.

As in other human activities, so in medicine in the modern era, science has become increasingly important. Yet it is clear that the translation of scientific discovery to clinical practice requires the interposition of technology. This is a two way process. It is often technology that makes possible scientific discovery, and medical practice itself prompts the development of new technology as well as suggesting problems for science. In fact a fair proportion of the science of medicine comes directly from clinical studies and the work of clinical scientists, whose ability to apply knowledge is vital to any success science may have in influencing medical practice. The interplay between these different but related activities emphasises the need for a close, harmonious, and creative relationship among scientists, technologists, and those engaged in the practice of medicine, something which as we shall see is not always as well developed in Britain as it should be.

There is a vast range and complexity of medical technology in routine use. Its applications may be diagnostic, or therapeutic, or in monitoring devices for both diagnostic and therapeutic purposes. They may also be preventive, remedial or to do with information systems.

Diagnosis begins in the doctor's surgery or clinic and has traditionally entailed using the stethoscope, invented in France by Laennec in the early nineteenth century.[1] There are now many different techniques available for clinical diagnosis. Inspection of organs has been made simple by the introduction in recent years of flexible instruments and it is now possible to introduce a fibreoptic instrument into any available orifice and be rewarded with a remarkable view.

The use of flexible sigmoidoscopes for example, permits the examination of the entire colon by physicians expert in this technique.[2]

Biopsy techniques have been of particular importance for medical diagnosis. One of the most ingenious devices, invented some time ago by an American army haematologist, Colonel WH Crosby, was a capsule for taking biopsies of the small intestinal mucosa, the lining membrane of the intestine where absorption occurs.[3] The capsule is swallowed on the end of a fine tube. A little knuckle of intestinal muscle is sucked into it, then a rubber sheet beneath the knife bulges up to release a spring and a piece of tissue is obtained. With a low power dissecting microscope, this technique at once demonstrates the difference between the normal appearance of the intestinal mucosa and the abnormal flat mucosa of an individual who has a sensitivity to bread causing coeliac disease. This can be done in an outpatient clinic during a morning and has completely eliminated the need for complex tests of absorption requiring hospitalisation that used to be necessary for diagnosis. It is an excellent example of how important simple low cost technology is for the practice of modern medicine.

Computer aided decision making in medicine is still relatively undeveloped but in the 10 years to 1983 the *Index Medicus* showed that the number of articles under "computers" and "decision making" more than doubled, an encouraging sign to those who seek to increase the accuracy of clinical diagnosis in this way.[4]

The next line of diagnostic technology is in the pathology laboratory. Blood haemoglobin levels and cell numbers have to be measured automatically in large and complex machines. The measurement of substances in body fluids also uses complex and expensive automated machinery so that a variety of tests of different substances in the blood can be rapidly provided. The use of radioactive tracers and of radio-immunoassay have also been of great importance in this. Histopathology and cytogenetics still rely on microscopical analysis and the use of the human eye, but the identification of different types of cell by using modern techniques, particularly the use of monoclonal antibodies to individual cell constituents, is promising to revolutionise this specialty. The use of DNA probes for the antenatal diagnosis of genetic disorders is one of the exciting aspects of modern medicine in which techniques of molecular biology are being applied to human problems. Until recently the identification of bacteria in the laboratory has been a time consuming business, with predominantly traditional techniques carried out by hand, but there is a new age of automation on the horizon and a fully automated bacteria identification system has recently been developed which is being introduced into microbiology laboratories.[5]

One of the important features of this increase in the use of automated machines for laboratory tasks has been the extraordinary rise in the numbers of tests asked for by clinicians. The nationwide numbers of samples sent to chemical pathology laboratories during the 1970s show a steep and linear increase. This reflects a commendable investigative zeal yet it is by no means certain that it has brought comparable benefits to the sick and suffering.

It is in diagnostic imaging that the most expensive techniques have been developed. Machines for radiological examination have always been expensive and complex modern equipment for ultrasonic examination is increasing in price yearly. But it was the introduction of computed x ray tomographic scanning that led to an escalation of costs of an entirely new dimension. The technique is particularly useful for the diagnosis and treatment of head injuries, a problem in both the young and the elderly, and in the management of cancer.

The latest development in this specialty is magnetic resonance imaging. This technique, which depends on the ability of a large magnet surrounding the body to interact the nuclei of atoms in cells with an applied magnetic field, allows the different tissues of the body to be made visible without recourse to radiation and there is, therefore, no radiation hazard. Nuclear magnetic resonance for imaging body organs, pioneered by ER Andrew in this country, is still in its development and assessment phase but it has already proved its value

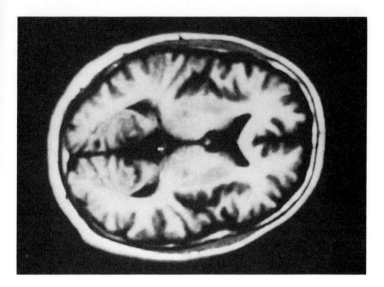

15 Magnetic resonance imaging of the human brain
(Courtesy of Professor R E Steiner, Royal Postgraduate
Medical School, London)

in providing images of brain and other organs that are vastly
superior to those obtained by other techniques.

But magnetic resonance imaging is not used only for
imaging. One its most exciting applications is for the study of
metabolic reactions of different organs in the body in vivo.[6]
At University College Hospital in London similar techniques
are being used to detect anoxia in the brain of newborn
babies.

Among therapeutic techniques surgery has been practised
since at least the time of the ancient Egyptians, and the use of
instruments to facilitate childbirth has a long history. There
are now lasers, cryosurgery, and machines that will dissolve
renal stones by sonication. These techniques, together with
the use of organ transplantation, heart-lung oxygenators,
renal dialysis machines and cardiac pacemakers have transformed the practice of medicine in the past three decades.
Techniques for the successful transfusion of blood and other
fluids have also been of vital importance for modern surgery,

as well as for resuscitation. They are essential for the replacement of blood loss after haemorrhage and the treatment of some varieties of anaemia associated with bone marrow failure.

Radiation therapy has been extended to include the use of neutrons produced by very expensive cyclotrons. Technology has always been a useful aid to obstetricians but the pioneering and wholly remarkable work of Steptoe and Edwards has now developed a reproductive technology reminiscent of Aldous Huxley's *Brave New World*, even if we do not yet have Bokanovsky's process or Podsnap's technique. Open heart surgery to undertake valve replacement has dramatically changed the lives of individuals who are otherwise doomed to a distressing death from heart failure, and artificial kidneys and renal transplantations have successfully extended the lives of sufferers from kidney failure for whom medicine previously had nothing to offer.

Anaesthetic techniques may be appropriately classified as therapeutic procedures. They include the use of machines of increasing complexity. There is a whole technology associated with the supply of anaesthetic gases, and anaesthetists are also particularly interested in monitoring techniques which are a sort of "automatic pilot" for the anaesthetist. It is perhaps worth recording here that anaesthetists are now the single largest specialist group in the National Health Service.

New techniques are also changing professional practices. Traditionally, operative techniques have been carried out by surgeons, physicians contenting themselves with diagnosis and the use of drugs. Now, however, radiologists are doing operations on blood vessels and with the advent of fibre-optics, physician-gastroenterologists are exploring the biliary and pancreatic passages, slitting the ampulla of Vater which leads these passages into the duodenum, and removing gallstones, something that was always the prerogative of the surgeon in the past.[7]

Monitoring devices are now available which can measure physiological changes in the human body over prolonged periods. They can be used either upon an ambulatory patient, to determine the effect of a drug on heart rate or blood pressure, for example, or in the intensive therapy unit where they have proved of particular value in the care of babies born prematurely. By using this sort of technology the blood pressure can be measured over a 24 hour period. This enables the investigator to study, for example, the circadian rhythms of blood pressure in normal people and in those with hypertension. The availability of computed analysis has been essential for this kind of study. The most important uses of monitoring techniques are in childbirth and in intensive care, and the successful survival of infants weighing no more than 500–700 g at birth may now be confidently predicted.

Preventive technology includes vaccines, the possible prevention of dental caries, and birth control. Despite the total eradication of smallpox throughout the world a decade ago by the World Health Organisation, using the technique introduced by Jenner in 1798, vaccination remains important as it is now possible, with modern biotechnology, to use the same method to incorporate other antigens that can induce immunity to other diseases.

Another interesting preventive technique is emerging in dentistry. Dental sealants are liquid plastic resins which are applied to the biting surface of the posterior teeth. Caries usually begins at the bottom of a fissure on the biting surface of the teeth, where bacteria ferment dietary sugar to produce acid and therefore caries. This can be prevented by the use of a dental sealant, the fissure being closed by the layer of clear plastic material which is resistant to acid, and which solidifies on exposure to light.

Birth control is perhaps one of the best examples of the use of both technology and science in medicine. Satisfactory mechanical methods of birth control, which have evolved immeasurably since the use of animal bladders and bits of intestine in the time of James Boswell, have been due to the use of new technology in the production of thin and reliably strong sheets of rubber. By contrast, the use of the rhythm method of contraception and of the contraceptive pill owe everything to Corner's careful scientific elucidation of the nature of the menstrual cycle and the discovery, in his laboratory, of progesterone.

Remedial and supportive technology have all kinds of important uses. As the years go by, life becomes increasingly dependent on prostheses and as so many people are living to an advanced age this is an important part of medical technology. The number of centenarians in the United States is currently considered to be as many as 12000 so there is a great opportunity to use technology in the service of the elderly.[8] At the same time the disabled and the handicapped deserve as much help as modern technology can give them.

Information technology also offers great opportunities for the future. In health education, as well as in the education of the individual patient with a specific complaint such as diabetes, there is much scope for the development of educational videos, computer programs, and films. Medical records sadly remains one of the problems of the National Health Service. Attempts at computerisation, photographic recording, miniaturisation, and standardisation are in their infancy. It is a part of medical activity which intelligently used modern information technology could surely improve.

So far as the provision of health services is concerned, one of the major effects of the development of technology has been on manpower. An army of technicians and other health personnel is now required to run the machines and carry out the techniques of modern medicine. At the beginning of the century, in the United States about 345000 people were estimated to work in health care and, of these, one in three was said to be a physician. By 1940 specialisation of the non-physician workforce was keeping pace with specialisation among doctors, for by then there were 27 new and recognised non-physician occupations, including physiotherapy, dental hygiene, radiological technology and so on. By 1976 the United States health workforce had grown to about 5.1 million and only one in 13 of these was a physician.[9] The allied health occupations (excluding nurses and nursing auxiliaries) contained 155 recognised specialities in 1976. The total number of staff employed by the NHS in the UK exceeds one million. There are approximately 29000 general practitioners, 38000 hospital medical and dental staff, an army of nurses and midwives (391000), a large number of non-medical scientific staff (65200) as well as ancillary (172000) and clerical and administrative staff (108000).

How has new medical technology developed and what has encouraged its development? The sequence of events that indicates that science leads to technological development and then to its application in practice holds true for the story of the development of antibiotics, vaccines such as those that have eradicated poliomyelitis, and currently for the application of the techniques of molecular biology to human problems. One may be led by these developments to conclude that in encouraging technological progress in medicine it is essential to support basic science. There is good evidence to support this view. Comroe and Dripps made a detailed study of the scientific basis for the support of biomedical science with particular reference to cardiac and pulmonary medicine.[10] They wished to examine the view expressed by President Lyndon Johnson and based on a study of how 20 important military weapons came to be developed, that too much basic research was being done, that life saving discoveries might have been made that were, in Johnson's words, "locked up in the laboratory," and that therefore there should be more targeted or mission orientated research. It was a viewpoint reflected in the Rothschild proposals for the organisation of government research in this country.

Comroe and Dripps first identified the top 10 clinical advances that they and a team of 40 other physicians considered to be the most important for their patients. They then identified 529 key articles that were considered to be essential for these advances. These were assessed as being either clinically oriented or not. Their conclusions were that 41% of the work judged to be essential for later clinical advances was not clinically oriented at the time that it was done. This is a powerful argument for the support of basic research but their study also shows that a large proportion of work considered important for advances in cardiac and pulmonary medicine was in fact clinically oriented. Furthermore, more than 15% of the key publications on the topic were concerned with the development of new apparatus, techniques, or procedures. Their work, therefore, also makes a compelling argument for effective research support in the clinical field as well as in technology. This is an important conclusion for those concerned with the support of medical research in this country. The Medical Research Council (MRC) has the responsibility of supporting the whole of biomedical research from the molecule to the community. Himsworth, a much respected secretary of the MRC, has recorded that in the mid-1930s Sir Frederick Gowland Hopkins, president of the Royal Society, protested publicly against the use of funds to support clinical scientists, and Himsworth records that in his own time he was not immune to attack for, as he put it, "wasting money on clinical research."[11] At a time when funds are increasingly constrained, there may well be attempts to hijack money that should properly go to clinical research. This would be unfortunate, for a study of the development of modern medicine shows how vital it has been to support clinical research and in particular to encourage brilliant and innovative doctors, who have the important responsibility of applying science and technology to medical practice.

There are many examples of the way in which pioneering medical practitioners have developed new technology. Renal dialysis machines were first developed by Willem Kolff, a Dutch physician who emigrated to the United States, and in this country it was Melrose, a surgeon, who pioneered the use of heart-lung machines, although in this case the MRC declined to support the work as being too technological. Charnley, an orthopaedic surgeon, was the innovator who made hip replacement operations possible. Dr Martin Wright of the Clinical Research Centre invented the machines we use to measure the flow of air in and out of the lungs, and he has also invented a number of accurate infusion pumps. His latest, the size of a wristwatch, is an effective artificial pancreas which will deliver insulin as required. In addition, the initial development of transplantation techniques was pragmatic and owes as much to the doctors who pioneered the use of renal dialysis and to Alexis Carrel's techniques of vascular suturing as to the brilliant work of immunologists in the laboratory.

The story of the development of fibreoptic instruments is perhaps worth recording in more detail, as it illustrates the interplay between the ideas of intelligent clinicians, the work of a brilliant innovative British scientist, and the extraordinary ability of the Japanese to exploit someone else's discovery. It began when a British gastroenterologist, Dr Hugh Gainsborough of St George's Hospital in London, met Harold Hopkins who was then working at the Imperial College of Science and Technology. Gainsborough, to use Hopkins's own words to me, was "pretty well appalled by the use of the old rigid gastroscope" which required the skill of a sword swallower on the part of both operator and patient. He asked Hopkins whether it would not be possible to have something flexible like a rubber gastric tube which could be swallowed much more easily. It was this suggestion that encouraged Hopkins to think about the matter. A few months later he formed the idea of a coherent glass fibre bundle for carrying an optical image along a flexible path. With his graduate student NS Kapany he was able to produce a successful image transmitting bundle and the work was soon published in *Nature*.[12] There were, writes Hopkins, many inquiries after the publication of this article, but sadly none from industry.

One, however, was from a British gastroenterologist, Dr (now Sir) Francis Avery Jones, who encouraged one of his young men, Dr Basil Hirschowitz, to follow up Hopkins's discovery. Hirschowitz had by now moved to Ann Arbor, Michigan, where he successfully developed a prototype. The next step was the production of a commercially viable instrument by industry but this was to prove much more difficult than the early experimental work. At first no individual firm in the United States or in Britain was willing to help develop the fibrescope. Finally, American Cystoscope Makers Inc agreed to make the fibrescope under licence but it was not until four years later that the first results from the use of commercial endoscopes were published in the *Lancet*.[13]

The remainder of the story, as is well known, belongs to

Japan. In 1962 Professor Tadayoshi Takemoto imported a commercially available Hirschowitz gastroduodenal fibre-scope from the United States. The moment was particularly propitious, for Japan at that time provided a particularly fertile field for the development of fibreoptic endoscopy. Japanese surgeons working in Toyko, concerned at the high incidence of gastric cancer in their community, and with the aid of the Olympus Company, had already developed a tiny camera attached to a fine cable that could be swallowed into the stomach for the purpose of early diagnosis. More than 1000 patients had been examined in Tokyo University by the use of this technique.

There was, therefore, in Japan a community of physicians and surgeons, as well as a commercial organisation, highly sympathetic to the use of new techniques in the investigation of gastrointestinal disease. It was in this favourable environment that Takemoto, together with the Machida Company and with Olympus, rapidly developed the new generation of fibreoptic instruments for endoscopy that have swept the world. The first endoscopes were on the market within a year of Takemoto's importation into Japan of the Hirschowitz instrument.

There are a number of lessons to be learned from these stories. First, that in the development of new technology a close association of innovative medical men with scientists and engineers, and particularly with those working in thrusting commercial enterprises, is essential; second, that there is often a compelling clinical need (in the case of fibreoptics a high incidence of gastric cancer); and third, that there should be a social milieu, as in Japan, where technology and applied science are highly regarded. There is also the vexed question whether, as the Science Policy Research Unit has put it, this country might profitably engage in a greater level of research forecasting.[14] They have concluded unequivocally, but with provisos, that the United Kingdom should attempt to bring its long term forecasting up to the remarkable level they identified in Japan.

Hopkins himself, asked why we were so sadly unable to

develop fibreoptics in this country, blames first the appallingly low standard of general and technical education in the commercial firms that existed at that time; second, the lack of risk capital; third, and above all, the lack of vision and confidence in what was possible from both the technical and commercial point of view.

Has anything changed since then? The successful development in recent years of computed tomography in this country and now of nuclear magnetic resonance suggests that it may have, but at the same time there is evidence that the British health care industry, if one excludes pharmaceuticals, is not at present rising to the challenge that the technology of modern medicine presents. Although the United Kingdom health care industry has, at least until recently, been in positive trade balance with the rest of the world, an analysis of the results of recent years is not encouraging, as it shows a persistent deterioration in the United Kingdom's position. This picture is not specifically a feature of medical equipment for it also applies to the whole field of scientific instrumentation.[15] Scientific officers who are responsible for the purchase of medical scientific equipment find the situation frankly depressing. Dr Harold Glass, senior scientific officer at the North West Thames Regional Health Authority, writes that most of the ultrasonic equipment he purchases is Japanese or American, as is virtually all the major biochemistry and haematology equipment. Microscopes are usually German or Japanese, and pathology equipment is becoming increasingly Japanese in origin. The major British x ray company, Picker Ltd, tends to incorporate large amounts of Japanese, Italian, and French electronics in some of its products. The most popular general purpose x ray table is imported from Belgium, the generators are manufactured in Italy and its sophisticated imaging and image processing equipment tends to come from the United States. The general picture from a British manufacturer's point of view appears to be becoming progressively worse each year. On the computer side, although major orders have been placed by health authorities with a British firm for patient administration systems, there is a continuing and increasing tendency to purchase many smaller similar systems from American manufacturers.

What is contributing to our lack of success? There appear to be a number of factors, which include British attitudes to technology, unsatisfactory relationships between industry and academe, a relatively small home market, and the influence of budgetary constraints in the National Health Service.

It is platitudinous to say that one of the major contributing factors remains the attitude to technology and applied science, but it must still be said. Medawar has pointed out that "Britain suffers from that most dangerous form of snobbism in science...which draws distinctions between pure and applied science...and which is at its worst in England."[16] In our schools any one who is "any good" is encouraged to do academic things, and engineering and applied sciences are regarded as lesser pursuits. This carries forward into university life and later into professional careers. It is a viewpoint reflected by the comment of a certain medical scientist that the award to Hounsfield of the Nobel prize for the introduction of computed tomography had been given for "mere technology." One is reminded of the immortal reply made to Brunel when he told a lady that he was an engineer, and she commented that she had mistakenly thought that he was a gentleman.

Medical attitudes may also tend to be against technology. The keystone of most doctors' philosophy is *primum non nocere* and so they are in general not the wild enthusiasts for new technology that some social analysts believe them to be. They usually follow the policy of being neither the first to start something nor the last to give it up. The medical reaction against new technology was perhaps best illustrated by the very strong initial opposition to the introduction by Sir John McMichael of invasive techniques of clinical investigation such as liver biopsy and cardiac catheterisation, which in fact soon became routine (see Chapter 13). Furthermore, among clinicians who are expected to replace an established technique with a new one there is often as much opposition as may be expected from a working man threatened with the obliteration of his job.

Yet there is more to the downgrading in our society of technology than the attitudes of academic or professional men. In an era when the threat of nuclear war is ever present, there has been a strengthening of the antitechnology lobby throughout the world. There is nothing new in the attack on technology. The dire predictions that were made when railway trains were introduced, Ralph Waldo Emerson's warning during the heyday of Victorian technological progress that "things are in the saddle and ride mankind" and Henry Adams's reactions to what he saw as the excesses of technology when he visited the Paris Exhibition in 1900, were later echoed by the disenchantment with technology expressed in Aldous Huxley's *Brave New World* and in Charlie Chaplin's film *Modern Times*, where the depersonalising effect of a contemporary production line was brilliantly depicted.

In recent years populists have sought to sow a mistrust of scientists and technology in the public mind. This has been accompanied by assaults on modern medicine by writers such as Illich[17] and the BBC's Reith lecturer for 1980, Ian Kennedy, as well as by doctors themselves. McKeown, among others, has argued that medical science and technology have been given too much credit for the improvements in the nation's health during the past century and in particular that the decline in mortality from infectious disease is due more to social change than to science and technology.[18] By contrast, he might now reflect that it is social change that has led to the current world epidemic of sexually transmitted disease and, in particular, to the tragedy of AIDS. Since epidemiologists are unlikely to succeed in changing sexual behaviour, it must be emphasised that it is only science that has anything to offer to the unfortunate sufferers from these unpleasant and sometimes fatal conditions, as is illustrated by the discovery that a specific retrovirus is associated with AIDS.[19] [20]

Whatever may be said about technology and medicine by populists, epidemiologists, cost analysts, and others, the one group that appears to be in favour is the patients whom we seek to help. This is even true in obstetrics, where there are many women's groups opposed to what they consider to be interference with nature. *Hospital Doctor* published the results of a survey of 1000 women giving birth at Queen Charlotte's Hospital with the arresting headline "Women give thumbs up to high tech birth."[21]

Apart from attitudes to technology there is considerable evidence that the relation between industrial laboratories and academics in bioengineering and medical physics has never been as well integrated as it has in pharmaceuticals. As regards medical equipment Brian Pullan, a distinguished ex-academic who has now founded his own successful business, has reflected on the reasons for this in a personal communication to me. Career structures and motivation, he points out, are very different in industrial and non-industrial environments. In universities and institutes of higher education the pressure is to publish completed pieces of work, gaining the most prominent position possible in the list of authors. By this means, prospects for acquiring grants and thereby publishing more papers and ultimately gaining promotion are improved.

There is consequently a reluctance on the part of academic researchers to allow a commercial enterprise to get involved before the work is complete and full academic credit has been gained. This results in delay in the commercial exploitation of ideas, a damaging release of key information to foreign competitors through freedom of academic communication, and, because apparatus has usually been made without the participation of professional engineers, an unnecessarily difficult problem of re-engineering.

By contrast, in the world of commerce there is a desire to get a product to the market place as soon as possible. Products are normally marketed as soon as they are judged to be saleable, and often contain many faults which are cured in later models. This has the commercial advantage that a quick return is achieved, and in addition later models make earlier models obsolete well before they have come to the end of their useful life, thus leading to renewed sales. This commercial approach, which is pursued to some extent by all companies, does not go down very well in academic circles.

Another cause of conflict identified by Pullan, which may result in ineffective collaboration, is that the academic usually tends to overvalue his ideas and often does not understand the very large gap between a single working laboratory prototype and a commercial unit. The latter has to be made in large numbers with a high reliability and with operating and service manuals, together with servicing, marketing, and sales support. All this costs money and highly skilled effort. The initial development, which is all that the academic sees, is a very small part of the overall task of commercial exploitation of an idea or invention. This simple fact is not widely appreciated outside industry.

There are, however, other more tangible influences upon the medical equipment side of the health care industry in this country. The first of these is the relatively small home market provided by the United Kingdom. By contrast with the medical equipment industry, the pharmaceutical market is booming and it is interesting that in pharmaceuticals there has never been the same separation between academe and industrial laboratories, as well as clinical practice, that Pullan describes. Contacts between research workers in commercial and academic laboratories have always been close, as is so clearly shown by the career of Sir Henry Dale who worked successively in a university, with Burroughs Wellcome, and with the Medical Research Council. Clinicians, particularly those who accept free rides on the Orient Express, have in fact been criticised for being too close to the pharmaceutical industry. It is, however, worth reflecting that it may well be that this proximity has contributed to the success of the drug companies in this country.

The home market for equipment and supplies is smaller than that for pharmaceuticals and smaller, too, than that in the United States, Germany, and Japan. This may be a reflection of the fact that these countries, as is well known, allocate a greater proportion of their gross national product to health than we do. The proportion of gross national product devoted to health in this country is about 6%, whereas it is more like 8% in other countries in Western Europe and 10% in the United States. So far as market size is concerned, however, the situation for our industry could surely be corrected by a more aggressive British approach to the European market. Whether British firms are sufficiently expert linguistically to achieve this is uncertain, as language teaching, like technology, remains another of the defective parts of our educational system. There is also to some extent a conflict of interest between the medical equipment industry and the National Health Service. Budgetary controls at regional and district health authority levels are a constraint on buying new technology, while the interests of industry demand, by contrast, a buoyant market. This is not to say that the NHS inhibits industry. The Department of Health and Social Security through its Scientific and Technical Services Branch has funds available to support new initiatives, which it has effectively done, and it also seeks to ensure that medical equipment should be safe and fit for its purpose.[22] More than 200 British Standards have now been established by the DHSS for medical equipment and supplies, and most manufacturers agree that only firms which comply with quality standards should be in the medical business. All this is to the good. Nevertheless, the situation in the NHS is quite different from that in a system of medicine controlled by the private sector and private insurance companies, where the cost of any new equipment or technology is simply added to the patient's bill. Medical technologies have therefore in the past been introduced, particularly in the United States, without real knowledge as to their cost: benefit ratio.

In examining the escalation of health care costs in the United States, it has been pointed out that the major root of the technology problem is the open ended reimbursement system which pays for almost anything recommended by health care providers.[23] Now, however, both the United States government, through its Medicare and Medicaid programmes, and the insurance companies are introducing an agreed series of investigations for therapeutic procedures which will be reimbursed only if the clinician follows the agreed procedure. We have not yet reached that point in this country as the stricter budgetary controls imposed in the NHS do not yet make it necessary. However, a move towards increasing private practice in this country would inevitably increase the use of technology and equipment in the private sector, which might well raise medical fees and costs without a proportionate increase in benefit to patients. Such a move would therefore require controls.

The continued concern with rising health care costs has, however, led many to conclude that it is technology that is the major cause of increasing expenditure. At the same time, terms such as "high technology medicine" or "expensive medical techniques" are used, implying that these techniques are the bogeymen in our health care system. In fact, they account for only a relatively small proportion of total health care costs, which are due immeasurably more to manpower and to the widespread use of minor and low cost technology throughout the entire health service. Such low cost technology, which is essential to the practice of modern medicine, tends to be neglected by contemporary analysts. Nevertheless, the simple replacement of porcelain for gold in the manufacture of dental crowns saves £26 a time, which at 25 000 crowns a year is £600 000.

Furthermore, if we look at the capital costs of even the most expensive medical techniques such as nuclear magnetic resonance, computed tomography, renal dialysis, and coronary artery bypass grafting, to say nothing of cardiac transplantation, they are very much less than comparable costs for extracting oil from the North Sea, communication by satellite, travel by Concorde, or the extraordinarily high expenditure on defence. One may well suspect that terms such as "high technology medicine" have a touch of the pejorative about them and may reflect, albeit unconsciously, the disenchantment view of technology rather than being solely the result of a concern with costs.

The Council for Science and Society has published the report of its working party on what it calls "expensive medical techniques," which it carefully does not define.[24] The vast majority of individuals working in health care would agree with the working party's view that assessment is necessary when new techniques are introduced. After all, the rejection of Jenner's work by Sir Joseph Banks was on the correct grounds that the technique of vaccination had not been validated. As the Council for Science and Society explains, there is room for improved methods of evaluation of new as well as of old techniques. There is a need for more specialist advice, more research, and a greater degree of consultation. But modern technology, whether it is expensive or not, does not emerge from the consensus of committees but from the innovative and fertile minds of individuals, and if we are to make progress in the future it is such individuals that we must cherish and encourage.

The Medical Research Council is not primarily responsible for undertaking programmes directed at commercially desirable objectives. Nevertheless, through its close association with the British Technology Group, Celltec, and directly with other commercial organisations, the MRC has a commendable record in encouraging new technology. The development of the techniques of molecular biology and of the use of monoclonal antibodies is largely due to the MRC's influence, particularly to the exciting work of distinguished scientists such as César Milstein at Cambridge. It is also worth recording that a simple method for measuring cholesterol in the blood, developed by a research officer at the MRC's Clinical Research Centre has been one of the top six money spinners of the British Technology Group (1981–82).[25] Nor is the MRC inactive in the equipment field. An automated machine invented by the divisions of clinical chemistry and bioengineering at the Clinical Research Centre, which will selectively measure up to 24 different blood constituents, has been developed to commercial production, sadly not with a British firm. It is now in use in the clinical chemistry department at Northwick Park Hospital.

So what of the present position? It is difficult to say whether there is enough venture capital available to sustain an innovative and successful medical equipment industry in this country, but there are many who feel that the root problem in Britain is not a lack of money for technological development but a lack, first, of ideas and, second, of that sort of fizzing critical mass that is immediately apparent if you visit Silicon Valley in the United States. A recent newspaper report suggested that there was not a single comparable critical mass in Great Britain today, which may be true as regards applied technology.

It is unquestionably not true, however, for medical research, where it is lack of money rather than lack of ideas that is currently the problem. The MRC's laboratories for molecular biology in Cambridge are effectively a Silicon Valley for this country in their subject and the current cuts in the MRC's budget are, therefore, a threat to some of the best scientific work being carried out in the world today. Since the development of much of modern biotechnology has derived its impetus from the work of these laboratories, to cut the MRC's funds is a short sighted policy. Equally, it is vital to the development of the National Health Service that we encourage the emergence of those innovative young people in the clinical field who can effectively apply scientific knowledge, and this too is threatened by the MRC's increasing inability to fund clinical research of high quality.

It has been repeatedly urged by those concerned with health care costs that new technology requires better evaluation, and the Council for Science and Society and others have proposed that there should be a central integrating body to coordinate this task.[23][26][27] In view of the problems I have mentioned, however, it would be preferable if such a body were to have the additional responsibilities of identifying promising future areas of applied research and stimulating new ideas, as well as fostering links between the academic world, the National Health Service, research, and industry. Whether such a body were to form part of a projected institute of medicine on the United States model, and what its relationship should be to the Department of Health and Social Security and the British Technology Group, would require further assessment. The idea, however, is worth exploring, as is the further suggestion that technology advisory groups should be set up in the National Health Service at regional and district level.

There is no reason to suppose that the pace of advance in man's technological environment will slow down. Already biotechnology promises to revolutionise medicine, not only in diagnosis and therapeutics but also in prevention. Voices will no doubt continue to be raised against technology, not just on grounds of cost but also because it is considered to be dehumanising. The old image of the caring, compassionate doctor has been replaced in some minds by that of a medical Dr Strangelove, in love with techniques for their own sake, his patients becoming mere bodies surrounded by machinery.

There is, however, no reason why medical technology, used with the compassion and understanding that is a feature of all good medicine, should be any more dehumanising than technology applied to travel or communication. Furthermore, the works of the great painters, musicians, and scientists of the past are surely no greater a reflection of the nobility of the human spirit than are the scientific and technical achievements of modern medicine. There is no human endeavour, other than the feeding of the hungry, to which the ingenuity of man can be better devoted.

NOTES

1 Laennec RTH. *De l'auscultation mediate*. Paris: JA Brosson and JS Chaude, 1819.
2 Matsunaga F, Tajima T. Sigmoidocamera and colonofiberscope. *Geka Shinryo* 1969; 11: 427–33. (In Japanese.)
3 Crosby WH, Kugler HW. Intraluminal biopsy of the small intestine: the intestinal biopsy capsule. *Am J Digest Dis* 1957; 2: 236–41.
4 Spiegelhalter DJ. Computer aided decision making in medicine. *Br Med J* 1984; 289: 567–8.
5 Tabaqchali S, Holland D, O'Farrell S, Silman R. Typing scheme for *Clostridium difficile*: its application in clinical and epidemiological studies. *Lancet* 1984; i: 935–7.
6 Anonymous. NMR monitors metabolism. *MRC News* 1982; 17: 4–5.
7 Cotton PB. Endoscopic management of bile duct stones (apples and oranges). *Gut* 1984; 25: 587–97.
8 Budd JH. Technological advances in medicine. *Postgrad Med* 1982; 71: 11–6.

9 Reiser SJ. Technology and the eclipse of individualism in medicine. *Pharos* 1982; **45**: 10–5.
10 Comroe JH, Dripps RD. Scientific basis for the support of biomedical science. *Science* 1976; **192**: 105–11.
11 Himsworth H. Thomas Lewis and the development of support for clinical research. *Pharos* 1982; **45**: 15–9.
12 Hopkins HH, Kapany NS. A flexible fiberscope using static scanning. *Nature* 1956; **173**: 39–41.
13 Hirschowitz BI. Endoscopic examination of the stomach and duodenal cap with a fiberscope. *Lancet* 1961; **i**: 1074–8.
14 Irvine J, Martin BR. *Project foresight: an assessment of approaches to identifying promising new areas of science.* Brighton: University of Sussex, 1983.
15 Schott K. Economic competitiveness and design. *Journal of the Royal Society of Arts* 1984; **132**: 648–56.
16 Medawar PB. *Advice to a young scientist.* New York: Harper and Row, 1979.
17 Illich I. *Limits to medicine. Medical nemesis. The expropriation of health.* London: Pelican, 1977.
18 McKeown T. *The role of medicine: dream, mirage or nemesis.* London: Nuffield Provincial Hospitals Trust, 1976.
19 Barré-Sinoussi F, Chermann, JC, Rey F *et al.* Isolation of a T-lymphotropic retrovirus from a patient at risk for acquired immune deficiency syndrome (AIDS). *Science* 1983; **220**: 868–71.
20 Gallo RC, Sarin PS, Gelmann EP *et al.* Isolation of human T-cell leukemia virus in acquired immune deficiency syndrome (AIDS). *Science* 1983; **220**: 865–67.
21 Fitchew J. Women give thumbs up to high tech birth. *Hospital Doctor* 1984; **C4** (34): 7.
22 Higson GR. Government help or government interference? *Journal of Physical Education* 1984; **17**: 335–6.
23 Banta D. Review of medical technology policies show need, opportunities for changes. *Hospitals* 1982; **1**: 87–90.
24 Council for Science and Society. *Expensive medical techniques.* London: Calvert's Press, 1982.
25 British Technology Group. *Annual report and accounts.* 1981–82. London: British Technology Group, 1982.
26 Jennett B. *High technology medicine. Benefits and burdens.* London: Nuffield Provincial Hospitals Trust, 1984.
27 Anonymous. High technology medicine: a luxury we can afford? [Editorial]. *Lancet* 1984; **ii**: 77–8.

12 Clinical research and the Medical Research Council

The Medical Research Council has the responsibility of promoting a balanced development of medical and biological research in this country. Throughout its history it has faced a dilemma in deciding the extent to which its support should be given to basic science on the one hand, or to clinical and applied research on the other. Not surprisingly, the council has from time to time been attacked by both wings of its biomedical constituency for its neglect or excessive encouragement of one or the other. In the 1930s, for example, a president of the Royal Society felt it incumbent upon him to protest at what he saw as the unwarranted diversion of the council's funds for clinical research work.[1] Yet at the same time Lord Moynihan, president of the Royal College of Surgions and most vociferous of generations of surgeon critics of the MRC, complained that the council took too lofty a view of clinical research and that it was out of touch with the needs and desires of clinicians. In the modern era the Rothschild proposals for the control of government funds for research and development reflected a similar concern. There has through the years been a constant undercurrent of opinion amongst clinicians that the council has been uninterested in applied clinical research, preferring the purer air of laboratory science. Contemporary commentators, for example Dollery in a recent Rock Carling monograph, have reflected the Moynihan view in referring to the "elitist philosophy of the MRC," as well as citing the views of

Harveian lecture given at the Harveian Society of London, 8 January 1986. *Quarterly Journal of Medicine* 1986; **59**: 435–47.

Health Department officials that "this elitist outlook meant that applied research was neglected."[2]

Yet the evidence of history shows that the MRC has a highly respectable record of support for clinical research in many topics and that from the beginning the council sought to encourage and foster clinical research in this country. It played a major role in developing the techniques of clinical trials. It supported and encouraged epidemiological studies in their early and formative days, in particular the work of Doll and Bradford Hill on the relationship between smoking and cancer of the lung. Furthermore, the council in the modern era has set up a well founded institute for clinical research at Northwick Park, a national venture which should surely be applauded by all concerned with supporting clinical research. The council has always encouraged the highest standards in both laboratory and clinic and it is sadly true that clinical research in this country had not always been able to achieve these standards. For its insistence on quality, however, the council surely cannot be faulted.

It was in fact a clinical problem that led to the foundation of a national agency for medical research in this country. In 1901 a royal commission was set up to inquire whether tuberculosis in man and in animals were one and the same disease. By 1904 the commission had concluded that it could not tackle the problem satisfactorily without carrying out research, and it therefore began experimental studies of its own, thereby becoming a research body endowed with funds from the public purse for the first time. Not everyone shared the view that medical research should be funded by government at that time but it was the Royal Commission on Tuberculosis that provided the stimulus to the foundation of the Medical Research Committee, which in 1920 became the Medical Research Council. In 1911 the commission issued its final report and in that same year Llord George, as Chancellor of the Exchequer, introduced the National Insurance Act which was effectively the precursor of the Welfare State. Among its many provisions, which included schemes for health and unemployment insurance, was that which arranged for sanitorium treatment for sufferers from tuberculosis. Sub-section (2) of section 16 of that Act established that one penny in respect of each insured person should be contributed to a fund for research to be carried out under the auspices of the insurance commissioners. A year later the departmental committee on tuberculosis recommended that the research carried out under the National Health Insurance Act should become the responsibility of a formally constituted Medical Research Committee. They made one further recommendation of major importance for the future – the work of the committee should not be restricted to the subject of tuberculosis.

So it was that a national organisation for the promotion of medical research was set up in this country. The committee, with its executive and advisory committees, was established in 1913 under the chairmanship of Lord Moulton of Bank, a law lord who was also a fellow of the Royal Society. At first the proceedings of the committee were somewhat leisurely and it was immediately apparent that an organising secretary of distinction was required. It was Gowland Hopkins, stimulated by TR Elliott, who suggested the name of Walter Morley Fletcher in early 1914. Hopkins knew Fletcher well. They had collaborated at Cambridge on muscle physiology and biochemistry and in 1915 they were jointly to give the Croonian lectures at the Royal Society. Fletcher had been instrumental in persuading his own college, Trinity, to support Hopkins at a critical stage of his career. Now, in those early days of the Medical Research Committee, Hopkins was an important member of the executive committee.

With Fletcher's appointment, the fledgling organisation began to establish itself. During the year that preceded the outbreak of war in 1914 the committee acquired the Mount Vernon Hospital in Hampstead intending to use the building for the establishment of its central research institute. Thought had been given to the use of some of the space for a research hospital as had been done at the Rockefeller Institute in New York, but considerations of cost led to the abandonment of this scheme. Nevertheless, the committee was particularly concerned to support clinical research and as early as March 1914 the names of Dr Thomas Lewis, who had been much influenced by the work of Sir James McKenzie, and of Dr TR Elliott, future professor of medicine at University College Hospital, had been put forward for consideration by the committee. With the outbreak of war, however, all immediate plans had to be set aside. The hospital in Hampstead was handed over to the War Office and the committee turned its attention to the problems of war. It was in fact the war that was to give the new committee its initial opportunity. Fletcher, in his later reports on behalf of the committee, drew attention to the way in which "the conditions of war had provided not only insistent demands for the application of the scientific method, but many exceptional opportunities at the same time for its easy and fruitful use."[3] Studies of infection, both bacterial and parasitic, the treatment of wounds, the problems of poison gas, renal disease among men in the trenches, and the introduction of effective statistical methods into military practice were all supported by the Medical Research Committee. There was also another problem of the first world war that was to be of great importance in the development of clinical research under the auspices of the MRC in this country, largely because of the individual who was recruited for the work. This was the condition of "soldier's heart" which was leading to increasing disability among military personnel condemned to the horror and hell of the trenches.

Sir William Osler, who had been a member of the original advisory committee, a short lived group irreverently referred to as "the forty thieves," had been one of those who in 1916 had proposed that a special hospital should be set aside for the study of diseases of the heart among soldiers. The War Office, however, initially opposed such special facilities and it was not until Osler, together with Clifford Allbutt, Sir James McKenzie, and Walter Fletcher himself, bearded Keogh, the director general of medical services, in his own den, that the War Office relented and Mount Vernon Hospital was designated for cardiological studies. Osler was a friend, admirer, and enthusiastic supporter of Fletcher and their mutual interest in medical history and in historical texts formed an important bond between them.[4]

From then on things went rapidly. Osler had written earlier in the year to Walter Fletcher expressing the hope that Dr Thomas Lewis could be induced to join in the work, and in April he told an American friend that Allbutt, McKenzie, and he himself had been appointed to select the staff for the Mount Vernon venture. There were to be four units. "Lewis has one," he wrote, "Parkinson and Meakins the others and we hope to get Fraser for the fourth."[4] And so it was that Osler was concerned in the appointment of Thomas Lewis to the full time service of the Medical Research Committee. This was an event of great significance, for Lewis was the first full time clinical research worker to be appointed in this country. It was also an important decision for him personally. He had just got married and as his widow later recorded, in responding to the council's tribute to her husband after his death in 1945, "He never forgot that it was through the Medical Research Committee that he was enabled to follow his star and I well remember how delighted he was to receive his first appointment under the Committee, which made his research work possible in consequence with the increased expenditure of married life."[5]

By the end of the first world war the Medical Research Committee had established a commendable reputation for its handling of research into wartime medical problems. Fletcher himself was knighted in 1918. He had now become the most powerful figure in the developing world of medical research in Britain. A number of important monographs and reports had been published and Fletcher was able to point particularly to the practical and financial value of the work on "soldier's heart," which he calculated was saving the Ministry of Pensions as much as £47000 per annum. In 1920, largely though the exertions of Sir Walter Fletcher, the Medical Research Committee was reconstituted as the Medical Research Council, but there was to be an important difference in its relationship to government authority. Instead of being administered by commissioners under the provisions of the National Health Insurance Act, it was now given a royal charter and came under the Privy Council. This established the Medical Research Council as a virtually autonomous body, which under Fletcher in the postwar years not only wielded increasing power in the allocation of the nation's resources in medical research, but also achieved a high degree of esteem in scientific circles as a result of the close links that were established with the Royal Society, to whose fellowship Fletcher had been elected in 1915. The Royal Society played a major role in the appointment of the members of the council in those early years.

Fletcher was a distinguished physiologist devoted to the scientific method and he was a strong supporter of the basic sciences throughout his years as secretary to the Medical Research Council. In addition, however, he believed in the ultimate applicability of science to practical problems. In his report for 1925, referring to the study of muscle function in which he and Gowland Hopkins had been such important pioneers in Cambridge, he wrote: "The studies of muscle function, which are almost notorious for their supposed uselessness to the student or physician, have laid down basic knowledge and are beginning to remove empiricism from practical studies of physical training and industrial labour."[6]

At the same time, at the beginning of the 1920s, the new council under Fletcher's guidance made a commendable effort to support and encourage clinical research, particularly in London. Research was supported in several London schools, the MRC's activities paralleling the initiatives then being taken in promoting the new academic professorial units, following Lord Haldane's report on the University of London. Thomas Lewis had great success in developing his own unit, which had been established at the end of the war at University College Hospital as the council's department of clinical research. Following a detailed review of Lewis's work in the late 1920s, the council recorded its view that: "It is not an exaggeration to say that the output of work for this centre in the last decade has constituted the central stream of progress made in these subjects anywhere."[7] But elsewhere the initiatives were not so successful. In the annual report for 1928-9, the council concluded that the teaching function of the academic units had been a success, but that the "heavy demand thus made upon the units in this work of teaching over the whole field of medicine have necessarily limited the volume of spontaneous and successful research coming from them in aggregate."[8] But above all, the units had not hitherto produced many men willing and able to devote themselves to a life of clinical research in experimental medicine. This last was the key to the future. There was an urgent need to establish a cadre of clinical scientists who would follow Lewis's lead. It was from the unit at University College Hospital that there were to emerge the pioneers of a new era. At the same time Lewis, who throughout his life committed himself to what he called "clinical science" with all the zeal of a Welsh nonconformist preacher, devoted his formidable mind to the future problems of clinical research.

In May 1929 he set out his conclusions in a memorandum of remarkable foresight to Sir Walter Fletcher.[9] He thought that the lack of progress on the clinical side of medicine and surgery was due not to any inherent difficulties in the subject but to a low standard of work and thought from a scientific standpoint; that this was the outcome of an almost constant association between clinical research work and the opportunistic atmosphere of practical work; and that to remedy this the council should set up an institute "within which the workers may be free from the distractions presented by the petty and mainly diagnostic problems of diverse and obscure cases, and in which they can settle down to a more profound and uninterrupted study of the natural history of selected diseases." His suggestions were considered by the MRC which did not think the moment then opportune; there was not then a sufficiently developed clinical academic community to support such a venture. But the council does appear to have acceded to his request that he be authorised to devote more time to the search for and training of suitable men and be empowered to make short term offers of six and twelve months at the rate of from £200 to £400 a year to two or, at the most, three young men for full time work over the period of the next few years. It was with such appointments to Lewis's unit that men such as Pickering, Wayne, and later John Squire were to begin their distinguished careers in clinical research. It was also in TR Elliott's university department of medicine at University College Hospital, alongside which Lewis worked, that Himsworth, Smirk, and McMichael came to be influenced by Thomas Lewis.

The council continued to debate the problems of clinical research during those years and in the report for 1929 Fletcher posed the question: "Is there a science of experimental medicine in which the actual material for study is the human patient, or is scientific work applied to physician and surgeon limited to the application in his art of scientific research worked out elsewhere in the laboratory and delivered to him for use?"[8] Lewis answered these questions in a long article, which was accompanied by a leading article entitled "Research Physicians," in the *British Medical Journal* of 15 March 1930.[10][11] He argued that there is "indeed a fertile science that deals primarily with patients and this must be encouraged to a more vigorous growth." He argued strongly for the creation and training of a group of workers who would devote their lives primarily to research, making disease as it occurs in man the centre point of their studies. He believed that clinical science had reached a stage where it should develop its own training ground for new recruits, and that it should also achieve independence and freedom. The *British Medical Journal* gave enthusiastic support and concluded: "The report of the Medical Research Council and Sir Thomas Lewis' clear analysis should go far to convince those who have at heart the progress of medicine in Britain, that some posts must be created for research physicians." It was well that the leading article paid tribute to the MRC for Lewis himself made no reference in his article to his service under the council, describing himself simply as physician to University College Hospital and omitting any acknowledgement to the organisation which had supported him for 14 years.

Fletcher, in a private letter to TR Elliott which was not in fact sent, complained with justifiable bitterness of Lewis's touchiness and manners and thought that he did not play fair, particularly in failing to acknowledge either his indebtedness to the council, or Fletcher's generosity in showing him copies of the council's annual report in proof, only to see the material contained within it used by Lewis before the report's publication.[12] Fletcher had been asked by Elliott not unduly to distress Lewis for he had by now had his first coronary attack. If Fletcher felt that Lewis was carrying disloyalty and ingratitude too far, he was a big enough man not to allow such matters to sway his judgement in continuing support for clinical research at University College Hospital.

In that same year, however, there were to be others who were to belabour the council for a supposed lack of concern with practical medicine. Lord Moynihan, in an address entitled "The Science of Medicine" on the occasion of the opening of the Banting Research Institute of the University of Toronto, attacked the council (who in his words "had approximately £500 to spend on research on every working day of the year") for its concern with mice rather than men, and for its temerity in even asking the question whether there was a science of experimental medicine.[13] To Moynihan the surgical art was a science in itself. He felt his own work in practical surgery deserved scientific recognition and, sadly, he deeply resented not being elected to the Royal Society.[14] In an indirect attack on Fletcher's own research interests, he stated: "In a standard textbook of physiology as much as a quarter of the text would be taken up with a discussion of the physiology of muscle, when in any textbook of medicine how many pages deal with the injuries or diseases of muscle?" In another address given at Guy's Hospital that same year Moynihan argued that "the Medical Research Council, which might exert so magisterial and so incisive an influence upon the progress of medicine, the very purpose for which it was founded, seems too busy with little things, too aloof from the day to day practice of medicine."[15] Two years later his fellow president, Lord Dawson of the Royal College of Physicians, joined Moynihan in attacking the MRC as well as the Royal Society for their supposed lofty attitudes to clinical research. "For many years past," wrote Dawson to Fletcher in December 1932, "there has not always been that warmth of feeling in the profession towards the Council which the work of the latter deserves."[16] Both he and Moynihan believed that the royal colleges had as much right to be consulted on matters concerning medical research as the Royal Society or the MRC.

Fletcher had little sympathy for fashionable practitioners who to their financial advantage hoodwinked the public with such transient crazes as ultraviolet light treatment, opsonic indices, and superstitions such as "status lymphaticus." He thought no more highly of college presidents. He replied with seven and a half closely typed foolscap pages, which to this day burn with the suppressed passion with which they were written. "You and Moynihan," he wrote, "the first two medical peers since Lister, have become figureheads of the practising profession, but you have not had the personal footing in the scientific world that Lister had, or that Osler and Allbutt had. Each of you have tended in fact to alienate scientific opinion by your new insistence that headship among successful practitioners is a qualification in itself for leadership in scientific work." He pointed out that the "profession" should not be looked upon as represented only by leaders in practice "whereas it truly includes all practitioners and hygienists as well as all the investigators in all the numerous fields of curative and preventive medicine and scientific work in genetics, laboratory biology, statistics, sociology and psychology." And if the Royal College of Physicians wanted to be consulted, what about the British Medical Association, the Royal Society of Medicine and the Scottish colleges? He pointed out further that the organisation of research was not the function of the royal colleges and that where they had been concerned, as in cancer research, their record had been lamentable. He also deplored Moynihan's public attacks on the Royal Society and the MRC and his "ignorant criticisms of British physiology" made in Canada. He concluded with four excellent proposals as to how the Royal College of Physicians might "whilst maintaining all its present ceremonial and dignity undertake more actively the task appointed to it."[17]

Fletcher's response on this occasion was uncharacteristically vehement. As Sir Harold Himsworth put it to me in a telling phrase, it was "hardly the sword play one expects from an experienced public servant." But in those early months of 1933 it was apparent to many of his colleagues and friends that Sir Walter was losing his customary resilience. He was much encouraged by a letter from his old friend and collaborator Gowland Hopkins, who wrote from Cambridge in February encouraging him to "see the whole thing in perspective and let it hurt you no more." Hopkins went on: "I think I understand the feelings of 'Distinguished Clinicians' just now. In this country they have been so long in the public eye as infallible augurs that the public think or has thought it is they who, standing steeped in wisdom by the bedside, think the great thoughts which advance medicine. But even the Man in the Street in getting better informed and Harley Street is feeling a new and more critical atmosphere. It is feeling chilly."[18] It was clear, however, that although Fletcher was undoubtedly in the right, the affair reflected a deeper malaise than was immediately apparent. Tragically, three months later he was dead.

When Edward Mellanby succeeded Fletcher as secretary, the Medical Research Council had become firmly established as an organisation of foremost importance in the scientific life of the country. The organisation was relatively small at that stage, however, and no one in 1933 would have foreseen the great expansion of the work of the council that was destined to occur during the next two decades. Mellanby, like Fletcher, had been closely connected with Gowland Hopkins in Cambridge, for it had been Hopkins who had stimulated his interests in nutrition and metabolism. He had later done pioneer work in the discovery of vitamin D and the abolition of rickets. As professor of pharmacology in the University of Sheffield, he had held an honorary appointment as physician to the Sheffield Royal Infirmary where for 13 years he had charge of his own beds. Mellanby therefore had a wider knowledge of clinical medicine than Fletcher and during his secretaryship there were to be important developments in clinical research, particularly in his own subject of nutrition.

248

He himself continued to conduct research, with the help of his wife, after his move to London. In 1933 the council, now committed to building up a staff of whole time clinical research workers, established a neurological research unit at the National Hospital for Nervous Diseases in Queen Square under EA Carmichael. Lewis continued to press the cause of "clinical science" in lectures and papers. He strongly supported the views of Sir James Paget, who had written: "I feel sure that clinical science has as good a claim to the name and rights of self-subsistence of a science as any other department of biology." In a series of papers and particularly in his Huxley lecture on "Clinical Science within the University" published in 1935, he argued cogently for the recognition of clinical science as a subject in its own right, urging the universities "to establish that branch of work that studies disease in living people as a science, by removing the obligation to engage in and teach the practical art, and by treating clinical science on precisely the same basis as the allied sciences, physiology and pathology."[19]

By now Lewis was perhaps becoming too successful in his advocacy for he provoked a powerful response from the president of the Royal Society, now Sir Frederick Gowland Hopkins himself. While Fletcher had been attacked by the clinical community in his final years, during Mellanby's early years as secretary the council was to be criticised by the scientists for its support of clinical research. In his anniversary address in 1934 Hopkins specifically referred to Lewis's argument that there was a great need for "a phalanx of trained clinicians who shall bring clinical science to a new pitch of scientific efficiency and hold it there." Hopkins expressed his own admiration for the brilliant contributions of Sir Thomas Lewis and Dr Edward Mellanby, but he thought that there would be relatively few disciplines other than cardiology or nutrition that would offer experimental opportunities of equal promise. He went further in stating that if support for clinical science became a national policy, the result might be the transfer to the ward and clinic of much of the financial support that might properly be enjoyed by research in the pure sciences ancillary to medicine.[20]

The MRC, however, was not to be deterred. In 1934 a new clinical research unit was set up at Guy's Hospital under the direction of one of Lewis's pupils, RT Grant, and in 1938 a short lived surgical research unit was established in Edinburgh. At the same time the council created six postgraduate studentships and four research fellowships. These posts were to be held by a distinguished group of young clinical scientists – who included JV Dacie – and several later became fellows of the Royal Society.

The ability of the MRC to encourage research in the universities was dependent on the development of effective clinical academic departments. Academic medicine had been slow to develop in London following the report of Lord Haldane's commission in 1913.[21] St Bartholomew's Hospital had appointed its first full time professor of medicine, Sir Archibald Garrod, in 1919 and by the early 1930s there were five full time chairs of medicine in London schools. The council noted with pleasure in its report for 1931–2 that Aberdeen University was reorganising its regius chairs in order to provide full time opportunities for teaching and research, and that other universities were following its lead.[22] There were then two developments which were of major importance to the council in providing opportunities for clinical research in the universities in the future.

The first was the opening of the British Postgraduate Medical School at Hammersmith Hospital in 1935. The new school attracted an outstanding full time staff in a range of clinical disciplines. Inspired by Francis Fraser, who had left Barts to become the first professor of medicine at the school, these individuals were able to devote their energies full time to postgraduate teaching, and particularly to clinical research. The council had no direct connection at the outset but in later years came to have a close and fruitful relationship with the Royal Postgraduate Medical School, as it later became (see Chapter 13).

The second development was the handsome endowment by Lord Nuffield at the University of Oxford of chairs for research and postgraduate teaching in medical science. Although clinical research matured more slowly than at

Hammersmith, the MRC's opportunities for promoting it at Oxford were immeasurably enhanced by the Nuffield chairs, which have attracted outstanding professors in the modern era. At the same time a department of clinical research was set up at Cambridge under the direction of the regius professor of physic.

At the time of the outbreak of another world war in 1939 the council was very much better prepared than its predecessor had been a quarter of a century earlier. Nevertheless, concerned that "the fruits of some promising research unrelated to war might be frittered away," the council in 1939, and again in 1940, emphasised the need for continuing its existing programmes of work, subject to whatever demands might be made for special investigations into particular problems in the national interest.[23] Wound shock again became a subject of study. The treatment of wound infection had already been markedly influenced by the introduction of the sulphonamides and was to be greatly improved by the use of penicillin as a result of the outstanding work that took place in Oxford. Professor Howard Florey had written to Mellanby within three days of the outbreak of war outlining a specific proposal for work on Fleming's penicillin with Ernst Chain. Mellanby responded on 8 September. "Provisionally," he wrote, "you can assume that we will give you £25 for expenses for this work and will remember your application for £100 expenses when the time comes." As Gwyn McFarlane has pointed out, there cannot be many government sponsored schemes that have had a smaller initial investment and a larger return.[24] It was in fact the Rockefeller Foundation who were to make a major contribution to this work. Sir Walter Fletcher's son, CM Fletcher, gave the first injections of penicillin to humans early in 1941 when working with LJ Witts as a young physician in the newly founded Nuffield department of medicine in Oxford.[25]

With the introduction of food rationing, nutrition again became an important wartime problem and RA McCance and Elsie Widdowson, both members of the council's staff, had provided important information in their classic monograph *The Chemical Composition of Foods*.[26] Other important contributions to the war effort by the MRC included advice on the treatment of tuberculosis and parasitic disease, the supply of satisfactory therapeutic substances for a nation cut off from Continental supplies, and the health of industrial workers. A particular feature of the MRC's work during the second world war was the setting up of personnel research committees, which did valuable work in advising the three services on the problems of men working in environments which were hostile not only in terms of the hazards of battle but also as a result of their exposure to situations of extreme and unusual physiological stress.

Sir Thomas Lewis was now nearing the end of his distinguished career and in 1942, concerned lest the prewar initiatives in clinical research for which he had been responsible might be lost, he sent to Mellanby a memorandum on clinical research when the war might end. The memorandum was accompanied by a letter thanking Mellanby for his good offices on behalf of a young man named Squire, then working with him. Lewis pointed out in his paper that "At the outbreak of war, there was in this country a group of young men highly trained in methods of research and strongly inclined to clinical investigation. *It was the most promising group of clinical research workers that the country has ever seen.*"[27] He went on to reiterate the need for a central institute for clinical science and outlined what was needed in terms similar to those he had set out in his 1929 paper to the council. Nothing further could be done in those dark days of war and Lewis did not live to see the council implement his ideas, for he died just before the end of the war in Europe.

Meantime a number of new clinical units had been created during the war, for example the burns research unit in Birmingham under the direction of Leonard Colebrook. In 1941, the radiotherapeutic research unit, directed by Constance Wood, was set up at Hammersmith where in the 1950s it was to develop into the cyclotron unit. This was the first of a series of units that were to benefit from the stimulating environment of the Royal Postgraduate Medical School. The council's wartime work on chronic pulmonary disease in south Wales coalminers was published in a series of reports between 1942 and 1945, and when the war ended the pneumoconiosis research unit was established at Llandough Hospital, Cardiff, initially under the direction of LJ Witts's young associate, CM Fletcher.

The two decades which followed the second world war were associated with a continuing and progressive expansion of the council's activities and new units sprang into being all over the country. Blood transfusion, endocrinology, dentistry, vision research, social medicine, tuberculosis, and the pathology of the skin were some of the clinical subjects supported by units.

In 1949 Sir Edward Mellanby was succeeded as secretary by Harold Himsworth. Himsworth had followed TR Elliot in 1939 as professor of medicine at University College Hospital and he had therefore been a young colleague of Sir Thomas Lewis. He had learnt at first hand of Lewis's unsuccessful attempt to persuade the council in the late 1920s to set up an institute for clinical and paraclinical research comparable to the preclinical National Institute for Medical Research, though he knew nothing of the 1942 memorandum at that time. Himsworth as a practising clinician was concerned to stimulate and encourage clinical research. At the same time, the implementation of the National Health Service Act in 1948 was to have important consequences for clinical research. The new Act gave ministers powers not only to conduct research but also to assist others to do so. A joint committee comprising representatives from the Health Departments and the MRC was soon set up under the chairmanship of Professor Sir Henry (later Lord) Cohen, and in 1952 their recommendations were accepted by ministers. There was to be a central organisation for the promotion of clinical research, the Clinical Research Board, established as part of the Medical Research Council, and extra funding was to be provided for this purpose at a later stage. At the same time, facilities for decentralised research were to be provided by regional hospital boards, boards of governors and hospital management committees. In this way, with the establishment of the Clinical Research Board, clinical research was recognised as a subject in its own right within the MRC. The

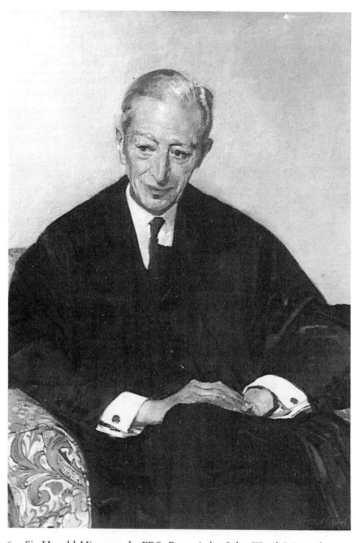

16   Sir Harold Himsworth, FRS. Portrait by John Ward RA in the council room of the Medical Research Council

254

first chairman was the distinguished Manchester neuro-surgeon, Sir Geoffrey Jefferson. It was also necessary to re-organise the way in which biological research work supported by the council was controlled, and at the same time the Biological Research Board was established.

The Clinical Research Board was to have an important influence in the next few years on the decision of the MRC to set up its own centre for clinical research. Sir Harold Himworth had been convinced by his own research experience that with the increasing development of techniques for investigating human disease a new era was opening for clinical research and that it would make an increasing contribution not only to the work of clinicians concerned with the care of patients but also to biomedical science in general. At the end of the second world war, when still professor of medicine at University College Hospital, he had learned with dismay of the decision of the council to move its National Institute for Medical Research from Hampstead to a site in Mill Hill surrounded by fields and totally isolated from direct contact with clinical and paraclinical research. He had at that time urged Sir Edward Mellanby and the then chief medical officer of the Department of Health, Sir Wilson Jamieson, both of whom he knew well from wartime work, to transfer the still unopened building at Mill Hill to the Agricultural Research Council, who were then needing a central institute, and instead to rebuild the national institute alongside a good non-teaching hospital such as the Central Middlesex. Both Mellanby and Jamieson were against the idea. Even if it had at that time been desirable, the building industry was at full stretch repairing bomb damage. Materials such as steel were in short supply and finance was difficult, so that when Sir Harold went to the MRC as secretary in 1949, he had abandoned any hope for a central institute for clinical research and he looked to individual research units to cover the council's needs in clinical research.

By the middle 1950s, however, experience with the working of MRC units was beginning to raise increasing doubts in his mind whether these, although admirable for many purposes, would in themselves enable the council to respond sufficiently to developments in clinical and paraclinical research. Necessarily clinical research is multidisciplinary but, units being guests in other people's houses, the freedom of the council to set up an adequate array of disciplines in response to developing needs on one site was necessarily limited. As a result a unit concerned with, for example, rheumatic disease was having to make do with a fledgeling PhD to meet its need for major biochemisty. In theory a unit should be able to obtain such ancillary support from the academic departments of the host institution, but unlike the heads of departments in an institute, as for example at the National Institute for Medical Research, the heads of these university departments were under no obligation to provide this. Moreover, although the council was always careful when setting up a unit to site it at a place where relevant work was in progress in the surrounding departments, the heads of these might change and their successors might well have quite different research interests.

So the idea of a clinical research institute began to be reconsidered by Sir Harold Himsworth himself and he was supported by the views of the then chairman of the Clinical Research Board, Sir Geoffrey Jefferson. A committee composed of clinical and paraclinical members of the council was therefore set up to review the MRC's provision for clinical research and to make recommendations. At the outset the committee members were sceptical as to whether any change in the existing arrangements was required, but they took exhaustive evidence from unit directors and they finally recommended unanimously that there were now compelling reasons for setting up an institute in which an adequate concentration of clinical and paraclinical research groups was brought together on one site, in association with a district general hospital. It was this report that formed the basis of the council's submission to ministers in 1959. With the warm support of Lord Hailsham, then Minister for Science, the concurrence of the then Minister of Health, and the provisional support of the Secretary of State for Scotland who expressed the view, routinely expected of all Scottish ministers, that any further institute of this kind should be set up north of the border, the plan was approved in principle.

The decision that the proposed centre should be associated with a non-teaching rather than a teaching hospital was made on the grounds that it would be difficult to have two bodies deciding research policy and competing for beds on one site. In those heady early days of the National Health Service the teaching hospitals still sheltered behind powerful boards of governors and were effectively administered separately from the remainder of the Health Service. The decision by a council sometimes thought to be too much orientated to basic science to link its clinical research centre with the work of a district hospital comprehensively serving a defined community must have been particularly welcomed by the Department of Health.

At first, thought was given to siting the projected centre at Chase Farm or at the Central Middlesex Hospital, but Sir John Charles, then chief medical officer at the Department of Health, pointed out that the North West Metropolitan Hospital Board, as it then was, was intending to build a new district hospital at Northwick Park near Harrow, as there were no effective hospital services in that area of outer London. The opportunity was therefore seized to build the new Clinical Research Centre at the same time as the district hospital and both the architectural design and the organisation of the Northwick Park site were to integrate the hospital and the centre as a single unit. It was an attractive and extensive site, with agreeable views of Harrow-on-the-Hill. Professor John Squire, director of the MRC's unit for experimental pathology at Birmingham University, had worked with Sir Thomas Lewis in his department of clinical research at University College between 1939 and 1942, and was therefore well known to Sir Harold and to the MRC. He was now appointed the first director of the projected centre. With characteristic enthusiasm and dynamic energy he got down to the problems of recruiting staff and designing the research centre, integrating its laboratories and wards effectively with the planning phases of the district general hospital. It was a herculean task carried out while he continued his departmental work in the University of Birmingham. And then disaster struck. In January 1966, during a visit to London, Squire developed angina. He hurried to his old medical school at University College Hospital in a taxi but tragically died there soon after his arrival. He was only 52. Squire, like Sir William Osler, was a man of great warmth of character who had to a high degree that indefinable quality that we call leadership.[28] There was no single man who could replace him and the council decided now to appoint both a director and deputy director as successors. Graham Bull, who had spent the early years of his research career at Hammersmith and was then professor of medicine in Belfast, took over as director and Richard Doll was appointed as his deputy. Until Doll's appointment as regius professor of medicine in Oxford they laboured together with the work of planning and recruitment and finally in 1970 the hospital and research centre were opened by the Queen.[29] The occasion was attended by a distinguished group including the then Secretary of State for Education and Science, Mrs Margaret Thatcher, Sir Harold Himsworth, the architect of the whole scheme, and the Bishop of Willesden, now translated to the Bishopric of London.

It was clear from the start that Northwick Park Hospital was to be entirely different from Hammersmith and other teaching centres in London. Whereas Hammersmith had built up an excellent reputation as a tertiary referral centre through the years and was providing first class training at postgraduate level, as were many of the London teaching hospitals, the work of the Clinical Research Centre was to be orientated to the study of those diseases which formed the bulk of the work of a district general hospital. It was also to develop a national role in the encouragement of clinical research. There was a fundamental difference in administrative structure. Graham Bull had proposed that the consultant staff of the hospital should be remunerated jointly by the health authority and the Medical Research Council, an arrangement similar to that of the Johns Hopkins University Medical School when it was set up in 1889. The health authorities concerned in the venture, however, refused and insisted that their own staff should be employed by them and under their control. They naturally had a concern that the district general hospital should effectively serve the community for whom they were responsible and they did not want Northwick Park to develop into another Hammersmith. Through the years the pattern of research work at Northwick Park has in fact closely resembled that envisaged by Sir Thomas Lewis in his 1929 memorandum to council. Northwick Park, with its district hospital providing an excellent service to the community and with 160 extra beds provided by the health authorities for research, has permitted the staff to concentrate on selected disorders.

It has regretfully to be said that the clinical research community in this country did not on the whole respond to the new MRC initiatives at Northwick Park with unbounded enthusiasm. The *Lancet* greeted the Northwick Park development in a leading article in 1969 with references to "mutterings about guinea pigs and monstrous white elephants."[30] Senior academics in medical schools, who should surely have supported any venture that sought to provide opportunities in clinical research to young investigators, were frankly critical and from the outset there were those, particularly in the universities, who thought that the Clinical Research Centre should not have been created, or alternatively that it had been set up in the wrong way. Despite the success of the Clinical Research Centre in developing a broad programme of clinical research which ranges from the molecule to the community, these prejudices still exist in the academic community of this country today. The *Lancet* has been more generous, commenting in a leading article on the centre's tenth anniversary in 1980 on its "excellent reputation for clinical research in psychiatry, dermatology, allergic asthma, anaesthesia and communicable diseases – to name but a few."[31] In 1985 in a further leading article on financial stringency entitled "The Distress of the Medical Research Council," the journal commented that "the Council's founding at Northwick Park of the successful Clinical Research Centre, with its commitment to the study of everyday medical matters in the community, is further evidence that the Council encourages research on the practical issues which confront the National Health Service."[32]

In the meantime the council has continued to support initiatives in clinical research in the universities, the projected institute of molecular medicine in Oxford being a particularly important new venture.[33] The council awards clinical research fellowships, programme grants and grants for projects, as well as giving travelling research fellowships for individuals who wish to work overseas. Clinical research professorships, which may be held at an individual university, have also been established in recent years and the third of these professorships has recently been awarded. Clinical research, however, no longer enjoys the special status that it had under the Clinical Research Board for in the early 1970s the MRC's board structure was reorganised into three major boards – Neurosciences and Mental Health, Cell Biology and Disorders, and Physiological Disorders and Systems. These boards were designed to combine both the basic scientific and clinical research interests of the council in these areas. Whether this development has had a deleterious effect on the MRC's funding of clinical research remains uncertain, but there is some evidence to suggest that council support for clinical research as opposed to basic science, has declined during the past decade in terms of the numbers of units it now supports throughout the country and in terms of the numbers of programme grants awarded to universities.

So what can now be said of the MRC and its attitude to clinical research through the years? If there are still individual clinicians who believe that the MRC is "elitist," that it is "out of touch with the needs and desires of clinicians," as suggested by Moynihan, or that applied research has been neglected, the evidence presented here must surely suggest the reverse. The MRC has always been interested in clinical research, has always sought to support clinical work and has established an institute specifically for this purpose. Furthermore the MRC has included clinicians amongst its council members, and clinical interests are reflected by the membership of the boards and grants committees. It is to these individuals that the clinical academic community should look to represent their interests at the MRC. Sadly, the clinical community on MRC council and boards does not always stand united. Clinicians are notorious for their hypercritical attitude to research proposals from other clinicians so that when clinical research projects are not supported by the council, it is not because the scientists have been unenthusiastic but because other clinicians have been critical. The future of clinical research under the auspices of the MRC depends entirely on the ability of the clinical research community to ensure that its work is satisfactorily supported by those of its representatives who serve the MRC.

Even though the financial squeeze may get tighter, clinical research will continue to enjoy the MRC's support providing that it maintains those high standards which Sir Walter Fletcher so rightly set from the council's earliest days.

NOTES

1 Himsworth H. Thomas Lewis and the development of support for clinical research. *Pharos* 1982; 45: 15-9.
2 Dollery CT. *The end of an age of optimism.* London: Nuffield Provincial Hospitals Trust, 1978.
3 Medical Research Committee. *Report.* 1916-17. London: Medical Research Committee, 1917. (Unbound volumes.)
4 Cushing, H. *The Life of Sir William Osler.* Vol 2. Oxford: Clarendon Press, 1925: 511; 523.
5 MS autograph letter, Lady Lewis to Dr Landsborough Thompson, 3 May 1945. MRC archives.
6 Medical Research Council. *Annual report.* 1924-25. London: MRC, 1925.
7 Medical Research Council. *Annual report.* 1926-27. London: MRC, 1927.
8 Medical Research Council. *Annual report.* 1928-29. London: MRC, 1926-27.
9 Typescript autograph letter, Sir Thomas Lewis to Sir Walter Fletcher, 31 May 1929. MRC archives.
10 Lewis T. Research in medicine: its position and its needs. *Br Med J* 1930; i: 479-83.
11 Anonymous. Research physicians [Editorial]. *Br Med J* 1930; i: 503-4.

12 Typescript letter, Sir Walter Fletcher to Professor TR Elliott, 17 March 1930. A line has been drawn through the letter and "not sent, W.M.F." written across the top of the page. MRC archives.

13 Moynihan, Lord. The science of medicine. *Br Med J* 1930; 2, ii: 779–85.

14 Bateman D. *Berkeley Moynihan, surgeon.* London: Macmillan, 1940: 342–3.

15 Moynihan, Lord. Surgery in the immediate future. *Br Med J* 1930; ii: 612–4.

16 Typescript autograph letter, Lord Dawson of Penn to Sir Walter Fletcher, 15 December 1932. Library of the Royal College of Physicians, London.

17 Typescript letter, not signed, Sir Walter Fletcher to Lord Dawson, 9 January 1933. Library of Royal College of Physicians, London.

18 Fletcher M. *The bright countenance. A personal biography of Walter Morley Fletcher.* London: Hodder and Stoughton, 1957: 285.

19 Lewis T. The Huxley lecture on clinical science within the university. *Br Med J* 1935, i, 631–6.

20 Hopkins FG. Anniversary address. *Proc R Soc B* 1934; 114: 181–205.

21 Royal Commission on University Education in London. *Report.* London: HMSO 1910–1913 (Chairman Viscount Haldane).

22 Medical Research Council. *Annual report.* 1931–32. London. MRC, 1932.

23 Landsborough Thompson A. *Half a century of medical research.* Vol 2. London: HMSO, 1975: 293.

24 MacFarlane G. *Howard Florey: the making of a great scientist.* Oxford: Oxford University Press, 1979: 300.

25 Fletcher CM. First clinical use of penicillin. *Br Med J* 1984; 289: 1721–3.

26 McCance RA, Widdowson EM. *The chemical composition of foods.* MRC Special Report Series No 235. London: HMSO, 1940.

27 Typescript autograph letter and memorandum, Sir Thomas Lewis to Sir Edward Mellanby, 11 June 1942. MRC archives.

28 Anonymous. John Rupert Squire [Obituary]. *Lancet* 1966, i: 157.

29 Anonymous. Opening of Northwick Park. *Lancet* 1969; ii: 884.

30 Anonymous. Northwick Park [Editorial]. *Lancet* 1969; ii: 787–8.

31 Anonymous. Ten years on the Watford Road [Editorial]. *Lancet* 1980; ii: 899.

32 Anonymous. The distress of the Medical Research Council [Editorial]. *Lancet* 1985, i, 25–6.

33 Medical Research Council. *Annual report.* 1984–85. London: MRC, 1985: 6–7.

13 Half a century of science and technology at Hammersmith

Fifty years ago King George V, in the year of his silver jubilee, formally opened the British Postgraduate Medical School at Hammersmith Hospital. It might so nearly not have happened. In the economic gloom of the 1930s it was remarkable that the founding fathers and particularly Sir Frederick Menzies, chief medical officer to the London County Council, had been able to persuade a reluctant Treasury and the council to part with enough money to enable the school to make a start.[1] The school, however, has never allowed financial stringency to affect its sense of ebullient self confidence, and in reading the contemporary accounts of that spring day in 1935 one senses still the high hopes and optimism that permeated the glittering gathering which greeted the King and which included the most distinguished medical men of the day resplendent in academic regalia. Sir Austen Chamberlain, brother of Neville and chairman of the governing body, told the King that the school was to have three main tasks: the continuing education of general practitioners, the training of specialists and, most important of all, the pursuit of research and the advance of medical knowledge. His Majesty graciously responded with the earnest hope "that the School, with its happy union of ward and laboratory, University and Local Authority, drawing students and teachers alike from all parts of our Empire...may prosper under God's blessing."[2]

Address given on 15 May 1985 in commemoration of the 50th anniversary of the opening of the Royal Postgraduate Medical School. *British Medical Journal* 1985; **291**: 1771–9.

Unquestionably the most important feature of the first years of the school was the quality of staff appointed and their wholehearted commitment to research as the major function of a postgraduate institution. Francis Fraser came from his chair at St Bartholomew's Hospital to be head of the department of medicine, George Grey Turner from Newcastle for surgery and James Young to obstetrics. EH Kettle also came from Barts as head of pathology, but he died in early 1936 and was succeeded by JH Dible. These men all attracted excellent younger staff as readers and assistants. Janet Vaughan was an early member of the pathology department, Ashley Miles was reader in bacteriology, and EJ King in clinical chemistry. Robert Aitkin was reader in medicine, Lambert Rogers in surgery, and Chassar Moir in obstetrics and gynaecology.

Francis Fraser, who had been deeply influenced as a young physician by his experiences in the United States, was the key figure among this galaxy of talent. He had worked as a clinical investigator with AE Cohn at the Rockefeller Institute in 1912–4, the period when Abraham Flexner's reports on medical education were the subject of intense discussion in academic circles.[3] He could not then have foreseen what was to happen at Hammersmith nearly 25 years later. In 1912 there were no full time clinical professorships in London. Fraser and other contemporaries at Rockefeller, such as Arthur Ellis, must have had great courage for they were consciously training themselves for full time posts in medicine that did not then exist. Academic posts in clinical medicine in London were only created after the first world war, when the recommendations of the Haldane commission were reluctantly implemented by the London schools. Fraser duly became professor of medicine at Barts in succession to Archibald Garrod in 1921 and at once set about creating there the type of university department envisaged by Flexner, with research laboratories associated with hospital wards. It was an uphill task at Barts. His young students could see Lord Horder arriving in his Rolls Royce and this aspect of a career appealed to them more than did the rigours of laboratory work. Academic medicine was slow to develop in

London, and in the 1930s there were still only five chairs of medicine. So when the opportunity of creating the new school at Hammersmith arose Fraser enthusiastically took up the challenge and it was he who established the principle of academic control of clinical facilities, with full time academic staff, on the American pattern.

Not everyone shared Fraser's view that the future of the school would depend on its ability to do creative research. Colonel Procter, the dean of those early years, held that the school was there for teaching only and that the new Nuffield departments in Oxford had been created to do research. It was a view of Oxford that has an echo in the modern era. Happily it did not prevail.

The idea that clinical departments required laboratories, however, was still not generally accepted in Britain at that time. HR Dean, professor of pathology in Cambridge, had advised that the school's laboratories should be entirely for pathology, since as he put it, "Physicians do not need to use laboratories." Fraser insisted that he must have his own laboratories or else he was no longer interested in the school. The result was the temporary building known as the lower medical corridor which is still there 50 years later.

In those early years before the last war the leadership of Francis Fraser and the enthusiasm and youth of the staff got the school off to a flying start. In medicine there were four assistants: Geoffrey Jennings, Charles Stuart-Harris, Guy Scadding, and Paul Wood. Scadding remembers that by comparison with today it was all very small scale in everything except the clinical workload. Fraser continued with the thyroid work on which he had been engaged at Barts, with the help of his technician, Arthur Latham. Scadding, who was given full charge of beds at the age of 28, recalls his studies of influenza during the 1936 outbreak, only three years after the discovery of the virus at Mill Hill. Fraser made available to him beds for all cases of influenza with lung complications. Wood was advancing cardiology with the simplest of equipment combined with astute clinical observations, and when an assistantship in medicine became vacant in 1937 Peter Sharpey-Shafer was recruited by Fraser to work as an endocrinologist. In pathology RG MacFarlane was writing his classic thesis on disorders of the clotting mechanism. He and Janet Vaughan were joined in 1937 by a young haematologist from King's, JV Dacie, whose enthusiasm for the subject had been stimulated by reading Dr Vaughan's book on the anaemias. All three were later to be fellows of the Royal Society. In surgery George Grey Turner was continuing his work on the management of oesophageal conditions.

In 1938 Robert Aitkin departed to the regius chair of medicine in Aberdeen and Fraser then made an appointment that was to have a major influence on the future research of the school. John McMichael was one of a group of academic contemporaries who had been inspired by Sir Thomas Lewis and who wanted to apply scientific methods at the bedside to the study of human disease. McMichael had spent three years at University College along with George Pickering, Harold Himsworth, Edward Wayne, and Horace Smirk from 1931 to 1934, the height of Lewis's career. In 1935 Fraser had tried to tempt him to join his new department, but McMichael was too well ensconced in Edinburgh and it was not until the readership became vacant that Fraser was able to attract him south. McMichael was impressed by Francis Fraser's leadership and he wholeheartedly supported his determination to create a full time academic department; so in the year of the outbreak of the second world war John McMichael joined the school.

And then it might all have come to nothing. On a gloomy Sunday morning, 3 September 1939, Neville Chamberlain, who had contributed so much to the foundation of the school as Minister of Health and had laid its foundation stone, announced the declaration of war against Germany. The dean, Colonel Procter, took the despondent view that the school should be closed down. Professor George Gask, however, then chairman of the school council and as professor of surgery at St Bartholomew's Hospital an ex-colleague of Francis Fraser, had the imagination and courage to insist that the school should continue. In particular he considered that with its equipment and laboratories it was in a strong position to pursue further research in wartime. Francis Fraser left to direct the emergency medical services in London, telling his new reader as he went, "Well McMichael, you just stay here because we have work to do." So it was that McMichael as reader became effective head of the department of medicine at the outbreak of war.

The war years were to have a highly significant influence on the future course of clinical research at Hammersmith, for the skeleton staff who remained rose magnificently to the challenge. Scadding and Wood went away to the war and McMichael was left with only Sharpey-Shafer and Bywaters. The hospital became a casualty hospital of 400 beds and, not being in central London, received the casualties that were dug out of bombed buildings at a late stage and often found with crush injuries. Among these unfortunates were many who went into renal failure and in 1941 Eric Bywaters published the first of a series of classical papers on crush syndrome and renal failure.[4]

A second important problem for the military was jaundice. At that time confusion existed between acute infective and serum hepatitis. Many soldiers, treated with arsenic at nearby clinics for sexually transmitted conditions, were developing jaundice. To investigate these problems John McMichael, whose MD thesis had been on liver disease, began to carry out liver biopsies in the early years of the war – the first liver biopsies to be performed in this country. Dible undertook the pathology and together with Sheila Sherlock, who later joined the department from Edinburgh, they were able to define the pathology of hepatitis.[5] This effectively established the school as a centre for consultation and they advised the American army in Britain on the problem of jaundice among its troops. Sheila Sherlock soon took over the liver work from McMichael, the first step in her career as an outstanding teacher and investigator in liver disease. Like Scadding, she was to be given full charge of beds at the age of 28.

The third important subject of research was McMichael's other major interest, cardiovascular physiology. It was obviously important at a time of war to know more about the

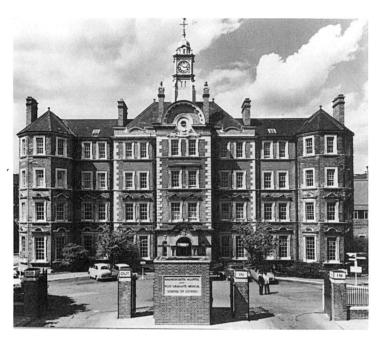

17   Hammersmith Hospital, London

effects of haemorrhage, and to do this a method of measuring cardiac output was essential. The acetylene method then in use was tedious. Sharpey-Shafer and McMichael were now stimulated by the paper by Cournand and Ranges, published in the United States in 1941,[6] to use cardiac catheterisation for the measurement of cardiac output. During this busy period in the department's activities they began their own studies and with Otto Edholm and Henry Barcroft clearly established the physiological reaction to blood loss.[7][8] There were, as McMichael has pointed out, no ethical problems with liver biopsies or cardiac catheterisation at that time, as the whole civilian population was anxious to help the war effort, and there was no lack of volunteers. There were those, however, who did express doubts on ethical grounds. Sir Thomas Lewis, hearing the first paper Sharpey-Shafer and McMichael gave to the Physiological Society at University College Hospital Medical School in December 1943, described their work as "startling" and hinted that they should abandon the procedure. Sir Henry Dale gave powerful and influential support: he argued that the accumulated experience of 394 cases, more than 100 of which were their own, established the safety of the procedure.[9]

The war firmly established the school's reputation for teaching. Numerous courses were held throughout this period in all subjects, but the international reputation of the school was established by the many Americans and Canadians who came to hear McMichael and his colleagues expounding what to all must have seemed a radical new approach to medicine.

In 1946 Sir Francis Fraser became director of the newly founded Postgraduate Medical Federation, and McMichael was now appointed professor of medicine. With the return of doctors from the war a series of other important appointments were made. JV Dacie took over the direction of haematology in that same year and soon afterwards Ian Aird was confirmed as professor of surgery. Later John McClure Brown became professor of obstetrics and gynaecology. Pat Mollison came to Hammersmith in 1946 with the task of directing the Medical Research Council's blood transfusion research unit, and with an honorary appointment to the department of medicine.

At this time the most important influence on the practice of medicine was the introduction of new antibiotics. This had, of course, been first achieved in Oxford, where CM Fletcher, as a young physician, had given the first injections of penicillin.[10] At Hammersmith there now began a period of expansion, which lasted for the next 20 years and which was associated with a flowering of the research effort that, despite everything, had been so effectively established during the school's first decade.

It was an era that was to be dominated by new technology. Biochemical techniques such as flame photometry and paper chromatography, mass spectrometry for the analysis of gases, metabolic balance studies, techniques for vascular imaging, and the introduction of radioactive isotopes into clinical investigation all had a major impact on the school's researches during those years. At the same time the school itself was to be concerned with the introduction of new techniques, some highly complex, of which the best example was the work of the department of surgery on heart and lung machines.

In the department of medicine McMichael set about the task of building a comprehensive department staffed by full time academics and covering an extensive range of medical specialties. He was to be greatly helped by the agreement made by the school with the Ministry of Health in 1951, which established that the school would provide the consultant staff to the hospital, while junior staff were paid by the National Health Service. He had a remarkable ability of bringing together some of the most outstanding men and women of their generation. He encouraged great intellectual freedom, but as CE Newman once remarked, it was a freedom that was never allowed to degenerate into licence.[11] He also greatly enhanced the quality of the Wednesday morning staff rounds, which Fraser had started, where the demonstration of intensive in depth studies of individual patients and their problems has continued to this day.

The work on acute renal failure continued. In 1946 AM Joekes joined Bywaters in the use of the first artificial kidney in Britain, which Kolff had given to Bywaters when he visited Holland after the war ended. It was a thankless task and Joekes remembers nostalgically "the full horrors of setting up the machine during the day and dialysing all night in an empty room on the north block using up to 2 grams of dry heparin to prevent clotting." When Bywaters left in 1947 to direct the Medical Research Council's rheumatology unit in Taplow the machine was given to the department of surgery. It was in fact to be temporarily superseded by GM Bull's work with AM Joekes and KG Lowe on the conservative management of acute renal failure, since they found they could get far better results from treatment with a high energy diet given by intragastric drip feeding, and with fluid restriction and careful attention to electrolyte balance.[12] Their work established the pattern of renal functional disturbance in this condition and effectively disposed of the "Trueta shunt" hypothesis then in vogue.

In hepatology Sheila Sherlock went on to establish liver biopsy as a routine procedure in this country. She pioneered the use of the cardiac catheter in studies of hepatic haemodynamics and metabolism and, with Summerskill and colleagues, described the clinical features of hepatic coma and its treatment with low protein diets and antibiotics.[13][14] Her group also achieved a remarkable first during the 1950s with the introduction by Margot Shiner of the technique of jejunal biopsy.[15] This was in part due to the school's relationship with the old Commonwealth countries at that time. The instrument she first used was Ian Wood's gastric biopsy tube, invented in Australia and brought to the haematology department at Hammersmith by a research fellow from Melbourne, Selwyn Baker. I Doniach provided the pathological expertise, just as Dible had done for the work on liver biopsy.[16]

McMichael's own work on cardiac physiology had established the nature of high and low output cardiac failure and now began to focus on the mode of action of digitalis and its possible primary effect in reducing venous pressure, a view that he modified after subsequent research.[17] He was joined in the early 1950s by JP Shillingford, who continued the physiological studies of cardiac function in health and disease, first in tricuspid incompetence. He went on to use dye dilution techniques for assessing heart valve function, but undoubtedly the best contributions were made in the studies of the haemodynamics of coronary artery disease and the development of the coronary care unit. For this work he was later to be given his own unit by the Medical Research Council.

McMichael had begun to study hypertension and was one of the earliest to treat patients with the newly discovered hexamethonium compounds. Brenda Morrison, Priscilla Kincaid-Smith, and later CT Dollery all joined in this work. McMichael himself, with his commitment to physiological studies, made no more than a start in the use of cardiac catheterisation for the diagnosis of congenital or valvular heart disease. After Paul Wood went to the National Heart Hospital in 1947 JF Goodwin did this with the enthusiastic cooperation of RE Steiner in the department of radiology. In later years the studies of the natural history of the cardiomyopathies were to be a major contribution of the clinical cardiology group.

Throughout this era a strong emphasis was laid on applied physiology. In pulmonary physiology there was outstanding work by WA Briscoe, who was followed by P Hugh-Jones, JB West, and EJ Moran Campbell. CM Fletcher, who succeeded John Crofton in respiratory medicine, was the only member of the department to adopt an epidemiological approach. With his colleagues he carried out comparative studies of bronchitis and emphysema in Britain and the United States. He also showed, in a mammoth study carried out locally, that stopping smoking was far more effective than treating bronchitis with prophylactic antibiotics.

In endocrinology Russell Fraser used the newly available radioiodine to study thyroid function. He also developed important research programmes in osteoporosis and calcium metabolism. Russell Fraser started the metabolic ward at the north end of the B block, with laboratory support from I McIntyre and the department of clinical chemistry. He was not the first to introduce the technique of pituitary implantation, but with GF Joplin he played a major role in developing this procedure in endocrinology. Russell Fraser's unit was the only one to lose a member of staff on what may be termed active service. In July 1966 Alice Dimitriadou died in a tragic helicopter accident while collecting samples from patients with thyroid disease near Bogota in Colombia.

RIS Bayliss worked on the newly discovered corticosteroids until his appointment to the Westminster Hospital in 1955. CL Cope was a meticulously careful student of adrenal steroid secretion for many years, and the excellence of his work continued after his retirement in 1968. He was a man of sterling integrity, sadly no longer with us. He thought that his last paper, published in *Clinical Science* in 1975 within a few days of his death at the age of 71, was one of his best.[18] J Vallance-Owen worked as Cope's senior registrar during the period that he was developing the use of the rat diaphragm for measurements of plasma insulin.

Undoubtedly the most impressive figure in these days in the 1950s was MD Milne. He had a scientific pugnacity and encyclopaedic scholarship before which all quailed. He did not get Conn's syndrome right first time, even though Cope and Garcia-Llaurado had found excessive aldosterone in the urine of his patient with so called potassium losing nephritis.[19] [20] But he became interested at the same time in nonionic diffusion, publishing his studies in the *American Journal of Medicine*.[21] This led, by a remarkable feat of scientific intuition, to his outstanding work on Hartnup disease and cysteinuria, in which he showed for the first time the jejunal transport defects for different amino acids in those conditions.[22] He went on to become one of those rare clinicians to be elected to the Royal Society.

It was an exhilarating era in the department of medicine. Its most exciting features were the revolution in the intellectual approach to medicine, an encouragement by McMichael of the young which was unrivalled in Western Europe, and the opportunity we all had to work in an atmosphere in which no established medical belief went unchallenged

Ian Aird, now firmly in charge of surgery, was, in McMichael's own words, undoubtedly a genius. His book, *A Companion in Surgical Studies*, was one of the most remarkable surgical texts ever written. He had an extraordinary vision and was far ahead of his time. When he became professor of surgery in 1947 he decided that his department should concentrate on two areas of research that he believed were vital for the future of surgery. One was a pump oxygenator to permit open heart surgery, the other renal transplantation. He had no experimental surgical facilities at Hammersmith and had to find space for himself in a floor of the old north block. But DG Melrose was set up to work at the Buxton Browne farm of the Royal College of Surgeons, where he successfully developed a pump oxygenator which could take over the circulation in dogs.[23] It was not easy to initiate studies in man but by 1954 the first operation had been carried out in a patient undergoing surgery on the aortic valve by WP Cleland, the pump oxygenator on that occasion being used simply to assist the circulation.[24] Open heart surgery, however, soon followed, particularly after the development by Melrose and his colleagues in 1955 of a method of producing elective cardiac arrest.[25] They worked closely with Goodwin and Steiner, whose diagnostic skills were essential to this endeavour. The cardiac surgery group at Hammersmith soon became world famous, and in 1959 the entire team was invited to Moscow to help develop open heart surgery in Russia

Meantime renal surgery was being developed by Ralph Shackman, and in the mid-1950s, after the commercial development of new and more satisfactory dialysis machines in France, the department reintroduced haemodialysis for the treatment of acute renal failure. Shackman and his colleagues were later to set up a unit for the treatment of end stage renal failure by dialysis, but this was not until after the pioneering work of Scribner in Seattle. Aird's dream of successful transplantation was to be realised at Hammersmith in the 1960s, but despite the early studies by WJ Dempster of experimental renal transplantation which Aird had stimulated, the first renal transplants were to be done not at Hammersmith but in Boston, Paris, and Edinburgh. The school's hesitation in exploiting early work in this field has to be accounted as one of its failures by any critical historian.

In the interests of historical accuracy it has to be said that operative surgery was not always Aird's own strongest suit, particularly in his later years. Nevertheless, he ensured that his department maintained the highest standards of practical surgery, and it was the part time staff who made the major contribution to this. WP Cleland, whose part in the development of cardiac surgery here was crucial, RH Franklin, who made major contributions to gastrointestinal surgery, carrying out the first operation for tracheo-oesophageal fistula in Europe, Peter Martin in vascular surgery, Geoffrey Knight in neurosurgery, and Selwyn Taylor in the surgery of the thyroid and parathyroid were all loyal and devoted members of Aird's department.

With the development of complex modern surgery, anaesthesia became vitally important in ensuring success, and anaesthetists were to become increasingly concerned in postoperative and intensive care. The work of Nunn and Payne, who both worked at Hammersmith on postoperative hypoxia, was particularly important. In the early years anaesthetists were members of the department of surgery, but anaesthesia achieved independent departmental status with the appointment of Sir Gordon Robson as professor in 1964. His researches in neurophysiology were to stimulate vigorous research developments in this subject.

The other major clinical department of that era was obstetrics and gynaecology. Robert Keller, future professor in Edinburgh, was Professor James Young's first assistant from 1937–9. J McClure Brown had succeeded Professor James Young at the end of the war, and his department was to make important contributions. Mollison carried out his early studies of exchange transfusion in haemolytic disease of the newborn, and Brown himself soon began to develop techniques for studying placental function. The department had a succession of readers and assistants during this period – Ian Donald and Norman Morris among them – who went on to greater things. At the same time Erica Wachtel was introducing new techniques of gynaecological cytology, and in operative gynaecology VB Green Armitage was one of those who pioneered tubal reconstructive surgery for women suffering from infertility.

There was no academic department of paediatrics in the early days of the school, but in 1954 the Institute of Child Health set up a readership at Hammersmith and Peter Tizard was appointed to the post. He soon established an international reputation for himself and his colleagues with his work on fetal resuscitation and neonatal physiology, and in 1964 he was awarded a richly deserved professorship. He went on to become professor of paediatrics at Oxford and his reader, John Davis, was subsequently appointed to the chair of paediatrics in Cambridge.

But if during those first three decades of the school's existence the clinical departments had established the school's international reputation for clinical research, this was due in major part to the collaboration and support they received from the departments of pathology, radiology, and medical physics, as well as from those Medical Research Council units that had been set up on the site. Nor should the workshop and its staff, so ably directed by Con Lorden, be forgotten, for they made major contributions to research throughout the school and they were closely associated with DG Melrose in his work on the development of the pump oxygenator. Both the library and the department of medical illustration have also given excellent support to the research activities of the school, often providing a service that went beyond the call of duty.

In many ways it has been the pathology departments that have been the scientific success story of the school. By the end of the war Lord Stamp and Earl King had emerged as professors of their respective subjects of bacteriology and clinical chemistry, and after Dible became emeritus in 1955 Dacie became professor of haematology and CV Harrison of histopathology. Increasing specialisation through the years led to the four departments becoming autonomous, though they still retained a rotating headship of pathology. The lunchtime clinicopathological discussions, a tradition brought from Barts by Fraser and Kettle, were in those days one of the most important features of the school. In histopathology AGE Pearse was pioneering the histochemical techniques that have made him a household name in so many laboratories throughout the world.[26] He was later to develop his APUD (amine precursor uptake and decarboxylation) cell concept, linking together the cells of that diffuse endocrine system that is a particular feature of the gastrointestinal tract and its associated glands. Doniach's work on the thyroid was by no means his only or even his major contribution; he was one of the most enchanting and generous of men and many of us in other departments turned to him for advice. It was also in pathology that George Popjak started his distinguished research career in lipid biochemistry in this country. He began with a bunsen burner in a corner of Dible's department.

In clinical chemistry Earl King was working on silicosis as well as setting standards for measurement that were to be increasingly important as techniques multiplied. Bill Klein's work on steroid chemistry was an important contribution to the department. McIntyre, initially concerned with divalent cations such as magnesium, went on to follow up the discovery of calcitonin by Copp and his associates.[27] With Pearse and his colleagues he investigated its localisation in the thyroid C cell. Nor should one forget the contributions of CE Dalgleish to paper chromatography. IDP Wooton continued to develop automated methods in clinical chemistry when he succeeded King as professor. He also played an important role in introducing computing at the school.

The other two pathology departments have a record of outstanding distinction. The department of bacteriology has an unequalled scientific record. It gave birth to two Medical Research Council units: the bacterial genetics unit of W Hayes, and DA Mitchison's unit for the laboratory studies of tuberculosis. It has three fellows of the Royal Society to its credit: Sir Ashley Miles, W Hayes, and Professor Naomi Datta, the pioneer of resistance factors in bacteria.[28] DA Mitchison, who succeeded Stamp as professor, made contributions to the school which went far beyond his own work. It was he who helped set Naomi Datta on her way. In addition, he was for many years the school's unofficial statistician, and there were many among us, in all departments of the school and at all levels of seniority, who turned to him for advice. Mary Barber, with her work on hospital infection, was a charismatic figure in the department until her untimely death in 1965.

The department of haematology, under JV Dacie's exacting leadership, set standards for this subject which have influenced the practice of haematology throughout the world. Dacie's own work on haemolytic anaemia, enshrined in his classic textbook, duly earned him his fellowship of the Royal Society. The department has a number of important firsts to its credit. One was the B_{12} assay. Mitchison drew DL Mollin's attention to the paper by Hutner and his colleagues in 1949 which showed that vitamin B_{12} was a growth factor for the green alga, *Euglena gracilis*, and this led to his successful development, with GIM Ross, of the first assay for vitamin

B_{12} in serum, a major step for those studying megaloblastic anaemia.[29] Other important discoveries have included Dacie's own demonstration, with JG Selwyn, of the importance of metabolic defects in the red blood cell in non-spherocytic haemolytic anaemia, [30] and the first description, with Oxford colleagues, of Christmas disease.[31] In the late '50s I was working with Mollin in that department, and we were able to show that the absorption of vitamin B_{12} is a function of the ileum, which was effectively the first time that absorption had been shown to be localised to a particular area of the small intestine.[32] A fifth department was added to pathology when the school appointed Professor AP Waterson to a newly established chair of virology in 1964. Particularly distinguished work was carried out on hepatitis virus by June Almeida when she worked in this department.

The department of radiology has been of great importance to the research achievements of the school. It was originally a department of the hospital under Dr Duncan White and it was not until the 1960s that the school began to take over responsibility for the consultant staff. RE Steiner, who had originally joined the department as a hospital consultant in 1950, became professor of radiology 10 years later and with JW Laws and FH Doyle created a department that was to be described by the *British Medical Journal* in later years as a "beacon light" to British radiology. All departments in the school owe a great debt to this department, which was particularly important to developments in cardiology. Equally important, however, were its contributions to hepatology, small intestinal disease, renal disease, endocrinology, and bone disease, to quote just a few examples.

The department of medical physics also made important contributions to imaging techniques. Some of the earliest brain scans were carried out at Hammersmith by JR Mallard and this department was vitally important to all who used radioactive isotopes in their researches, as many did.

The development by the Medical Research Council in the postwar years of several units on the Hammersmith site was an indication of the increasing importance of the school in clinical research in this country. The radiotherapeutic unit, moved to Hammersmith during the war, evolved into the cyclotron unit after the cyclotron first produced a beam in 1955. It was the use of short lived isotopes from the cyclotron that enabled JB West and CT Dollery to carry out their classical studies on ventilation and blood flow in the human lung.[33] More recently Mary Catterall has conducted her careful trials of neutron treatment at Hammersmith. Court-Brown worked at Hammersmith in the Medical Research Council's radiation sickness unit and carried out the studies that established the importance of radiation in causing myeloid leukaemia in patients with ankylosing spondylitis. Mollison's Medical Research Council blood transfusion research unit was housed in the hut between C and D blocks, and he and his colleagues, between 1946 and 1960, did for blood transfusion what Dacie had done for haematology. NB Myant's lipid research unit was set up after Popjak left in 1962, and distinguished work was later done on the relation of hyperlipidaemia to atheroma.

By the 1960s the school had become, in the words of historian Noel Poynter, "the most advanced and successful medical school in the British Commonwealth. It was," he wrote, "an example of what can be achieved when the restrictions imposed by tradition and vested interests are loosened. This Institution with its brilliant record has been of tremendous value in radically changing the attitudes of British doctors to medical education and the way it should be organised."[34]

There then occurred two events which were to be landmarks in the history of the school. The first was the tragic and untimely death in 1962, by his own hand, of Ian Aird, that lovable but wayward genius; the second was the retirement in 1966 of Sir John McMichael. A fellow of the Royal Society, knight bachelor, Wellcome trustee, and the recipient of numerous honorary degrees and other distinctions, he had become a towering figure in the school. In nearly 30 years at Hammersmith he had not only served the school with great devotion, but had also had a greater influence on British academic medicine than any one of his contemporaries.

RB Welbourn, who succeeded Aird as professor of surgery,

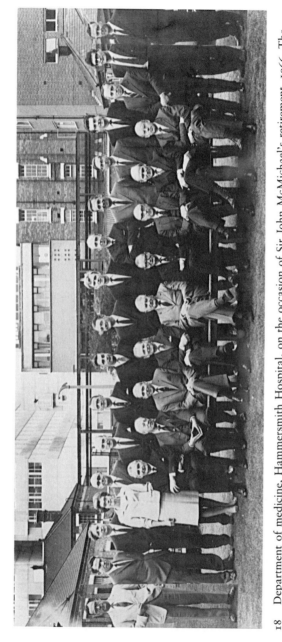

18 Department of medicine, Hammersmith Hospital, on the occasion of Sir John McMichael's retirement, 1966. The future professors of paediatrics in the universities of Oxford (Sir Peter Tizard) and Cambridge (Professor John Davies) are also included

inherited the excellent experimental surgery facilities that had now been built in the cyclotron building with the help of the Wellcome Trust, and at the same time the school obtained further support for a floor at the top of the new Commonwealth building for the department. The two main areas of surgery were to be linked by a bridge named in memory of Ian Aird. Welbourn believed in advancing knowledge through the careful study of surgical patients and by using the special opportunities provided by surgical operations to study normal and abnormal structure and function. He organised clinical trials for the treatment of breast cancer and made important contributions to the study of patients with Cushing's syndrome, phaeochromocytoma, and the neuro-endocrine tumours of the gut. He particularly encouraged plastic surgery under James Calnan, who did important work on lymphoedema. In orthopaedics Charles Galasko carried out extensive studies on skeletal scintigraphy. He was subsequently appointed to the chair of orthopaedics in Manchester. Welbourn firmly believed in the value of research as the best education for a surgeon and he encouraged many younger members of his department to undertake research.

In October 1966 I undertook the daunting task of continuing in the steps of Fraser and McMichael. I had been a house physician with Sir John in 1952 and had subsequently worked in the department since 1954. For five years I was seconded to haematology to work with DL Mollin. After Sheila Sherlock's departure to become professor of medicine at the Royal Free Hospital in 1959 I had taken over gastroenterology and developed a unit for the investigation and treatment of small intestinal disease. The work on sites of absorption in the small intestine continued. Later GR Thompson carried out the first studies of vitamin D absorption in man. RH Dowling investigated the important question of how the small intestine adapts to resection or disease, work that he continues as professor of gastroenterology at Guy's Hospital; Soad Tabaqchali, now professor of medical microbiology at St Bartholomew's Hospital, began her definitive studies on how bacteria affect absorption in the small intestine. Graham Neale was the outstanding clinician of this group.

There were now wider issues to be considered. The first was the commitment to teaching of the department of medicine. With increasing specialisation in different subjects a need for specialist rather than general courses developed, and in 1968, under the direction of Graham Neale, the format of teaching was changed from courses in general medicine alone to short courses covering a wide range of specialist subjects.

At the same time it was clear that Britain was no longer the imperial power of which George V had been King Emperor in 1935. The school had many links with the United States, Canada, and other Commonwealth countries such as India. A particularly fruitful exchange had been set up with the University of California in Los Angeles. With encouragement and support from the Wellcome Trust, DA Warrell was seconded to Zaria, northern Nigeria, where he developed his interest in snakebite. There were also important exchanges with the University of the West Indies, where Hughes studied cerebral lupus erythematosus. But it was now time to become European. Dollery had been secretary and later president of the newly founded European Society of Clinical Investigation and many of us were members. In Germany there was a Pearse Club. The gastroenterology group had established cordial links with the department of Professor JJ Bernier at St Lazare in Paris. Phillipe Bordier from the Centre du Metabolism Phosphocalcique at Lariboisière held a part time lectureship in the school.

With the help of the British Council the school's courses were advertised in many European countries. They were an immediate success and brought increasing numbers of postgraduates from Europe. The department of surgery followed suit and also began to attract European postgraduates. At the same time the department of medicine introduced a scheme of inviting a distinguished European clinical scientist as a visiting professor for one week during each of the year's three terms. In this way important links were created between the school and some of the best clinical research workers in

Europe, and the development of a group of European clinicians at senior level, all of whom knew each other well, was further encouraged.

The overall direction of research in the department of medicine also needed reconsideration. Sir John McMichael, in the open day address that he gave on the school when he retired in 1966, showed a diagram of how he then viewed the relations between the different departments. His commitment to clinical physiology was expressed by his view, a reflection of Sir Thomas Lewis's philosophy, that every physician should be a physiologist.[35] It all depended, of course, on what you meant by physiology. But by now it was clear that there were scientific lacunae within a school that sought to be in the forefront of clinical research.

We then needed doctors who were pharmacologists, biochemists, cell biologists, and immunologists just as now we need clinical molecular biologists. Sir John had set the scene for future developments in clinical pharmacology, and in the new Commonwealth building, opened by Her Majesty the Queen in the year of his retirement, he had ensured that there was space for CT Dollery to pursue his interests in pharmacology. Dollery's extraordinary energy had led him into a variety of activities during his earlier career, starting with hypertension with McMichael and including the studies of the lung using isotopes produced by the cyclotron with JB West already referred to, as well as the investigation and treatment of hypertensive and diabetic retinopathy with Eva Kohner and Graham Joplin. He was now focusing his attention on clinical pharmacology. At the same time Sir Charles Stuart-Harris, one of the department of medicine's original assistants who was then chairman of the medical subcommittee of the University Grants Committee, told us that there was a real need for a department of clinical pharmacology that could train the teachers of the future. In 1969, with the help of the Wellcome Trust, Dollery was appointed professor of clinical pharmacology with his own independent department. It was an excellent move, which has been fully vindicated by the extraordinary success of the department in training a whole new generation of professors of this subject.

Research in the department has included studies of the relations between different drugs when multiple prescriptions are given, and more recently the pharmacology of adrenaline and noradrenaline and of the prostaglandins.

Several members of the school were also interested in the possibility of developing a department of biochemistry, but this proposal failed on the grounds that there was no apparent postgraduate student body. We therefore turned to the creation of multidisciplinary groups that would bring biochemistry and clinical medicine together. This led to the formation of the endocrine unit under the joint direction of Russell Fraser and Ian McIntyre, again with support from the Wellcome Trust. In addition, individual research teams were to recruit biochemists to their strength, as both Milne and Sherlock had done earlier.

The third subject that required examination was immunology. It was a subject that was burgeoning but it had been little exploited in the school at that time, except in the department of haematology where Sheila Worlledge was carrying out excellent serological work in the blood transfusion laboratory, and in the department of clinical chemistry, where JR Hobbs was studying immunoglobulins. The first of our European visiting professors to the department of medicine, the late Professor JF Heremans of Louvain, played an important role in stimulating interest in immunology in the school. His lectures to the department of medicine were given every morning for a week to more than 200 people. Soon after his visit CL Cope retired. It might have been possible to develop the subject within programmes of research in the department of medicine itself, but we decided instead to create a new department within the division of pathology and Cope's readership was transferred to pathology for the purposes of creating a chair. Robert Steiner as chairman of the academic board did sterling work in providing support for this development and Peter Lachman was the first professor. He has since been elected a fellow of the Royal Society. In the meantime DK Peters had joined the department of medicine from the Welsh National School of Medicine in succession to OM Wrong. His renal interests and his close association with Lachman led to a series of important studies on the role of complement in renal disease.[36] Peters went on to pioneer the use of plasmapheresis in the treatment of renal disease associated with antibodies to the glomerular basement membrane. His work has had important implications for other immunological diseases, in particular for the treatment of myasthenia gravis.[37] In gastroenterology WF Doe, a young Australian now professor of medicine at the National University of Canberra, was studying gut immunology and he too derived considerable inspiration from the new department.

There was a price to pay for the move away from traditional clinical physiology, still dominant in many academic departments of medicine in Britain. JB West left in 1969 for California, depriving us of one of the world's best respiratory physiologists. The previous year EJ Moran Campbell had been appointed to the foundation chair of medicine in the new school at McMaster, where he created an outstanding department.

Another opportunity arose to develop a multidisciplinary group crossing departmental boundaries when RHT Edwards, who had trained with Moran Campbell but was now working on muscle physiology in the department, obtained financial support from the Jerry Lewis Foundation to put up a building on a vacant rooftop to house his own research, and that of Dr DK Hill from biophysics, as well as the studies of muscle biochemistry that Victor Dubowitz, Tizard's successor, was carrying out in children with muscular dystrophy. This highly successful group continued until Edwards succeeded CE Dent in the chair of human metabolism at University College Hospital in 1977.

Other influences during the period of the late 1960s were bringing departments together. The different cardiology groups, for example, formed themselves into a division. Haematology had originally been part of the department of pathology and its members did not care directly for patients. Dacie's patients with paroxysmal nocturnal haemoglobulinuria, whom he always himself painstakingly transfused with red cells washed in saline, were usually admitted under the care of a physician. McMichael in his later years, however, gave beds within the department to haematology, and with the building of the leukaemia unit to house the clinical work of the Medical Research Council unit directed by DAG Galton, haematologists were increasingly to be seen on the wards, and Sir John Dacie himself would now conduct ward rounds. In this way haematology at Hammersmith became a clinical as well as a laboratory discipline, an essential step in the development in recent years of the bone marrow transplantation programme.

Russell Fraser's retirement in 1974 led to a reappraisal of the research direction of endocrinology. Dr SR Bloom, then at the Middlesex Hospital, was making a name for himself in the measurement of the newly discovered gut hormones using radioimmunoassay and he now joined the department of medicine. Like DK Peters he was appointed at the age of 30. He at once joined up with AGE Pearse and Julia Polak in histochemistry to form the team that has been so successful in the subject of regulatory peptides. New radio-immunoassays were developed for measuring these substances and immunocytochemical techniques made it possible to identify the types of cells associated with their secretion. This made possible the study of the pathophysiology of peptides such as vasoactive intestinal polypeptide and entero-glucagon, as well as many other substances, for the first time.[38] The group has a number of important firsts to its credit. Professor RB Welbourn, with his interest in endocrine surgery, collaborated fruitfully with this team, and the department of surgery contributed important expertise in experimental surgery.

In 1977 DK Peters was chosen to succeed me as professor of medicine. I had been asked by Sir John Gray, then secretary of the Medical Research Council, to consider becoming director of the Medical Research Council's Clinical Research Centre at Northwick Park in succession to Sir Graham Bull. It was a difficult decision. At Northwick Park, however, there would be an opportunity to develop new initiatives in clinical research in this country, particularly in molecular medicine and cell biology. Furthermore, I had been professor of medicine at Hammersmith for 11 years and from the point of view of the school there was an opportunity to appoint someone younger and better than myself. In addition, it was clear that the type of work carried out at Northwick Park, with its emphasis by the Medical Research Council on the work of a district general hospital and service to a defined community, was entirely complementary to the very high quality tertiary referral work that through the years had come to dominate clinical activities at Hammersmith.

My acceptance of the Medical Research Council's offer was obviously right for the department of medicine, which has gone from strength to strength. Immunological medicine has, naturally, been encouraged. There has also been a commendable zeal for the promotion of infectious disease as a clinical specialty. Dermatology has had a much needed research boost, and a geriatric department, at first headed by Professor M Hodkinson from Northwick Park, was set up. Gastroenterology continued to carry out distinguished work, initially under the direction of V Chadwick, who has now been appointed to Horace Smirk's old chair in the University of Dunedin.

In radiology the development of modern imaging techniques for diagnostic purposes has accelerated in both quality and quantity. Professor Allison has succeeded his now legendary predecessor who continues with support from the Medical Research Council to direct the school's excellent work on the exploitation of magnetic resonance imaging. Allison himself has developed techniques of interventional radiology, particularly in the treatment of vascular and malignant disorders. Other imaging techniques have included the work on positron emission tomography in the Medical Research Council cylotron unit, which has recently been rewarded by the promise of a new machine.

The characterisation of the calcitonin gene was the result of a collaboration between McIntyre and the molecular biologist RK Craig, working at the Middlesex Hospital, [39] but in other respects molecular biology has perhaps been slow to develop in clinical research at Hammersmith. Its importance in the modern era, however, was recognised by the appointment of Professor Lucio Luzatto to the chair of haematology, where he carries out distinguished work on the molecular genetics of glucose-6-phosphate dehydrogenase deficiency. Both the presence of Professor Beverley Griffin in virology and the recent acquisition of a distinguished microbial geneticist as professor of bacteriology strengthen molecular biology in the school. The school's European connections have been encouraged not only by Professor Luzatto's appointment, but also by Professor Attilio Maseri's acceptance of the Sir John McMichael chair of cardiology in the school in succession to JP Shillingford. Professor LH Blumgart's innovative and original work in hepatobiliary surgery has stimulated the department, which he now heads. There have also been changes in the department of histopathology, where Professor NA Wright's studies of cellular kinetics are achieving international distinction.

The importance through the years of good administration by the office of the dean deserves special notice. CE Newman, who began his decanal career as Colonel Proctor's assistant, provided a quality of self effacing integrity at a time when the school was growing, and he ensured that none of the giants who were his colleagues ever got their hands in the till at the expense of another. Selwyn Taylor was an excellent courtier when Her Majesty the Queen opened the Commonwealth building in 1966 and he presided over important changes in the school. Finally, MPW Godfrey provided the school with inspired leadership during the most difficult period of its history and brought it through stronger than ever. Dr DNS Kerr bravely continues in his distinguished footsteps.

Hammersmith has been, as Richard Crossman once said on a visit as Secretary of State, "a triumph of the human spirit over adversity." It is a place where there is always a fizz of excitement that gives a champagne quality to every day. Some years ago a Swedish visiting professor to the department of medicine wrote afterwards to tell me that he had never been anywhere where there was such a glow of enthusiasm for clinical research. Yet accustomed as he was to Sweden's immaculate clinical facilities, he could only bewail the fact that the work had to take place in such inadequate surroundings. He went on to comment that it must have been intentional so as to show the students from the Third World how much could be done with how little. Happily this era is coming to an end with the approval of the building plan for the new hospital and the immediate start on the first stage.

So we come to today and the beginning of a new half century. The opportunities for clinical research have never been so challenging or exciting. We stand at the threshold of an era when it will be possible to treat virus diseases, unravel the causes of cancer, understand the biology of mental illness, and probably introduce gene treatment. There is, therefore, even more need now for this school, with its commitment to clinical research, than there was 50 years ago.

NOTES

1 Newman CE. A brief history of the Postgraduate Medical School. *Postgrad Med J* 1966; **42**: 738–40.
2 Anonymous. British Postgraduate Medical School. Opening by the King. *Br Med J* 1935; i: 1044–5.
3 Corner GW. *A history of the Rockefeller Institute 1901–1955*. New York: Rockefeller Press, 1964: 98; 106; 258.
4 Bywaters EGL, Beall D. Crush injuries with impairment of renal function. *Br Med J* 1941; i: 427–32.
5 Dible JH, McMichael J, Sherlock SPV. Pathology of acute hepatitis. *Lancet* 1943; ii: 402–8.
6 Cournand A, Ranges HA. Catheterisation of the right auricle in man. *Proc Soc Exp Biol Med* 1941; **46**: 462–6.
7 McMichael J, Sharpey-Schafer EP. Cardiac output in man by a direct Fick method. *Br Heart J* 1943; **5**: 33–40.
8 Barcroft H, Edholm OG, McMichael J, Sharpey-Schafer EP. Post-haemorrhagic fainting. *Lancet* 1944; i: 489–90.
9 McMichael J. Forward. In: Veral D, Grainger RG, eds. *Cardiac catheterisation and angiocardiography*. Edinburgh: Churchill Livingstone, 1962.
10 Fletcher CM. First use of penicillin. *Br Med J* 1984; **289**: 1721–3.
11 Newman CE. John McMichael. *Postgrad Med J* 1968; **44**: 5–6.
12 Bull GM, Joekes AM, Lowe KG. Conservative treatment of anuric uraemia. *Lancet* 1949; ii: 229–34.
13 Sherlock S. Hepatic vein catheterisation in clinical research. *Proceedings of the Institute of Medicine of Chicago* 1951; **18**: 335–42.

14 Summerskill WHJ, Davidson EA, Sherlock S, Steiner RE. The neuro-psychiatric syndrome associated with hepatic cirrhosis and an extensive portal collateral circulation. *Q J Med* 1956; **25**: 245–66.

15 Shiner M. Jejunal biopsy tube. *Lancet* 1956; i: 85.

16 Doniach I, Shiner M. Duodenal and jejunal biopsies. II. Histology. *Gastroenterology* 1957; **33**: 71–7.

17 McMichael J. Dynamics of heart failure. *Br Med J* 1952; ii: 525–9; 578–82.

18 Cope CL, Loizou S. Deoxycorticosterone excretion in normal, hyper-tensive and hypokalaemic subjects. *Clin Sci* 1975; **48**: 97–105.

19 Evans BM, Milne MD. Potassium-losing nephritis presenting as a case of periodic paralysis. *Br Med J* 1954; ii: 1067–71.

20 Cope CL, Garcia-Llaurado J. The occurrence of electrocortin in human urine. *Br Med J* 1954; i: 1290–4.

21 Milne MD, Scribner BA, Crawford MA. Non-ionic diffusion and the excretion of weak acids and bases. *Am J Med* 1958; **24**: 709–29.

22 Milne MD. Disorders of intestinal aminoacid transport. In: Code CF, ed. *Handbook of physiology. Alimentary canal.* Vol 3. *Intestinal absorption.* Washington DC: American Physiology Society, 1968: 1309–21.

23 Melrose DG, Aird I. A mechanical heart-lung machine for use in man. *Br Med J* 1953; ii: 57–62.

24 Aird I, Melrose DG, Cleland WP, Lynn RB. Assisted circulation by pump oxygenator during operative dilatation of the aortic valve in man. *Br Med J* 1954; i: 1284–7.

25 Melrose DG, Dreyer B, Bentall HH, Baker JRE. Elective cardiac arrest. *Lancet* 1955; ii: 21–2.

26 Pearse AGE. *Histochemistry.* London: J and A Churchill, 1953.

27 Ashwini Kumar M, Foster GV, McIntyre I. Further evidence for calcitonin. A rapid-acting hormone which lowers plasma calcium. *Lancet* 1963; ii: 480–2.

28 Datta N. Transmissible drug resistance in an epidemic strain of Salmonella typhimurium. *J Hyg (London)* 1962; **60**: 301–10.

29 Molin DL, Ross GIM. The vitamin B_{12} concentration of serum and urine of normals and patients with megaloblastic anaemia and other diseases. *J Clin Pathol* 1952; **5**: 129–39.

30 Selwyn JG, Dacie JV. Autohaemolysis and other changes resulting from the incubation in vitro of red cells from patients with congenital haemolytic anaemia. *Blood* 1954; **9**: 414–21.

31 Biggs R, Douglas AS, Macfarlane RG, *et al.* Christmas disease. *Br Med J* 1952; ii 1378–82.

32 Booth CC, Mollin DL. The site of absorption of vitamin B_{12} in man. *Lancet* 1959; i: 18–21.

33 West JB, Dollery CT. Distribution of blood flow and the pressure-flow relations of the whole lung. *J Appl Physiol* 1965; **20**: 175–83.

34 Poynter FNL. Medical education in England since 1600. In: O'Malley CD, ed. *The history of medical education*. Los Angeles: University of California Press, 1970: 235–50.

35 McMichael J. The postgraduate medical school: the present situation. *Postgrad Med J* 1966; **42**: 740–3.

36 Lockwood CM, Rees AJ, Pearson TA, Evans DJ, Peters DK, Wilson CB. Immunosuppression and plasma exchange in the treatment of Goodpasture's syndrome. *Lancet* 1976; i: 711–5.

37 Pinching AJ, Peters DK, Newsom Davis J. Remission of myasthenia gravis following plasma exchange. *Lancet* 1976; ii: 1373–6.

37 Bloom SR, Polak JM. Regulatory peptides and hormone-secreting tumours. In: Booth CC, Neale G, eds. *Disorders of the small intestine*. Oxford: Blackwell, 1985: 376–97.

39 Allison J, Hall L, McIntyre I, Craig RK. The construction and partial characterisation of plasmids containing complementary DNA sequences to human calcitonin precursor polyprotein. *Biochem J* 1981; **199**: 725–31.

14 Clinical science today

Clinical research as we know it in Britain today had its origins in France and Germany during the nineteenth century. It was in Paris that the modern medical clinic was born and in Germany that there developed academic departments in clinical subjects in the universities, headed by professors who had their own laboratories and assistants and who prosecuted research.[1] British clinical science was also greatly influenced by events in the United States where both philanthropy and the example of the German universities were to play an important role in the development of modern academic medicine. The period of expansion that followed the ending of the American Civil War was associated with the growth of new industries that were vitally important to the emergent economy of the modern era. These developments of modern capitalism led in turn to the progressive accumulation of riches by an elite group of industrial entrepreneurs who included Johns Hopkins, a railway developer, John D Rockefeller, whose fortune was based on oil, and Andrew Carnegie, the formidable steel magnate. With enormous wealth at their disposal all turned to philanthropy and both Hopkins and Rockefeller, through the benefactions they made to the institutions that bear their names, were to play a pivotal role in the development of medical education and research in the United States. The German pattern of organisation of medical teaching and research was taken to the

Adapted from an address given to the Medical Society of London on 13 January 1986 and from the presidential address to the British Medical Association on 25 June 1986. *British Medical Journal* 1986; **293**: 23–6.

United States by the first professors at the newly founded Johns Hopkins Hospital Medical School in 1889. Many of them, including Osler and William Welch, had studied in Germany. The German system was reflected in the foundation of the clinical centre associated with the Rockefeller Institute when it was established in New York City in 1901. It was also the German model of medical education that so deeply influenced Abraham Flexner, whose report on medical education in the United States in 1910 revolutionised the American medical schools and played a major role in stimulating clinical research in the modern era.

In Britain clinical research developed more slowly. There had been some excellent clinical studies during the eighteenth century (see Chapter 1). During the nineteenth century there were still examples of outstanding achievement in clinical research in this country, Bright's work on renal disease and the studies of Addison and Hodgkin being examples, but despite Lister's innovations, Sir James MacKenzie's pioneering work, and the studies of Manson and his pupils, British medicine in general fell behind that in the Continental schools. In the early years of this century, however, Archibald Garrod published his pioneering work on biochemical genetics and there were then two developments that were to be of major importance in the creation of opportunities for clinical research in this country. The first was the establishment of full time chairs in clinical subjects in the medical schools following the report in 1913 of the Royal Commission on University Education in London, chaired by Lord Haldane.[2] The commission had been greatly influenced by the evidence given by Abraham Flexner and Sir William Osler, first professor of medicine at the Johns Hopkins Medical School and by then regius professor in Oxford. With their experience of developments in medical education in the United States at that time, both strongly commended the German pattern of medical education to the commission which responded by recommending that a limited number of full time chairs be established by the University of London in the medical schools in the capital. Garrod, at St Bartholomew's Hospital, was the first to be appointed in 1919, but he left to succeed

Osler as regius professor in Oxford before taking up his post. The second was the foundation of the Medical Research Council, originally the Medical Research Committee, to whose service Sir Thomas Lewis was to be recruited in 1916 as the first full time clinical research worker in this country. Under the aegis of the Medical Research Council Thomas Lewis was later outstandingly successful in creating the unit for clinical research at University College Hospital. It was Lewis who was the forerunner of what we understand as clinical research in Britain today.

Before the opening of the British Postgraduate Medical School at Hammersmith in 1935 and the setting up of the clinical school in Oxford a year later, clinical research in the universities and medical schools made only a faltering start. As in the United States, however, philanthropy was to be of great importance in encouraging medical education and research. The Oxford clinical school, now so outstanding, owes its origins to the success of the Morris motor car, for it was the benefactions of Lord Nuffield that enabled the University of Oxford to establish its first clinical chairs. In July 1936 Lord Nuffield had heard Sir Farquhar Buzzard, then regius professor of medicine at Oxford, deliver his presidential address in the Sheldonian Theatre to the British Medical Association, an address in which he had made an eloquent plea for the establishment of a postgraduate clinical school.[3] Nuffield was immediately persuaded. Always a man of action, he did not delay and by the end of the year the Oxford chairs had been founded. It was in that same year that another great and influential philanthropic venture, the Wellcome Trust, was also established.[4]

Clinical science today includes a wide range of subjects from epidemiology to studies of individual patients in depth and the laboratory analysis of specimens or tissue. It also entails the study of experimental models of physiology and disease in animals where necessary. Lewis in his time believed that clinical science was a specialty and a discipline in its own right in the same way as pathology or physiology. He considered that the clinical scientist should not primarily be concerned with the day to day problems of clinical practice,

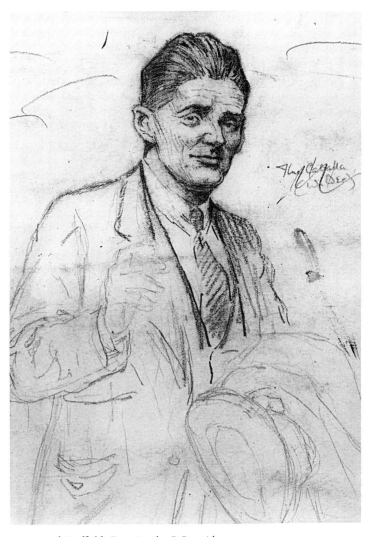

19   Lord Nuffield. Drawing by B Partridge
(National Portrait Gallery, London)

where clinicians devoted their energies to the diagnosis and treatment of often obscure cases. The routine diagnosis and treatment of patients should, he believed, properly belong to such practising clinicians, but the clinical scientist should be in charge of his own beds and laboratories and there concentrate on the study of the natural history of selected diseases.[5]

Lewis's view of clinical science has been overtaken by a number of important developments in this country. A generation ago clinical research was still predominantly the preserve of university departments of medicine, surgery, and pathology. Since the end of the second world war, however, clinical research has greatly widened its scope as a result of the emergence of new subjects. Many have been associated with the development of new technology – for example, cardiac surgery, organ transplantation, intensive care, modern molecular genetics, imaging techniques, and all the technologies that now govern diagnostic departments of pathology. Epidemiology was greatly stimulated by the pioneering work of Doll and Bradford Hill, and subjects such as community medicine, geriatrics, social psychiatry, and general practice are now making a significant contribution to clinical research in this country.

Specialisation has also had a particularly important influence on clinical research. Instead of the wide ranging interests of the clinical investigator of Lewis's time most modern clinical scientists are brought up to the practice of a clinical specialty. Such individuals have increasingly tended to look to scientists in the basic sciences for help in their research, so that clinical science does not stand alone, as Lewis envisaged. Since Lewis's day there has also been a dramatic change in the nature of clinical research. Lewis was an advocate of the school of clinical physiology and it was physiology that was the driving force of his own work. His views had an important influence on a whole generation of his successors and to this day the Medical Research Society, which Lewis founded, remains greatly influenced by a physiological view of clinical research, which still permeates the activities of too many departments of academic medicine in the universities. The situation in clinical research has been markedly changed in recent decades by the scientific revolution that has overtaken biology and medicine with the impact of the new pharmacology, immunology, biochemistry, and particularly by developments in molecular and cell biology.

Why is there a need for clinical research? So far as the nation is concerned support for basic scientific research is an obvious requirement and is very easy to justify in view of the extraordinary success of British biologists in winning Nobel prizes. The distinction between basic and clinical or applied research, however, is a sterile debate. As Pasteur put it: "Il n'existe pas des sciences appliquées, mais seulement les applications de la science."

We need clinical research for four main reasons. Firstly, as part of the life sciences it contributes to the overall body of scientific knowledge from fundamental studies of man in health and disease. Secondly, it develops and applies advances in the basic sciences and in technology to the effective investigation and treatment of human disease. Thirdly, clinical research has the responsibility of maintaining a constant assessment of both new and existing methods of clinical practice. Finally, it ensures that teaching at both undergraduate and postgraduate level does not degenerate into dogma.

Those who actually do clinical research in Britain, the clinical scientific community, include the staff of university departments that are concerned with clinical teaching in medical schools and the scientists and clinicians who work in the institutes or units of the Medical Research Council. These individuals, if they are to carry out effective clinical research, require laboratories, staff, and equipment to support their work. Clinical staff of the National Health Service also make a significant contribution to clinical research. Such individuals, if they work in a teaching hospital, or at an institute such as the Clinical Research Centre at Northwick Park, may have their own laboratories, but for the most part NHS staff do not have laboratories of their own. For this reason, if they are to undertake research, they often collaborate closely with colleagues in paraclinical departments such as pathology or radiology. Many NHS staff and university departments also cooperate closely with the pharmaceutical industry in carrying out drug trials, which are of particular importance to the Committee on Safety of Medicines. The NHS is the sector where most clinical research should be orientated to the critical assessment of new and existing methods of practice, a topic that requires constant attention and is accorded too little importance by most health authorities in this country. Nor should one forget the medical staff of the armed services who have always made an important contribution to clinical research. Military work on tropical disease and naval studies of the hazards of diving have been particularly good examples.

Financial support for the clinical research community in this country is derived from a number of different sources. The government makes a major contribution through its support of biomedical science. It does this not as in so many countries through its Health Department, but through the Department of Education and Science. As far as government funding is concerned medical science is, therefore, part of science as a whole rather than being associated directly with the Health Department. The Secretary of State for Education and Science receives recommendations on scientific funding from the Advisory Board for the Research Councils, which has the responsibility of allocating the science budget to the various national research councils, Science and Engineering, Agriculture and Food, Economic and Social Science, the Environment, and the Medical Research Council. The board is also responsible for allocating money to the Royal Society, the Natural History Museum and, to a small extent, to the London Zoo.

The total allocation for science for 1984–5 was £550 million, of which £117.2 million was given to the Medical Research Council.[6] By international standards, and certainly by comparison with North America, the British government's commitment to biomedical science is, therefore, relatively modest. The government's support for clinical research also includes research carried out under the auspices of the Department of Health and Social Security but the majority of this work is orientated to health services research or health economics. In addition, regional health authorities have a certain limited budget for the support of research at district level and most of this is allocated for clinical research. The laboratories of the Public Health Laboratory Service, a nation-wide organisation with a specific responsibility for the control of infectious disease, play an important role in the national research effort in microbiology, and in the epidemiology of communicable disease.

The contributions of the pharmaceutical industry to clinical research in Great Britain are difficult to quantitate. Yet it is clear that the laboratories of the major industrial concerns are vitally important particularly in drug and vaccine development. Several of these laboratories, for example those at the Wellcome Foundation at Beckenham in Kent, have an important commitment to basic as well as applied research.

One of the most significant features of British clinical research, and in this it contrasts with other European countries such as France, is the major importance of the private foundations for the support of both basic and applied research. The Wellcome Trust, which receives the profits from the pharmaceutical company, the Wellcome Foundation, disburses more than £20 million per annum for bio-medical research at present as well as supporting veterinary research and the study of the history of medicine. The trust now, in 1986, anticipates a virtual doubling of this income to more than £40 million per annum as a result of the release to the open market of a proportion of its shares in the Wellcome Foundation.

The Wellcome Trust has been so important to clinical research in this country that it is worthy of special consideration. Sir Henry Wellcome, founder of the great pharmaceutical enterprise which bears his name, died in London in 1936. Wellcome was a product of that same technologically exciting and entrepreneurial American society of the later years of the nineteenth century that had given Rockefeller and Carnegie their opportunity. Originally an American from the midwest, Wellcome had worked at an upcountry

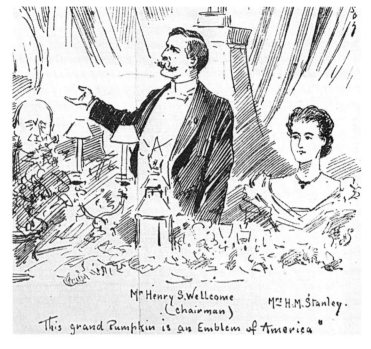

Mr Henry S. Wellcome
(chairman)

Mrs H.M. Stanley.

"This grand Pumpkin is an Emblem of America"

20   Sir Henry Wellcome at the American Society's Thanksgiving
dinner, Cecil Hotel, London, November 1896
(Wellcome Institute Library, London)

drugstore owned by an uncle and he had been a travelling
drug salesman. In 1880, however, struck by the commercial
opportunities opening up in Great Britain, he formed a
partnership with Silas Burroughs with the intention of introducing into Britain the manufacture of ready made pills,
which he called "Tabloids," a new technology at a stage of
active development in the United States. It was an immensely
successful venture. Silas Burroughs died in 1895, and when
Wellcome followed him to his Maker more than 40 years later
he controlled one of the largest industrial fortunes in this
country. The puritanical son of a missionary father, he was,
like John D Rockfeller, imbued with a moral responsibility
towards his fellow men and their misfortunes, and it was this

that guided many of his actions throughout his long life. At his death he left his entire fortune and his commercial enterprises to trustees who were to continue to control his business as sole shareholders. The Wellcome Trust, created under the terms of his will, has had a major influence through the years on medical and scientific research as well as on tropical medicine and the study of the history of medicine. The trust has been of extraordinary importance to a whole generation in this country. It has given a start in their careers to many young men and women. It has provided vitally important support to our universities and medical schools during the recent period of severe retrenchment. Without the trust's imaginative schemes for the support of clinical research fellows, senior lectureships, special awards to prevent individuals joining the "brain drain," and linked appointments for basic scientists working in clinical departments the position in the medical schools today would be nothing short of disastrous. For whole departments the enthusiastic encouragement of the trust and its officers has been of vital importance in the development of new initiatives. The trust has invariably been more receptive of new ideas than other grant giving bodies in this country and is always prepared to look at novel ways of doing what needs to be done. Within its elegant premises in Regent's Park it tends to lend a more understanding ear to the problems faced by research workers than do more formally constituted bodies. For those working overseas, in Thailand, India, East Africa, or Belem, the trust has given support that has often been far more than merely scientific. As the director of the trust has pointed out: "A flexible, relaxed, helpful body is of great importance to those who seek funds." The academic community of this country is particularly fortunate that the Wellcome Trust has been just such an organisation.[4]

There are many other charitable organisations that have been of great significance in the support of clinical research. The Imperial Cancer Research Fund, the Cancer Research Campaign, the British Heart Foundation and the Leukaemia Research Fund support a wide range of clinical research in their respective specialties. There are also many smaller trusts concerned with specific diseases such as multiple sclerosis, rheumatism, cystic fibrosis, coeliac disease, and so on. Together with the major foundations, these charitable organisations contribute almost as much per annum as does the government through its support for the Medical Research Council. Such funds are particularly important in providing an essential buffer to research workers seeking support for their work, as well as acting as a source of income complementary to that available from the government.

There is a general impression that resources for clinical research are declining in this country. The question, however, is not simple. The answer depends on a number of factors which include the proportion of money available in our community between the private and public sectors, the relationship between the support for basic science and that for clinical research, and the support being given to universities where the majority of clinical research is carried out. Recently, however, it has been the progressive erosion of support for the universities, as a result of deliberate government policy, that has caused the most serious problems. By 1990, if present policies continue, it has been estimated that the universities will have suffered a 30% cut in real terms in a decade. This is a disastrous situation, a total rejection of the views of a previous Tory prime minister, Benjamin Disraeli: "Upon the education of the people of this country," he stated, "the future of this country depends." The government's policies are having a major impact on medical schools at present and murmurings about closures are already being heard. These are matters that should greatly concern all members of the medical profession for we share a loyalty to our medical school and to the teachers who guided our first faltering footsteps in medicine. Some of us are in serious danger of losing our alma maters. University clinical staff, with their undue responsibility for teaching and clinical care in our medical schools, must give priority to these activities and the nationwide swingeing reductions in academic staff which have taken place are unquestionably leading to a reduction in the amount of time and energy that can be devoted to research. There is evidence in Britain that this is being reflected by a reduction not just in morale but also in requests to the Medical Research Council for support for clinical research, particularly from the young and from new recruits. The university, as a place of "light, liberty and learning," to use Disraeli's phrase, is increasingly under attack.[7]

Until now, the one budget that was preserved against cuts was the research budget. This is no longer the case. In recent years there has been an increasing reluctance on the part of the government to support science in Britain as effectively as is necessary to maintain this country's scientific position in a competitive world. The Advisory Board for the Research Councils has pointed to the serious consequences of the government's policy of not funding pay awards beyond the percentage set by the government itself and to its failure to fund superannuation or restructuring costs; and has shown that the decline in the exchange value of sterling leads to uncontrolled increases in the level of international subscriptions to bodies such as the European Molecular Biology Organisation. Furthermore, no account is taken by government paymasters of the additional equipment costs made necessary by the increasing sophistication of science. Twenty years ago the best electron microscope cost about £12 000. Nowadays it costs between £250 000 and £1.5 million depending on the type. At the same time any research director seeking to develop the techniques of molecular biology in his institution knows how much more expensive a postdoctoral assistant or scientist is now than even a few short years ago.

These rising costs are inevitable in modern medical science, and since the current funding of the Medical Research Council takes little or no account of them the overall result has been an erosion of the total research capacity of the council. During the past two years its boards have been unable to fund a considerable proportion of research projects graded "alpha" and even those which have been funded have often received less support than requested. The total number of project grants in 1984–5 had to be pruned by 19%, and in the units and institutes of the Medical Research Council equipment grants have been severely curtailed and in some instances totally withheld.[6] The Save British Science Campaign has dramatically highlighted the government's shortcomings, particularly in relation to the shrinking support for basic science. There is no doubt about the current unease afflicting the scientific community in this country. Within a few weeks of its foundation in early 1986 the Save British Science Campaign attracted the support of 1500 scientists, of whom 50 were fellows of the Royal Society and eight Nobel laureates.

The sad feature of the erosion of government research support, which is a reflection of an overall government commitment to reduce public spending so that taxes may be reduced, is that it is probably not what the public wants, particularly in respect of medical research. The charitable sector of medical research funding is increasing every year, suggesting that the average citizen is favourably disposed to medical research. Yet the British system, which incorporates the funding of medical research within an overall budget for science and which, therefore, effectively insulates the medical research budget from political pressure, may well be unable to reflect this public will as far as medical research funding is concerned. The lobbying of members of Parliament, for example, might conceivably result in an overall increase in scientific funding but there would be no guarantee that the Advisory Board for the Research Councils would channel such an increase in funding into medical research and no further guarantee that the Medical Research Council would then devote that money to clinical research. This is particularly galling at a time when the prospects for clinical research have never been so challenging or exciting.

So far as government support for research is concerned the Medical Research Council unquestionably requires additional resources. Where are they to come from? The inescapable conclusion is that the government should reconsider its priorities. Government support for defence research projects accounts for as much as half of the United Kingdom expenditure on research — vastly greater than the 10% figure for Germany or 33% for France. This is an intolerable position for a European island, no longer a great power, off the north coast of a great continent. As members of a noble profession whose work depends on research we must persuade our legislators to change their policies. Scrutator, writing in the *British Medical Journal*, took the academics to task for not being more passionate about it all.[8] Perhaps, though, we "rather bear those ills we have, / Than fly to others that we know not of? / Thus conscience doth make cowards of us all."

The one resource that is not declining either in quality or quantity in medicine is the young. Most European countries are producing more doctors than they need and the grim spectre of unemployment has already begun to stalk the wards of even our best hospitals. This is at a time when the intellectual quality of entrants to medical school has never been higher. After their period in medical school this remarkable galaxy of talented scholars should emerge as eager to discover as to cure. Unfortunately, this does not seem to happen as frequently as it should. It remains uncertain what happens in medical schools to turn an open and inquiring mind at entry into a conformist junior resident who wants to get into practice as quickly as possible, but it may in some way be a reflection of the organisation of university departments responsible for clinical teaching in this country.

The organisation of clinical academic departments of medical schools in Britain is quite different from that in the United States where for the most part university departments follow the pattern established after the implementation of the recommendations of Abraham Flexner's report.[9] American departments are very much larger, they provide academic staff with more time for research, and they are comprehensive. The professor in the United States university department of medicine or surgery for example, is not only head of the specialty subjects within his field, but also chief of service of the hospital department. With the help of senior staff acting as attending consultants, the routine investigation and treatment of patients is undertaken by the residents and interns (registrars and house staff). They are responsible to a chief resident who reports to the head of department, as chief of service. Other specialty units within the department, for example, gastroenterology, cardiology, and infectious disease, are led by university staff and their head often holds the rank of professor himself. With his staff, he provides both a service in his subspecialty and acts as a consultant throughout the hospital. This system ensures that the academic members of the university clinical department are not overwhelmed by clinical commitments, and many American academics spend no more than a month or two a year as attending physicians. Clinical academic staff in American schools, therefore, have greater freedom than their counterparts in Britain to develop research interests with a strong laboratory base. They also have access, through the National Institutes of Health and the wealthy American charitable foundations, to richer sources of research funds. This has sometimes led to an overemphasis on basic science at the expense of clinical, but at the same time it has been the strength of the American pattern of medical education and of its commitment to clinical research. It is also a system within which new initiatives can rapidly and readily be undertaken.

In Britain the situation is different. At the end of the first world war, following the report of Lord Haldane's royal commission, the universities began to establish clinical academic units in the medical schools headed by full time professors, who were debarred from private practice. Osler, in his evidence to the Haldane Commission had called for "an active invasion of the teaching hospitals by the Universities." What in fact was achieved, however, was no more than a bridgehead. In contrast to the situation in the United States, the academic units were single firms in a particular specialty and they existed alongside hospital units already established in the teaching hospital by men working part time, who also undertook private practice. The professors were, therefore, not heads of service in their subject and they had no control over other specialty interests except for those they controlled in their own unit. This arrangement has had unfortunate consequences. Since professors tend to breed other professors, the British system perpetuates the specialty interests of the existing professors, to the detriment of the development of new subjects. This explains why so many

academic departments have persisted for so long in encouraging clinical physiology at the expense of the new
science. Vicariously, however, the professors were able to
influence events beyond the confines of the academic unit by
encouraging the teaching and research activities of their NHS
colleagues, but the academic departments remained relatively
small and the average professor in a clinical medical school
was a far less powerful patron of the young than his American
counterpart. In addition, after the establishment of the NHS
in 1948, the academic departments became increasingly
responsible for the work of the NHS and for the routine work
entailed in the investigation and treatment of individual
patients. This led to an unfortunately competitive spirit
between academic and NHS staff in many teaching hospitals.
Gradually, however, academic staff increased – a trend that
has now been dramatically reversed. At the same time the
successful teaching hospitals have established effective links
between academic and NHS staff, sometimes by creating
joint university/NHS appointments. In fact, in medicine now
it is rare to encounter an NHS clinician in a good teaching
hospital who is not only a successful practitioner, but also the
head of his own research team. Furthermore, the NHS has
agreed to fund, in certain universities, clinical chairs in
specific subjects.

The only exception to the Haldane model of the academic
department in Britain is the Royal Postgraduate Medical
School at Hammersmith Hospital (see Chapter 13). Stimulated by Sir Francis Fraser, first professor of medicine at the
school, Hammersmith developed a system that paralleled
that in the American schools. The school made an agreement
with the health authorities that the consultant staff of the
hospital would be full time academics, holding positions in
the university, whereas the junior medical staff, like the
American residents and interns, would be paid by the hospital.
This arrangement effectively established the professor in the
major clinical departments as chief of service on the American
pattern. The heads of subspecialty units, however, did not
have the same freedom as their American counterparts, firstly
because they were not so lavishly provided with staff and

secondly because the total responsibility for their subspecialty rested on them. They also provided an emergency take service at least once a week in rotation with other units. The Hammersmith model has been particularly effective in providing opportunities for clinical research and for the training of medical teachers. It is still, however, a model in which the major emphasis has been on the investigation and treatment of individual patients and it is for this reason that Hammersmith has established a reputation for tertiary referral work and the exploitation of new and complex technology.

Although clinical departments in the universities have served this country reasonably well through the years, particularly in teaching, there is evidence to suggest that in the next few years taking us to the twenty first century they may be increasingly unable to adapt to the challenges facing clinical research in the modern era. There are in the British system factors which provide a constant resistance to change. One of the major problems facing clinical research today is the orientation of the National Health Service and the medical schools to a "systems" approach to medicine. In the NHS medicine is practised according to specialties that are system orientated. There are cardiologists, gastroenterologists, neurosurgeons, and so on, and this is a reflection of a centrifugal fragmentation of the older subjects in medicine into more and more parts. The medical schools follow this pattern so that undergraduate curricula are often designed to a "systems" model which follows NHS specialties. At postgraduate level the royal colleges with their commitment to higher training follow the same specialty and systems model. Clinician scientists tend simply to line up their research alongside this "systems" model. The problem for those who are trying to influence clinical research in the modern era by applying modern biomedical science to clinical problems is that the scientists who are recruited, whether they be clinical or non-clinical, are not interested in an approach by systems. Science, in contrast to the divergence evident in clinical practice, has not been fragmenting but is converging. The Nobel laureate Arthur Kornberg perceived this paradox when he pointed out that the most profound development in medical science "is the confluence of many discrete and previously unrelated medical science subjects into a single unified discipline. Anatomy, physiology, biochemistry, microbiology, immunology and genetics have now been merged and are being expressed in a common language...by reducing structures and systems into molecular forms," he went on, "all aspects of body form and function blend into a logical framework."[10]

This development is reflected by the desire of the modern breed of clinical scientists to be unshackled from a rigid "systems" approach. An individual interested in type 1 immunological responses, for example, may be investigating allergic responses in skin, gut, and lung. A clinical molecular biologist interested in growth factor genes is concerned with patients with atheroma, the genetics of the insulin receptor in diabetes, and may also need to study the molecular biology of Wilms's tumour of the kidney, to say nothing of his involvement in the cloning of an oncogene. A clinical scientist interested in collagen disorders, initially a dermatologist, may find himself investigating berry aneurysms of the brain, as they too may be due to an abnormality of collagen synthesis. A cell biologist interested in organelles may have to study liver, gut, blood vessels, and leucocytes. For such individuals – and they are all examples of actual clinician scientists who have worked at the Clinical Research Centre at Northwick Park – there is a need for institutions and academic departments that are free from the fetters of system and organ orientated approaches to clinical science.

There is also the question of time. The modern clinical investigator who wishes to be internationally competitive in molecular or cell biology can afford to spend only a limited amount of his time in the clinic, perhaps not more than 20%. It is essential that he build up his laboratory work, usually in association with a multidisciplinary group that includes basic scientists, who will have no respect for him if he is simply one of those clinicians who nod into the laboratory once a week and inquire how things are going. The present structure in the medical schools, with their orientation to a system based curriculum, may be effective in subjects orientated to diagnosis and therapy, such as departments of surgery and radiology. It is, however, too inflexible to allow the development of clinical scientists who have enough freedom to do what they want or to develop new approaches rapidly. The present models available for clinical research in this country are unlikely to be adequate for the future. Flexible organisations are urgently required in which as well as studying the traditional specialty subjects, clinical scientists have the freedom to develop their own ideas in their own way untrammelled by an overwhelming NHS commitment.

It is against this background that we must consider how the Medical Research Council has sought to encourage clinical research. The MRC has not always got things right throughout its history. It was parsimonious in its dealings with Howard Florey in the development of penicillin and it did not want to be involved in the reproductive technology introduced by Steptoe and Edwards. But I do believe that through the years the British public has had good value for the money that has been invested in the MRC. It has great achievements to its credit. It is a national institution whose high international reputation is fully deserved and of which the nation should be proud. British work in molecular biology and in a great many other topics of biomedical research, which include the contributions to modern epidemiology of men such as Sir Richard Doll, indicates that in terms of research achievement per pound spent the British public is getting good value for its money.

Approximately 60% of the MRC's budget is allocated in house – that is, to its units or to its major institutes, the National Institute for Medical Research at Mill Hill, the Clinical Research Centre at Northwick Park and the Laboratory of Molecular Biology in Cambridge. Much of the remaining 40% of the MRC budget goes in programme or project grants to universities and their staff, which are awarded on a competitive basis by the various research boards of the council and to awards for training at home and abroad. At the same time the council provides support within universities to exceptional individuals by giving them their own unit, the staff then being appointed and remunerated by the MRC. The unit for the study of molecular haematology at Oxford, under the direction of the Nuffield professor of medicine, Professor David Weatherall, is just such an example. Sir Thomas Lewis's outstandingly successful department of clinical research at University College Hospital was another example of MRC support for a distinguished clinical scientist at unit level.

It is to Lewis's vision that the modern generation owes the establishment by the MRC of its own centre for clinical research in association with the district general hospital at Northwick Park. The hospital at Northwick Park, opened in 1970, provides a comprehensive service to a defined community in Harrow. It is a district hospital of 800 beds, of which 160 are allocated to the MRC for research purposes. These beds are available for the study of "the natural history of selected diseases," to use Sir Thomas Lewis's phrase. The Clinical Research Centre model is, therefore, quite different from that in the universities in this country. It has made no attempt to duplicate the tertiary referral work so well carried out at Hammersmith. The facilities at Northwick Park have been particularly valuable in encouraging long term studies of commonly encountered human diseases, as originally envisaged by Lewis (see Chapter 12). The programmes of research include studies of the biology of the brain in schizophrenia, alcoholism and its prevention, vascular disease, sexually transmitted disease, obesity, allergy, arthritis in children, diarrhoeal illnesses, and diseases as banal as the common cold, for the MRC's common cold unit in Salisbury is an important outstation of the Clinical Research Centre. Northwick Park provides a unique environment in which clinician scientists, in close association with basic scientists, can develop laboratories which are independent of NHS requirements, which can be used flexibly, and where new developments are not governed by the need to subscribe to a particular curriculum, as is the case in both undergraduate and postgraduate schools of medicine.

In the present climate of financial stringency, however, it seems increasingly uncertain whether the nation can afford to support two major institutions undertaking clinical research – one at Hammersmith and the other, only five miles away, at Northwick Park. For this and other reasons a recent report to the Medical Research Council has recommended that the Clinical Research Centre should now be merged, on one site, with the Royal Postgraduate Medical School, a suggestion that would bring together a major activity of the University of London in clinical research as well as that of the MRC.[11] It would also merge the high technology approach of Hammersmith with the commitment to the study of common diseases in the community that has been so uniquely developed at the Clinical Research Centre. The report has received strong support.[12] There has naturally been some scepticism as to whether this laudable aim may ever be achieved. For the future, however, the multidisciplinary model of clinical research that the council has developed at Northwick Park, where there is close association between different research groups, must at all costs be preserved for future generations, particularly now when we live in an era of research that has never been so challenging.

In the coming decades it is possible that gene therapy may become a reality and there is no doubt that genetic disease will be preventable to a considerable extent. We may well also begin to unravel the biology of the brain in chronic mental illness. We shall certainly witness the introduction of effective antiviral agents. Both hepatitis and measles should be eradicated and we shall increasingly know what motivates a cancer cell. In addition we may well understand how to prevent coronary artery disease. But we must always remember in words written a century and a half ago: "In research the horizon recedes as we advance…and research is always incomplete." In some senses the research worker is constantly in search of the Holy Grail, but mercifully now and again he finds it.

There is little doubt that the state of clinical research in this country is better than it was 25 years ago. In many medical schools it has immeasurably improved, and it now enjoys a high reputation both in Western Europe and in the United States.

So why is it that among university professors in traditional clinical subjects in this country, and elsewhere, there appears to be a general spirit of gloom and depression about the current state of clinical research?[13][14][15] Perhaps they believe with the poet that "Nothing's so dainty sweet as lovely melancholy." But there is more to it than that. The medical academic community in this country does not want to be relegated to the fourth division at a time when opportunities have never been so exciting, the tools provided by basic science so powerful, or the challenges of human suffering so much in need of the application of the scientific method. University departments have been hard hit by the swingeing cuts in financial support for our universities, to which I have already referred. There are also economic problems which have resulted from the financial disparity that has developed between academic staff and those who work for the National Health Service. One of the major constraints to the recruitment of young clinicians to research has been the introduction, with the best intentions, of the system of extraduty payments for junior clinical staff of the National Health Service. There is no longer comparability in salary between trainees in clinical science and their clinical colleagues in the Health Service – to the serious disadvantage of the scientist trainee. He cannot claim extraduty payments from the university or research council for the time spent doing laboratory work into the small hours, or writing papers on the results of his work. At senior level a similar disparity in salary between clinical academic staff and NHS staff has been created. National Health Service staff who work full time are now permitted to do limited private practice for their personal gain. This has encouraged a change of attitudes among academic staff. There has long been a tradition in Britain of academic staff working full time, and if they see private patients and charge fees the fees go either to their own department or to the medical school. Now as a result of the government's encouragement of a nationwide increase in the private sector individual academics, particularly surgeons, obstetricians, and gynaecologists, are seeking to do private practice for personal gain, a development which will be to the

313

further detriment of clinical research in this country. While Dr Johnson reminds us that there are few ways in which a man can be more innocently employed than in the getting of money, the Bible warns that the love of money is the root of all evil.

There is also the problem of training. In a previous generation, the clinical investigator who had had a firm grounding in physiology as a medical student could decide to attack a problem in clinical physiology and simply get going. He now requires further postgraduate training not only in research techniques but also in new subjects, and this has to be undertaken in addition to postgraduate training in his chosen clinical discipline. He then has to follow that uncertain road which lies between studies of laboratory animals on the one hand, and the more lucrative pastures of clinical and private practice on the other. He has to learn to be sufficiently thick skinned to pay scant attention to the views of scientists who say that he is not a proper scientist, and to those of his clinical colleagues who say he is not a proper clinician. To undertake postgraduate clinical training to the level required for the acquisition of specialist registration, to do an MSc or PhD degree, as well as postdoctoral work, often overseas in a laboratory of basic science, is the sort of careeer that the new breed of clinician investigator has to follow. It is a daunting prospect and only the most dedicated are now succeeding.

Other influences have also been at work in recent years to inhibit the investigative zeal of the young. It is unlikely that there has been any reduction in the overall ability of medical students, for the inquiring spirit of the human mind is unlikely to vary from one generation to another. It is more likely that in terms of the recruitment of young clinician scientists it is environmental influences rather than inherent ability that determines attitudes. Perhaps one of the most important of these has been the attack on elitism. Science is associated with an elite, elitism is incompatible with egalitarianism, therefore, in an egalitarian society, science is suspect. For this and other reasons science has been attacked, particularly following the development of nuclear weapons, and populists have at the same time sown a deep mistrust of scientists in the public mind. Modern technology has been under attack and medicine has been portrayed as unfeeling, losing sight of the needs of the suffering individual. Undoubtedly we have been passing through a phase when some of these criticisms have rubbed off on young medical students and there has been a feeling among them that relevance is all important – the desire to cure and care more praiseworthy than to investigate.

The achievements of clinical science, and particularly of university clinical departments, have also been criticised. The incursion of the university into undergraduate teaching hospitals in London, even where no more than a bridgehead has been established, has not been considered an unmixed blessing by some of the more old fashioned consultants.[16] A more serious and significant critique of clinical science in this country, however, was made by Lord Platt, a retired professor of medicine who had been president of the Royal College of Physicians, in his Harveian oration for 1967 entitled "Medical Science – Master or Servant?"[17] Platt accepted that the application of the scientific method had brought much benefit to the investigation of bodily function and of disease, but he considered that academic clinical departments had hardly been responsible for any of the revolutionary advances in therapy of the previous 40 years. He argued that there had been "far too great an emphasis on clinical measurement and a positive obsession with measuring what are now called *parameters* of chronic organic illness to the neglect of other more important problems." He acknowledged that "some real discoveries have been made in academic clinical departments, often in the field of rare diseases such as primary hyperaldosteronism," but he went on to complain "that the accurate study of function in chronic obstructive disease of the lungs, the kidneys and the liver has sometimes seemed more akin to an absorbing hobby than a therapeutic exercise." He thought that too little attention was given to subjects such as mental illness, to the relationship between physician and patient, and to taboo subjects such as sex education. Altogether he was reflecting the view that clinical research should be relevant, a notion succinctly put by AP Herbert:

> I love the doctors, they are dears,
> But must they spend such years and years
> Investigating such a lot
> Of illnesses that no one's got?

Although a single correspondent congratulated his lordship on his "brilliant account of the misdirected efforts now wasted on certain types of clinical research," it is fair to say that Platt's Harveian oration caused an outcry from many of the clinical academic professors of that era. WS Peart, in particular, responded with the comment that the medical academic units were a very recent acquisition in many schools, but he admitted that the lack of biochemical and pharmacological training for doctors had been a major drawback. He pointed out to Lord Platt that he was "grievously wrong in contrasting the understanding of patients and their needs with the scientific aims of medicine. We can keep out the dangerous fools attached to machines," he went on, "as long as we can let in the wise men." Furthermore, he asked what on earth Lord Platt had been doing about it all, since he had himself been a professor of medicine for many years.[18]

The Royal Society of Medicine responded by founding a Barnes lecture to describe and discuss the contributions that clinical academic departments had made to the practice of medicine, and the inaugural oration was a spirited defence of clinical academics by KW Donald.[19] Further defences of the system were offered by RV Christie, who had headed the medical academic unit at St Bartholomew's Hospital, in his Harveian oration in 1969, and by LJ Witts, first Nuffield professor of medicine at Oxford, whose title was "The Medical Professorial Unit."[20][21] Nevertheless, it is possible with hindsight to grant that there was more right on Platt's side than was apparent to his opponents. There had been too much clinical physiology and not enough study of the basic nature and natural history of human disease, the major function of clinical science as defined by Lewis. There had been, and still is, too much emphasis on the rare and the esoteric. In addition few academic clinical departments were sufficiently flexible to react rapidly to the changes brought about by the new science, a situation that the present cuts in university expenditure are doing little to relieve.

For the future, however, the most important issue is the survival of clinical research. As biologists we can perhaps take heart from evolution, and as scientists we are incurably optimistic. Clinical research is a tender and delicate organism requiring constant care and attention, but as with all other species two attributes are vital: the capacity to adapt to changing circumstances and the ability to reproduce. I believe that clinical science has demonstrated remarkable adaptability. It has already adapted to cuts – which are not always a total disaster, since they can enable some effective pruning to be done, and there are few universities or research institutes that do not have some dead wood. It is also increasingly adapting to the new science.

But is the clinical research community reproducing itself? Here the most important factor is the recruitment and support of the young. We need, as Sir John McMichael once put it in a memorable phrase, to have the young upon our shoulders, not trample them under our feet. It is for their elders to lead by example and for their teachers constantly to encourage a questing frame of mind, something at which Sir George Pickering so greatly excelled.[22] But in the final analysis if you want to encourage clinical research and you are a professor or a research director what do you actually do? You pick a good man at as young an age as you can, you give him all the support he needs, and you let him get on with it.

NOTES

1 Booth CC. The development of clinical science in Britain. *Br Med J* 1979; i: 1469–73.
2 Royal Commission on University Education in London. *Report*. London: HMSO, 1910–13 (Chairman Viscount Haldane).
3 Buzzard EF. And the future. President's address to the British Medical Association. *Br Med J* 1936; ii: 163–6.
4 Hall RA, Bembridge BA. *Physic and philanthropy*. Cambridge: Cambridge University Press, 1986.

5 Lewis T. The Huxley lecture on clinical science within the university. *Br Med J* 1935; i: 631–6.
6 Medical Research Council. *Annual report*. 1984–85. London: MRC, 1985.
7 Booth, C. Better a commitment to health and research than to missiles. *Br Med J* 1986; **293**: 23–6.
8 Scrutator. The week. *Br Med J* 1986; **292**: 1536.
9 Flexner A. *Medical education in the United States and Canada*. New York: Carnegie Foundation for the Advancement of Teaching, 1910.
10 Kornberg A. Cited by Wyngaarden JB. The role of government support in biomedical research. Symposium on Molecular Biology and Medicine, Estorel, Canada, September 1985.
11 Clinical Research Centre Committee. *Report to the Medical Research Council*. London: MRC, 1986 (Chairman Sir Michael Stoker).
12 Booth CC. The Stoker report and the future of Northwick Park. *Lancet* 1986; i: 372–4.
13 Dollery C. *The end of an age of optimism*. London: Nuffield Provincial Hospitals Trust, 1978.
14 Oliver M. The shrinking face of clinical science: where are tomorrow's research workers? *Eur J Clin Invest* 1979; **7**: 1–2.
15 Wyngaarden JB. The clinical investigator as an endangered species. *N Engl J Med* 1979; **301**: 1254–9.
16 Fowler PBS. Landmarks in medicine. *Br Med J* 1985; **291**: 1719.
17 Platt, Lord. Medical science: master or servant? *Br Med J* 1967; ii: 439–44.
18 Peart WS. Medical science: master or servant? *Br Med J* 1967; ii: 616.
19 Donald KW. The contribution of clinical academic departments to the advancement of medicine. *Proc R Soc Med* 1971; **64**: 303–11.
20 Christie RV. Medical education and the state. *Br Med J* 1969; ii: 385–90.
21 Witts LJ. The medical professorial unit. *Br Med J* 1971; ii: 319–23.
22 McMichael J, Peart WS. George White Pickering. *Biographical Memoirs of Fellows of the Royal Society*. Vol 28. London: Royal Society, 1982: 431–49.